www.CancerFreeAreYouSure.com

 Facebook.com/cancerfreeareyousure

CANCER FREE!

Are You Sure?

Jenny Hrbacek, RN

PUBLISHER'S NOTE:

The authors, editors, contributors, and publisher have made every effort to ensure the completeness and accuracy of all information contained in this book and we assume no responsibility for inaccuracies, omissions, or inconsistencies.

The information given herein is strictly for informational purposes and to increase knowledge. It is not meant to diagnose or treat or a substitute for consulting with your physician. The confirmation of a cancer-free or cancer status is to be done of your own recourse and we are not liable for damages. This book is an account of our own experiences and provides information that may be of value to others. In the event that you utilize this information of your own free will to achieve your personal health goals, we assume no responsibility.

We are not officially endorsing the included labs, practitioners, or any additional services or treatments that they may offer. The information is provided solely for your education and reference in contacting them. We are exercising our freedom of speech, freedom of press, and freedom of religion as provided by the first amendment of the United States Constitution.

The overall contents of this book and statements made have not have been evaluated by the FDA.

It is imperative that you consult a qualified practitioner if you feel that you have cancer.

Hrbacek, Jenny
Cancer Free! Are You Sure?

| ISBN-13: | 978-0-9913688-7-7 |
| LCCN: | 2015930598 |

| Editing: | Mary Budinger, Business Results LLC |

| Published by: | New Voice Publications |
| | Irvine, CA |

Dedication

This book is dedicated to all those who have or will be touched by cancer, and to my Lord and Savior, Jesus Christ, who planted the seed for this work, provided the title, and opened doors every step of the way.

Acknowledgments

I thank all of the practitioners and labs who shared their time and knowledge with me. I thank my friends, especially Misty May, Bobbie Hood, and Angela Lavespere who provided support. And I thank my editor, Mary Budinger, who without her knowledge and skills, this book would not be all that it is. I thank Sue Hurst for her careful final read of these pages before they went to the publisher. And I thank my husband, Dean, who loves and provides for me so that this work could be accomplished.

What Others Are Saying About This Book

When I first met Jenny it was like a light from heaven came shinning in my door. She is so full of life and zeal to reveal truth about how to find answers about what your current health status is really like through functional testing not normally provided for by the standard medical office.

As a clinical practitioner since 1992 in the Houston area, I have seen every type of person, all different races, ages from 2 weeks old to 92 years, and every condition for which doctors can give a disease label. One thing I am thoroughly convinced of and that is: we need people to know and understand how to properly test for dysfunction and not waste time or money on the traditional testing just to look for a disease label. Disease treatment and testing is outrageously expensive and bankrupting our country and our Medicare/Medicaid system.

Wellness care is now becoming popular as a catch phrase because people have become more concerned and educated about the topic. The United States has sunk very low on the totem pole of healthy countries; we now rank 37th in the world. The reason for my passion in wellness care is much similar to that of Jenny's. At age 25 I was told I would spend the rest of my adult life by the age of 40 in a wheel chair because of an autoimmune disease of arthritis in my spine called ankylosing spondylitis. At age 55 – and not in that wheelchair – I have much to say from my own experience and that of my patients about wellness care. My wife Amy and I have owned and operated the Nutrition and Health Center in Houston for 20 years now. We strongly suggest that functional tests that are best for you.

Since the largest cancer treatment center in the world is in the Houston area, we see a number of cancer patients. Historically I can tell you the survival rates of those patients who follow the traditional treatments of chemo, radiation and aggressive surgery are low. Those who implement a diligent lifestyle of healthy change in everything from eating more fresh, whole, organic foods to exercise and supplementation with quality nutritional supplements are definitely longer lived.

Through the years, the people we see who combine chemotherapy, radiation and surgery with lifestyle and diet changes typically astound their doctors when test results come back so much improved. We hear of doctors' comments like: "Your white blood cell levels are not dropping below the safe levels as often indicated with the treatment."

I've documented many testimonies of people on a journey to greater health just like you in my book, *The Trinity Diet*. Food is more spiritual than you ever realized and you can learn more about how to live an abundant life that is available through the way God made us to live. Enjoy the journey to abundant health!

– Steve Steeves, CCN, ND
Author, *The Trinity Diet*

⌘⌘⌘

The title, "Are You Sure," could be the title for many aspects of our life journey.

When faced with unknowns, what do we do with them? Some use curiosity and courage to dispel the unknown; many do not know what to do and fear prevents them from going any further, so they wait it out and take their chances. For many, fear is based on our lack of knowledge about the situation.

Just imagine being able to address, "Are You Sure" with the maximum peace and assurance possible. Imagine having someone to help you pursue the answer to this question who has the wherewithal to provide you emotional support, curiosity, and courage to dispel the unknown.

Well, this is now available to you with Jenny Hrbacek, RN. Jenny has fought the battle of cancer and knows, first hand, what the journey is about. In other words, "been there, done that, got that T-Shirt."

With the work that Jenny has done in providing tools that can detect cancer early, you have the best possible resources one could have. She has gained the vitally important first-hand experience and knowledge to provide you the support, encouragement, and expertise needed for you to address "Are You Sure?" and move forward rather than living in fear.

Consider the tragedy of those who have had cancer for years and didn't know it. I invite you to examine the information presented in this book.

Wouldn't it be worth taking the opportunity to see if you can move from "Are You Sure?" to that peace of mind state, "I Am Sure!"

– Paul Bennett
Dallas, Texas

⌘ ⌘ ⌘

I began my cancer journey in January 2009 with my annual mammogram, which lead to a sonogram, MRI, biopsy, and finally results.

My cancer was Triple Negative, Stage 1. Stage 1 – good; Triple Negative – not so good – rare and very aggressive, the doctor said. And it's just not as common so we do not have as much data on it.

My mom had gone through cancer 7 years before so I somewhat knew what would be in store for me.

I had the bi-lateral mastectomy surgery and during my 6-week recovery, I found out that Jenny Hrbacek had also been diagnosed with breast cancer and had the same surgery by my doctor and plastic surgeon. I had known Jenny and her husband through my work. Five weeks after my surgery, I went to see Jenny and that visit started our very special, friendship-filled, faith-filled, fight-filled, and even a little (and more) fun-filled walk together. I am so thankful I had Jenny on my cancer journey. (My husband called us "Bosom Buddies!")

Jenny and I attended a cancer support group together one day and I was overwhelmed and actually astonished to hear how many women in the room were there with a second or even third recurrence. There were only about 5 or 6 out of 50 women there who were going through this for the first time. After the meeting, several of us talked in the parking lot and I said I was NOT coming back because this was not the "support" I needed.

I also remembered finishing my treatment and my doctor saying that I was done and I could go back to my "normal life." I hit a real time of depression as I finished my treatment because I felt my "normal life" had resulted in cancer.

I remember Jenny bringing me a book one day, *Beating Cancer with Nutrition*. She was so excited! She told me, "This book empowers us! It's not just what they are doing but what we have to do."

I joined Jenny in visiting Dr. Ray Hammon in Rowlett, TX. I took the Greek test and have retested as well. Over the past 3 years, I have been "stable" and considered "in remission." At my last oncologist visit, my numbers were the best they ever were! I continue to fight the fight with my changed diet, exercise, and supplements, as well as reducing my stress level. It's not always easy and I am definitely not perfect but I do want my body and immune system to be strong enough to fight the cancer cells.

Jenny's medical knowledge as an R.N. was invaluable to me. She taught me to take control of my numbers and challenged me to do my part. Her passion in wanting me and others to be healthy is terrific and she stays on me even today, years later! I use the testing in this book to monitor my health.

I join Jenny Hrbacek in the cancer fight and in taking control of our health by good nutrition, supplements, and doing all we can do for this body that God has created for us so perfectly. This is all we can do and our dear Lord will take care of the rest.

Thank you Jenny and Dr. Hammon! You are truly a blessing to me and I am so grateful for your knowledge, passion, and loving care for me and so many others.

– Karen Glynn
Sugar Land, Texas

⌘⌘⌘

The doctor told me I had stage 4 cancer that had metastasized from my breast to my bones and down my vertebrae, to my ribs and into my pelvic and pubic areas, and even into some of my organs and lymph nodes. I had between 3 weeks and 3 months to live. Surely this was a mistake! How could this happen? I have never smoked. I have always been good to people. I cried out, "God, I have served you all my life. This can't be right!"

At the young age of 45, with one daughter married, one in college, and a son of 14 now, the doctors were telling me I was facing death.

For one year, I fought the greatest battle of my life, both in the spiritual and the physical realms. Today I am standing whole, healthy, and cancer free. This was accomplished without the use of chemo.

I met Jenny in the fall of 2013, after my diagnosis and cancer battle, and we made an immediate personal connection. I felt her compassion and desire to help others and I knew that our meeting had not been by chance. Oh how I wish that I would have had the information that she shares in this book many years ago. It is not necessary for cancer to go undetected as mine did. Cancer is an awful disease and this book contains instruments that you can use to find it early and be victorious. I pray that you will find enlightenment and direction within its pages.

– Shirley Williams
Marathon, Texas
Author, *Stage 4 Cancer Gone*

⌘⌘⌘

I consider my friend Jenny Hrbacek one of the reasons I can call myself a "cancer survivor," having had extensive treatment and recovery from HER 2 Triple Negative breast cancer in 2010 and 2011.

I first met Jenny at a "Survivors Offering Support" (SOS) meeting in the spring of 2011. I had just been through the traditional medical treatment regime of discovering breast cancer through a biopsy, which led to chemo, then double mastectomy surgery with complete reconstruction, followed by 6 weeks of radiation. Imagine my surprise when I heard Jenny speak at the SOS meeting and tell all assembled that what I had just experienced was no guarantee that cancer would not return. And, even further, that there were many new exciting alternative medicine therapies now available. Jenny challenged the audience that night with the question: "Your doctor tells you your cancer is cured, but can you really be sure?" My first thought on hearing Jenny was to think I guess I chose to believe my doctors. I thought, "I have been assured by my doctors I am now cancer free. I have already been through all of this. It would have been good to know about these new choices before I went through everything I have been through but that is all past now." I kept all of the information Jenny gave everyone that night thinking I would never again need it.

In September of 2013 I felt a continuous pain in my sternum and left breast, the same breast where the original tumor was discovered and removed. Test confirmed that my breast cancer was back and had metastasized. After 3 years of educating myself about breast cancer and good health in general, I knew my first round of traditional treatment had failed me. It was time to link back up with Jenny again.

Jenny has been a tireless advocate for my care and a fearless warrior on my behalf. As Jenny fights to win her own battle with breast cancer, she has dedicated her considerable life energy to my fight and others as well. Some people are closer than a sister. What Jenny has discovered and brings to this book is the result of her dedication to our fight and to anyone who may get that dreaded call to announce: "You have cancer." Cancer is an evil thing. What Jenny has researched and brought to these pages is invaluable when you have a big fight on your hands and short time to figure out just where to go and what to do. As you read through this well researched book, I know you will be amazed at what the doctors never tell you. It takes a fighter like Jenny to dig it all out for us. I pray you will be as blessed by this book and Jenny Hrbacek as much as I am.

– Darnell Richards
Sugar Land, Texas

Foreword

A world without cancer is possible. I collaborated for many years with Dr. Tsuneo Kobayashi in Japan. He is a molecular biologist who has shown us how, with early detection of cancer, the world could be nearly cancer-free. Many years ago, Dr. Kobayashi realized the imaging method of detection was too coarse to detect tumors until they were well established. He achieved a major breakthrough in developing a new marker system that grades your cancer outlook on a scale of 1-5. His rating of 5 is the equivalent to what in the United States is typically called a stage 1 cancer. In other words, when you top out on the Kobayashi scale, your problem is just now visible for the first time in the American system.

Dr. Kobayashi's patients undergo his annual cancer test, not because the doctor is trolling for business: Ah ha! A lump – sign up this person for chemotherapy and radiation, ka chink! No, Dr. Kobayashi wants his patients to avoid getting to that point. His annual cancer test is a very effective way of showing people their degree of risk, whether they are inching closer to that day when they would get a diagnosis, at which point someone will want to make money treating them with toxic 60-year old chemicals. To prevent the arrival of a diagnosis, he uses more rest and less stress, cuts sugar out of the diet, adds more nutrient dense food and exercise, and uses several methods of detoxification including infrared sauna and herbs to enhance the immune system.

In the last 25 years, Dr. Kobayashi has treated more than 20,000 early stage patients. He treated another 2,000 mid-to-latter stage patients who subsequently went into long term remission and had an average life span after treatment of 7 years. In comparison, the average life span of traditionally-treated breast cancer patients "in remission" is 4.5 years and for metastatic prostate cancer patients it is around 2 years.

For years, many of us packed our patient's blood samples in dry ice and shipped them to Dr. Kobayashi in Tokyo. It was not a perfect system; sometimes customs officials caused delays that meant the sample had to be thrown away. However, Dr. Kobayashi's work has been embraced by other pioneers in the development of true early detection testing. Many of the tests described in this book are built on the foundation that he laid and some of them are just as capable now of that kind of early detection, although they are newer and have not had time to accumulate the proven data that annual testing combined with a program of natural prevention can virtually eliminate clinical cancers.

As doctors, we take the Hippocratic Oath where we swear we will "first do no harm." It is a good phrase for patients to keep in mind because sometimes business managers can make oncologists forget that. So for you as a patient, it means that after you have read Jenny's book and you move forward and take an early detection test, DO NOT take that test to your oncologist and let them do harm. Dr. Kobayashi and many others have proven that the body will bring early cancer tests back to safe normal levels if you do the kinds of things Jenny takes time in this book to spell out.

We all have cancer cells in our bodies. Cancer cells and pre-cancerous cells are so common that nearly everyone by middle age or old age is riddled with them. If we have got a strong immune system, we will have no problem because those cancer cells will be disposed of every day. But if our immune system doesn't work right, we can have problems. And even then, some of those cancers will go away on their own without any interference from modern medicine. Cancers require more than mutations to progress. They need the cooperation of surrounding cells, hormones, and a number of other factors. As some researchers have said, it is interesting to know why we get cancer, but it is far more interesting to know why we don't get cancer!

The hero scientist who defeats cancer will likely never exist. Cancer is an intricate, potentially lethal collaboration of genes gone awry, of growth inhibitors gone missing, of hormones and epigenomes changing, and rogue cells breaking free.

Early detection should not be used as a means to shuttle people into surgery, radiation, and chemotherapy. Mainstream treatment for cancer is usually a waste of time and money, yet amazingly no one in academia ever mentions how easy it is to bring PSA into safe ranges and keep it there for life. And recently, a study conducted at the University of Michigan Medical School found that for women, genetic tests, advanced imaging, and having a strong fear that cancer would develop in their second breasts makes it more likely that women will choose to have a "preventive" double mastectomy even if the procedure does not improve their odds of survival. No one ever tells us how *not* to develop breast cancer.

Early detection means you have to get serious about the kinds of things Jenny talks about in the last 3 chapters of this book. Detecting cancer – after the fact – is not as good a course of action as using an early detection test to predict risk and take actions to head off a diagnosis.

We must learn how to live cancer-free through the use of old fashioned nutrition, targeted supplements, and therapeutic modalities such as homeopathy, acupuncture, microcurrent, laser, pulsed electromagnetic fields, craniosacral therapy, and stress reduction techniques.

Our world is full of heavy metals, devitalized foods, fungal infections, pollutants, endocrine disrupting chemicals, carcinogens and more. I am convinced that only with sensitive cancer screening tests can we motivate ourselves to achieve the level of health our body needs to keep the daily errant cells inside us from coalescing into a cancerous mass.

Jenny Hrbacek tells you about the many early detection tests for cancer available to you today. No one needs to be in the dark about whether cancer is getting foothold in their body. And if you do have a diagnosis, Jenny spells out to how obtain personalized treatment that is proven to be more effective than the standard cookie cutter treatment most cancer patients are told about.

We have managed to poison our planet. If you want to avoid that cancer diagnosis, you need a friend like Jenny Hrbacek to give you the bigger picture your oncologist likely is not able to give you. She will inspire you to make the diet and lifestyle choices necessary to be cancer free.

> – Garry F. Gordon, MD, DO, MD(H)
> Director of F.A.C.T. (Forum on Antiaging and Chelation Therapy) The world's largest alternative medicine online discussion group for health professionals.
> (www.gordonresearch.com)

⌘⌘⌘

Dr. Gordon received his Doctor of Osteopathy in 1958 from the Chicago College of Osteopathy in Illinois. He received his honorary M.D. degree from the University of California Irvine in 1962 and completed his Radiology Residency from Mt. Zion in San Francisco, California in 1964. For many years, he was the medical director of Mineral Lab in Hayward, California, a leading laboratory for trace mineral analysis worldwide. Dr. Gordon is a co-founder of the American College for Advancement in Medicine (ACAM). He is former Founder/President of the International College of Advanced Longevity, Board Member of International Oxidative Medicine Association (IOMA), advisor to the American Board of Clinical Metal Toxicology (ABCMT), and a full-time consultant for Longevity Plus, a nutritional supplement company. With Morton Walker, D.P.M., Dr. Gordon co-authored *The Chelation Answer. How to Prevent Hardening of the Arteries & Rejuvenate Your Cardiovascular System.*

Preface

I wrote the book I wish I had available to read years before I was diagnosed with cancer and definitely before I submitted to surgery and chemotherapy. These were invasive treatments that I can't reverse. My goal is for you to know that there are other options that your health provider may not offer or know about – options that can complement cancer treatment or help you prevent a formal diagnosis. If I had known about the tests that I tell you about, I could have had a heads-up years before my 2009 diagnosis, a warning that cancer was growing in my body.

The decisions that you make concerning your health will have profound effects on how the remainder of your life will play out. If you have received a cancer diagnosis, I encourage you to slow down, do research, and explore all your options. I know it is hard to slow down once you have been told you have cancer growing in your body. However, the reality is that it usually has been growing there for a long time and in most cases it is really worth your while to take a little time to look beyond what your physician has recommend. Better yet, do explore beyond what is presented in this text. This is what I found in my search; your journey may lead you down a different path. Be open to where God may lead you.

I am so thankful that you have picked up this text. You are already on a path that not many follow. May we go down that path together, so you can determine what is right for you.

May God bless our relationship together as we begin this journey.

– Jenny Hrbacek, R.N.

TABLE OF CONTENTS

Part 1 – Tests to Detect Cancer: Early Detection

Part 2 – Tests to Detect Cancer: Non-Early Detection

Part 3 – Functional Tests: Providing Early Warning Signs

Part 4 – Additional Information to Consider

CANCER FREE!

Are You Sure?

Chapter 1

Introduction

So you have been told that you are "cancer free," but are you sure? Did you just have your annual physical, with the standard lab work, and receive a clean bill of health? What if there were tests you could use to detect cancer before it was big enough to be felt or scanned by a machine – before a tumor is discovered and you have been told it has been growing silently for 8-10 years? What if there were steps that you could take to see cancer coming early and knock it out before it becomes something really big and life-threatening? In this book, you will learn about information that will empower you to take control of your health.

A diagnosis of cancer resonates fear in most people. I have been there so I can tell you the fear of dying, the fear of losing life as you know it, can be irrevocably changing. The thoughts of enduring painful and expensive treatments, losing body parts and hair . . . all that and more come instantly come to mind. Those fears have a way of pushing almost every other thought out of your head. You rush into surgery because you want the cancer out of your body as fast as the nearest doctor can yank it out. You endure months of rigorous treatments. When all is said and done, however, you may come to find out the cancer is back. And if it has spread, that is called a metastasis and that kills 90 percent of patients.

For many cancer patients – and I am one – the treatment of the tumors is not the cure. That can sound like a radical idea for some, so I'll say that again. Cutting out a tumor does not cure cancer. Some people get lucky and live long enough to die of something else, but many do not.

More Americans die of cancer every 18 months than have died in all the wars the nation has ever fought. The National Cancer Institute tells us that less than 66 percent of people diagnosed with cancer are "survivors," meaning they were still alive 5 years after their diagnosis. An estimated 580,350 precious souls died of cancer in 2013.[1] A report released by the World

Health Organization (WHO) in early 2014 said the forthcoming rise in cancer worldwide is an imminent "human disaster." Christopher Wild, director of the International Agency for Research on Cancer, put it succinctly:

> We cannot treat our way out of the cancer problem. More commitment to prevention and early detection is desperately needed in order to complement improved treatments and address the alarming rise in cancer burden globally.[2]

The first occurrence of cancer is generally easier and more successful to treat than most recurrences, especially when the cancer has metastasized. Once that happens, the outlook is often downright bleak. In the words of the National Cancer Institute:

> Although some types of metastatic cancer can be cured with current treatments, most cannot. Nevertheless, treatments are available for all patients with metastatic cancer. In general, the primary goal of these treatments is to control the growth of the cancer or to relieve symptoms caused by it. In some cases, metastatic cancer treatments may help prolong life. However, most people who die of cancer die of metastatic disease.[3]

Often cancer is not caught until it has spread into the lymph nodes, bones, or other organs, making recovery much more difficult.

So, if you have received conventional cancer therapies, how do you know that after your first rounds of treatment are over, you are as cancer free as your doctor says you are? I learned the hard way that you usually don't know and your doctor doesn't really know. And standard cancer treatments may actually raise the odds significantly that the cancer will return. You can be in the dark while cancer cells are re-gaining a foothold somewhere in the body until they have built a fortress big enough to be seen on the scans that are part of the routine check-ups. By then you have a BIG problem.

Or perhaps you have seen family, friends, and business associates spend time and money to undergo cancer treatments and you don't want to go through that. If you could find out that cancer was developing inside you, much sooner than when it is eventually detected with symptoms and standard scans, would you? A lot of people would. With an integrative physician, they can learn to make lifestyle changes and greatly reduce the odds of hearing the words, "Sorry, its cancer, and we need to get you into surgery and chemo right away."

You need to know if cancer cells are circulating in your body. Whether you have been diagnosed with cancer or you just wonder if cancer is about to strike you, there is a better way of finding out than what is usually recommended. Most of the tests doctors tell you about are designed to find cancer much later than the tests I will tell you about.

I learned it the hard way, but you can learn it the easy way – I've bundled it all up for you in this book.

My name is Jenny Hrbacek. I am a registered nurse (RN) from the big state of Texas. I was diagnosed with breast cancer using standard lab tests, biopsies, and scans commonly used in the United States today. At the time of my diagnoses, I seemed perfectly healthy and life was good. I had no idea how my life was about to change. As a patient, I was compliant and completed the recommended treatment protocol, and then I was congratulated and declared as having "no evidence of disease," meaning "cancer free" for now.

I expected my treatments to cure me, as my cancer was caught fairly early according to the commonly accepted indicators. It seems that the candles were still warm on my celebratory cake when I discovered, despite what my oncologists had told me, that I was walking around with microscopic cancer cells still circulating quietly in my blood. Further, because of the initial cancer and the treatments I had been exposed to, I was at a higher risk of having a recurrence for a more aggressive form of the cancer. I was not cancer free at all.

The familiar 3-pronged approach of surgery, chemo, and radiation was developed after WWII. As decades went by, there was an explosion of technological advances – science was even able to map the human genome – but how cancer is treated has not significantly changed. In 1971, President Richard Nixon declared a war on cancer with the signing of the National Cancer

Act. Since then, some $100 billion has been spent on cancer research with little success in terms of "finding the cure" and reducing deaths.

Conventional cancer treatment has become big business offering a poor end product. As the 2014 WHO report showed, the rocketing cost of responding to the "cancer burden" has reached the point it is measurably hurting the economies of rich countries and is beyond the means of poor ones. The report also said about half of all cancers were preventable and could have been avoided if current medical knowledge was acted upon.

It is heart breaking to witness the pain and suffering that cancer brings and I want to help.

I discovered many tests that can detect the presence of cancer cells even before signs or symptoms develop. The science behind these tests is compelling. Today, I use these tests to monitor my cancer status and the effectiveness of the therapies and lifestyle changes I have implemented to keep me on the path to health.

This book tells you about 9 early detection tests that are more sensitive than the tests that have become standard procedure, and 16 tests that can provide early warning signs. It is possible for you to have peace of mind, even if you have a family history of cancer. Each test is broken down into easy to read sections providing information on the cost, mechanisms of operation, benefits, limitations, and other important facts about each test. Some of the tests are available without a physician and are simple enough to be performed at home. Others are more complex and require the guidance of a trained clinician. Several tests even offer information that is invaluable in formulating a personalized cancer treatment plan by identifying the best targeted therapies for each patient.

Most cancer patients finish their treatment and then are put in what I call the "wait, watch, and wonder" program. Your physician waits a few months and then calls you in to watch for overt signs of cancer. Meanwhile, you are left wondering if they are going to find more cancer and if you are really cancer free. I don't recommend you wait, watch, and wonder, unless you have a death wish.

In the search for solutions, I found that some exciting, simple, and great options exist. And we desperately need them because our lives are at stake – we are not winning the war on cancer. There is almost no effort nationally or globally to prevent this disease. Oh yes, they tell us to stop smoking. But since only 18 percent of Americans smoke, that leaves 4 out of 5 people with no prevention tools other than vague admonishments to eat better and exercise more. Good luck with that.

Cancer is a wily beast. It hides but we have gotten better at finding it. Good early detection tests are key. Early detection tests are available, legal, and sometimes even covered by insurance, but you won't usually find them at your local doctor's office. You have to know where to find them. I will tell you.

And as a bonus, I will tell you some really important things – things I wish I had known when I was diagnosed – about treatment side effects, the accuracy of scientific studies, what "survival" really means, how tiny tumors too small to be seen on a scan can begin the process of metastasis, why famous people don't fare any better than you and me with American cancer treatments, and why cancer cures can be toxic. I will tell you what one food you never want to touch if you are serious about fighting cancer. I will invite you to take a closer look at the advertisements designed to influence your thoughts, opinions, and choices concerning cancer treatment. Cancer is big business – you don't have to be a mindless cog in the big revenue stream.

You will discover that there are some very good integrative oncologists out there, years ahead of their colleagues, who have impressive track records. Also that there are clinics using methods to support the immune system and rid the body of cancer without the organ damage, immune system damage, and other harmful side effects that result from chemotherapy and radiation. And who knew there were cancer consultants who have been successfully guiding patients for years through the maze of conventional, complementary, and alternative options?

In the Resources section, you will find websites, books, videos, and reports you can access.

In a cherished interview with Charlotte Gerson, daughter of Max Gerson who pioneered the use of dietary therapy for the treatment of cancer and chronic diseases, Charlotte explained that cancer treatment, to be successful, must address toxicity and deficiency. Food can be used as medicine to correct those deficiencies. I can confidently say that I would have made very different treatment decisions at the time of my diagnosis had I known the information contained in this book. And my cancer could have been detected even earlier, long before an oncologist could see a small tumor on my test films.

It is my prayer that this book will give you and your loved ones accurate, superior, and life changing information. It's a big world out there! You have the right to choose, so choose responsibly. Educate yourself. The decisions you make can save your life or the life of someone you love.

You *can* take control of your health. Get tested and have peace of mind. If you have had cancer in the past, consider one of these tests to verify or reduce the possibility of a recurrence before your next oncology appointment or scan. Patients who have chosen integrative therapies may use these tests to determine which treatments are working. Anyone whose previous therapy has failed them may use several of the tests discussed to formulate a new targeted plan. And for those of you who are just wondering if you could have cancer, get tested!

May God bless and direct you,

– Jenny Hrbacek, R.N.

Beloved, I wish above all things that thou mayest prosper and be in good health, even as thy soul prosperpereth.

– 3 John 1:2 (KJV)

Footnotes

1   National Cancer Institute. SEER Fact Sheet: All Cancer Sites.
     Retrieved January 15, 2015 at: www.seer.cancer.gov/statfacts/html/
     all.html.
2   Hume T, Christensen J. WHO: Imminent global cancer 'disaster'
     reflects aging, lifestyle factors. CNN.com. February 5, 2014.
3   National Cancer Institute. Fact Sheet: Metastatic Cancer.
     Retrieved January 19, 2015 at: www.cancer.gov/cancertopics/
     factsheet/Sites-Types/metastatic.

Chapter 2

Jenny's Story

Cancer does not respect your schedule, not the least little bit. When I received the diagnosis of breast cancer in April 2009, I was forced to find time in the next few months for six surgeries, four rounds of chemotherapy, a PET scan, an MRI scan, a nuclear heart scan, two CT scans, a bone scan, and more doctors' appointments and lab tests than anyone should endure in a lifetime. All because of a little 1.9 cm tumor, something as small as a penny.

At the time of my diagnosis I was a perfectly healthy 47-year-old female, or so I thought. And I should know, right? I am a nurse.

I never had a problem with needles until they were aimed at me, and very quickly I began to feel like a walking pin cushion. Today, I can't even count the number of times that I have been stuck for blood draws and infusions. And the whopping big medical bills – I had insurance with a $10,000 deductible plus a 20 percent co-pay. One hospital bill alone was roughly $35,000.

The lack of control over my life was also a new experience. And with it came a pronounced loneliness. My husband would leave for work, the kids would head off for school, and my dear friend Jacque would show up to take me to a doctor's appointment or help with dressing changes. Even with the multitude of cards, casseroles, and support from family and friends, I felt so alone when I would lay my head on the pillow at night. In the darkness it was just me, my prayers, my faith, and the cancer.

My official diagnosis was: "Invasive ductal carcinoma of the right breast with lobular features. Pathology staging of T1A N1A M0, Stage IIA, ER/PR positive, HER-2 negative, and negative for BRCA1 and BRCA2 mutations."

From the moment I was told I had cancer, I felt an uncontrollable urgency to get rid of it and quickly! I kept picturing myself on a train ride that I did not remember buying a ticket for. What I did not understand at that time, was that the ticket that read "*All Aboard - breast cancer, Jenny Hrbacek*" had been slipped into my back pocket 7 or 8 years before. I would learn later that cancer starts developing almost a decade before it is usually discovered.

Just a few days after that diagnosis, I had the double mastectomy that I believed would get rid of the cancer. I chose the mastectomy because I wanted to alleviate the possibility of having cancer in the other breast. Also, the breast surgeon and plastic surgeon said lumpectomies require radiation – that's protocol. They explained that the radiation damages the breast and makes any future reconstruction very difficult.

I selected a talented plastic surgeon who specialized in reconstruction at the time of the mastectomy. The thought of being bare-chested haunted me. My plastic surgeon showed me photos of his amazing work as well as let me interview several patients. I never thought of myself as a person who would ever have a plastic surgeon, but somehow the thought of replacing cancerous tissue with nice implants didn't seem so bad.

Upon waking up from the initial surgery I received a report that all of my lymph nodes were clear. Unfortunately, 10 days later, I received the revised report that one lymph node had a 2.4mm seed of cancer cells. Suddenly, the game plan changed. The National Comprehensive Cancer Network (NCCN) guidelines called for immediate removal of all lymph nodes under my right arm, followed by chemotherapy. The NCCN also listed radiation as an option. Thank goodness, my breast surgeon, plastic surgeon, and my heart said "no" to radiation. I questioned why it would be safe for me to have radiation while the radiation techs are wearing radiation exposure monitors and protected by heavy aprons and steel plated walls.

I agreed to four cycles of chemotherapy. I received Taxotere® and Cytoxan®. My hair fell out and I ended up in the hospital for five days in reverse isolation due to a temperature and a low white blood cell count. One of the most shocking things about my hospital stay was that I was only allowed to eat processed food. That meant no apples, cucumbers, or even lettuce on a hamburger. Thank you to my husband and friends who were able to sneak contraband fruits and veggies past the nurses' station. Four weeks later after my next chemo infusion, I again had a spike in my temperature. Rather than call my oncologist and the hospital, I took two Tylenol and left it to the Lord. My temperature returned to normal the next day.

I read the side effects of the chemotherapy drugs that I was being given. Most of them sounded as bad if not worse than the original 1.9 centimeter tumor in my right breast. The possible side effects of heart, kidney, and liver damage as well as the development of other cancers, didn't sound appealing. As I sat one day receiving a chemotherapy infusion, I looked around the room. The lady across the aisle from me was on oxygen due to heart damage caused by a listed side effect of her chemotherapy, and the man to my left was so weak that he needed a walker to stand due to heart damage from his chemotherapy. I looked diagonally across the room and watched a young teenager with a brain tumor eating French fries and drinking a soda. He followed that with a bag of cookies. Believe me, I have nothing against cookies; I have eaten my fair share of them in my life time. However, in my new reality, I looked at things from a cancer patient's perspective.

I had learned that the PET scans that are used to diagnose tumors involve a radioactive tracer with sugar injected into the vein. Cancer cells use sugar for metabolism and growth, so they absorb the radioactive sugar and glow on the scan, thus revealing cancer cells/tumors. The thought of this young man eating French fries that break down to sugar, followed by a sugary soda and cookies, broke my heart. I decided to keep my mouth shut for the moment and reached for my IV pole and walked over to the patient snack area. There I found a vending machine full of cookies, crackers, chocolate, etc. It is well known that sugar feeds cancer cells and damages the immune system. If I could find this information after a few hours of Internet research, why didn't the doctors and staff at this major cancer treatment facility know this? I could not understand why the facility did not have educational posters up around the room and have healthy snacks available for the patients receiving chemo.

I knew these patients must want to live or they would not be subjecting themselves to these harsh treatments and suffering through the side effects. I felt certain these patients would be happy to receive any information that could help them in their journey to restored health. I gathered several research studies, books, and supplements to take to my next appointment with my oncologist. I had a list of questions and felt armed with good data. The nurse saw me carrying a container of dehydrated wheat grass powder, Essiac® tea, a few other supplements, nutritional studies, and several books into the small exam room and placing them on the counter to discuss with my doctor when he came in. She said, "You can't bring all of this stuff in here." I smiled and told her that I felt certain that the doctor would want to know what I was taking and would be interested in my nutritional concerns during treatment. But I was wrong.

My oncologist also agreed that I could not bring in such material. He was more concerned with the report of my white blood cell count and the calendar to schedule my last chemo infusion. I gifted him the copy of *Beating Cancer with Nutrition* by Patrick Quillin that I had purchased for him. He actually tried to give it back to me and said I could not be giving him gifts. I was stunned. He seemed shocked that I was trying to understand the disease process and told me that most of his patients don't ask many questions. I continued. I told him it would be nice if they provided some healthy snack options in the vending machine. After a short pause, he said, "Well, I am not in charge of the vending machine." I thought to myself, well then you are not in charge of me either. That was the end of oncologist #1. I cringe every time I see one of the television commercials promoting how much they "care" at this huge oncology facility.

So, it was on to oncologist #2. Even though I had completed my agreed upon treatment protocol, I felt that I should be followed by an oncologist and I wasn't going back to oncologist #1. Oncologist #2 was at least willing to hear me out and added a few things to my protocol to counteract some of the side effects that were brought on by the chemotherapy. I was put on the schedule to see her every six months.

I had joined a breast cancer support group. We talked, had parties, exercised, and enjoyed monthly speakers. I learned that approximately half of the women in the group had experienced a recurrence of their original breast cancer. They seemed satisfied with their medical care. They showed up wearing pink survivor caps, usually with a wig. It seemed like every month there would be an announcement that another woman was back in treatment with a recurrence. It was starting to make sense why the oncologists want patients to come in for checkups every six months. They know that completion of the NCCN treatment protocol often leaves patients with a weakened immune system and with a high risk of recurrence. They know that the surgery, chemotherapy, and radiation that they are offering are not a cure, but only a treatment – which can be repeated for additional revenue.

That's when I set out not to be a statistic. I was determined to build up my damaged immune system. At one of our cancer support group meetings, I met a new friend, Faye. She gave me the direction that I had been praying for. After hearing her out, I made an appointment at the Integrative & Functional Health Center in Rowlett, Texas where she was a patient. I made the four hour drive to be evaluated and by the end of that day, I was empowered and had taken the first steps to take back control of my health. I had dug my heels in and refused to live from oncologist appointment to oncologist appointment, praying for them to pronounce me cancer free for a few more months.

My heart breaks for anyone that has to live with the anxiety associated with regular cancer checks with their oncologist. I receive several emails a month asking me to pray for someone that is going to one of those "cancer check appointments;" here is one:

Pray for Neil tomorrow for a 5 year cancer free checkup.
We won't know results until next week.
Thanks for praying!
Love, Kathy and Neil

The detailed information contained in this book is about the journey that began the day of that four hour drive to meet with Dr. Ray Hammon of Integrative & Functional Health Center and R.G.C.C. USA labs (Research Genetic Cancer Center). I learned about very sensitive blood tests that are available, but not offered by the mainstream oncologists in the U.S. I also learned that not only can we put men on the moon and build tiny microprocessors, but we can detect and harvest cancer cells circulating in the blood.

It was now eight months after my surgery and I was sporting two new beautifully reconstructed breasts. I was on a mission to strengthen my immune system. I had clean margins and a clean scan, but after seeing that half the women in my breast cancer support group had experienced a recurrence – some of them two or more recurrences – I wanted to be sure I would stay cancer free.

Dr. Hammon said we should first perform a blood test to see if cancer cells were indeed still circulating in my body.

He uses R.G.C.C. in Greece for the test where they utilize a patented process to harvest and grow in vitro (petri dish) any remaining circulating cancer cells that may be in my blood. If the lab was able to find any cancer cells, the test also included sensitivity testing for chemotherapy drugs and many herbs and vitamins. In other words, the test would tell me which drugs and natural substances would work for me and which would be a waste of time and money. My insurance company would not pay for anything that was not both FDA approved and part of the NCCN cancer treatment protocol. This did not matter to me; I got out my check book and paid for the test. I had to know if I had any circulating tumor cells in my blood from the primary breast cancer. I was determined not to have an oncologist order a PET scan – with its dose of sugar and radiation – and give me any more bad news.

The results shocked me. "You have the highest level of breast cancer cells of anyone who has come through these doors," Dr. Hammon told me.

My hair had not even grown back yet from the chemo. What happened to the "clean surgical margins" and the "clean CT scan"?

I really thought the test would show I was cancer free, that this test would come back with "0" circulating tumor cells (CTCs) present in my blood. After all, I had completed surgery with clean margins and received four rounds of very toxic chemotherapy. But the test showed 14.2 cells per 7.5 cc of my blood. It confirmed my biggest fear that I was just like the other women attending the cancer support groups. I had circulating cancer cells from the primary tumor looking for a new place to set up shop. I was surprised to learn this since my oncologists had released me from treatment and put me on a six month check-up program.

Integrative & Functional Health Center immediately referred me to oncologist #3, Dr. Jairo Oliveras, M.D., where I was told that with such a high number of CTCs, I should begin more chemotherapy immediately. I refused. He said he would give me 90 days to get my CTC count down below 10, using nutrition, exercise, and the natural substance sensitivity testing that I received through Dr. Hammon. If I was able to do it, he would support me. Dr. Oliveras looked me sternly in the face and told me to do everything that my sensitivity test had indicated and make strict lifestyle changes – including intravenous vitamin C, and an extremely low sugar, no processed food diet. I agreed and made an appointment to see him in a little over three months. I immediately got on the personalized natural substance program indicated on my test. Many of the items included in my protocol were available at the local health food store. I was grateful he had the ability to consider the body's ability to heal when given the proper support.

The "father of medicine," Hippocrates, said, "Let food be thy medicine and medicine be thy food." I did and found it really works for cancer. I came to see that my processed food diet was lacking so many of the herbs and nutrients that have been proven to have anti-cancer properties. I learned that I could take responsibility for my health and change my future.

Wow! Three months later, it felt so good to walk into the next appointment holding a lab report that read: "Jenny Hrbacek, CTC 5.5 / 7.5 cc of blood." Not only did I meet his goal of lowering my count below 10, but I was at 5.5! I continued with my protocol and in another 90 days, my CTC was down to 2.9. Amazing! I did that without expensive and toxic chemotherapy.

I was beginning to understand how thousands of people have handled their cancer with natural therapies. The book stores and Internet are filled with their testimonies. I had to learn more. I spent the next 3 years attending integrative cancer conferences. I found myself sitting in lecture halls filled with physicians who had dedicated their practices to combat cancer with less toxic therapies while supporting the body so that it can heal. I talked to every attendee who would talk with me and I scoured the exhibit halls during the breaks. I took copious notes. I was able to interview doctors from across the U.S. and around the world. Wow, I have met some amazing physicians. I had read Suzanne Somers book, *Knockout*, but I never thought I would get to meet many of the doctors she interviewed. These people are more than just a chapter in a book, but real people who are actively networking to learn as much as they can to help their patients. I have to tell you, I was like a kid in a candy store. Like a sponge trying to soak up every detail that I could absorb. These doctors used terms and tools that I did not learn about in nursing school and had not heard of during my personal cancer treatment. I had to learn what seemed like a new language and approach. I still have a hard time believing the average person does not have access to the information that I learned. You have to work hard find it. It was during this time of research that I discovered more about what cancer really is and that it can be detected early using many different tests. Tests that I wish I had known about years before my diagnosis.

It is important to know that when cancer cells duplicate, they make errors in their DNA. These mutating cancer cells require a multifaceted and targeted approach. There are brilliant biologists, scientists, and doctors working far from the shores of the United States and right here in our country, without the benefit of the billions of dollars that are raised from groups like the American Cancer Society. They are providing real results and a targeted, less toxic approach to cancer treatment. I am so excited to be able to share this information on a larger scale.

I ask that you set aside the information that you have received from pharmaceutical marketing, the media, and the big money machine that operates in the cancer industry. Think outside the box. Your health or the health of someone that you love will benefit from what you learn.

⌘⌘⌘

When I got the initial diagnosis, I was fearful. It all came at me so fast. I thought I was being given accurate and complete information about all my options. I let the surgeon remove my breast tissue because I had an overwhelming desire to get the cancer out of my body. I believed I was getting rid of my cancer and the possibility of any future breast cancer. What I learned later is that research shows that there is no substantial increase in life expectancy in women who have had a lumpectomy versus a mastectomy.

Before Dr. Hammon, no one had talked to me about the fact that removing breast tissue did not mean that breast cancer could not pop up somewhere else in the body. Mastectomies and lumpectomies do not necessarily get rid of the cancer because they do not deal with the compromised immune system and the left behind circulating tumor cells (CTCs) that allow cancer to spread. It is the metastasis that makes cancer so fatal.

I look back on the decision process to have a double mastectomy with more clarity now. I see that I based my surgical decision on information that was incomplete at best. I am still profoundly sad that no one corrected my false belief that by having all of the breast tissue removed, I would never have to deal with breast cancer again. How many times had I verbalized that wish to my healthcare professionals?

What I know now is that science has shown that tumors over 1-2 mm have a blood supply and the cancer cells have a pathway to the blood stream through this blood supply and the lymphatic system. So all I did was increase the chance that a breast cancer cell would turn up later in some place other than breast tissue. That's not a good thing to have happen. When doctors find the primary cancer in other organs, it becomes metastatic stage 4 cancer. The information I had been given was that surgery with clean margins took care of the cancer – end of story. But it is not.

From the first day of diagnosis and continuing throughout the entire treatment process, I kept asking about my immune system. If it is true that every day the human body produces upwards of 10,000 cancer cells and the immune system routinely kills them, why did my immune system falter and let the cancer cells multiply and grow into a tumor that was discovered years later? I was repeatedly told that it was bad luck and that there was no need for cleanses, vitamins, or a diet change.

I was later told by all my oncologists that the taking of oral contraceptives had fueled the cancer cells because lab test showed the cells to be positive for estrogen receptors. Oral contraceptives contain synthetic estrogen. Every morning I was feeding the breast cancer cells when I took the prescription given to me by my gynecologist to ease the side effects of menopause. I should have done my own research and not filled that prescription.

If you are wondering what happened to oncologist #2, let me take a step back and fill you in. At a follow up appointment with her, she noticed my tumor markers were up several points; however, they were never above normal even when the tumor was first discovered. Tumor markers are done with a blood test that measures substances produced by tumors. She said that she wanted to order a CTC (circulating tumor cell) test because of the tumor marker increase. I asked her what we would do if I had some CTCs. She said that we would do a PET scan to determine were the cancer had spread. I said okay to her CTC test. She handed me a lab slip and I was told to make an appointment in the next few days to have my blood drawn. I found out that she was sending my blood off for a CELLSEARCH test; it is performed by Janssen Diagnostics, a U.S. company that is a subsidiary of Johnson & Johnson and is the only U.S. FDA approved CTC blood test.

The following day, I had my first appointment with Dr. Hammon at the Integrative & Functional Health Center. He drew my blood for a different CTC test. This vial of blood was sent to a laboratory in Greece. I spent several days in Rowlett, Texas, and had three IV infusions of high dose vitamin C before returning home to Houston and having the CELLSEARCH test drawn.

About two weeks later, I received the result from both CTC tests. The test result from CELLSEARCH found "0" CTCs. And as I explained earlier, the test from Greece found 14.2/7.5 cc of blood, a large number of microscopic cancer cells growing and circulating in my blood.

I asked oncologist #2 how the Greece lab test could find a large number cancer cells in my blood while the CELLSEARCH test that she ordered said that I was "cancer free," especially since she suspected something was not right because of the increase in my tumor markers. She said she was not familiar with the Greece test and dismissed its positive result. She did say there was no need for a PET scan because her test, the CELLSEARCH test, will not pick up cancer until it has metastasized to another organ and she would continue to monitor my tumor marker labs.

Being a nurse, I was not satisfied with her dismissive answer and wanted to understand the big discrepancy. I wanted to know what my CTC was when I had the original 1.9 cm tumor. To my surprise, she told me that oncologists do not perform the FDA-approved CTC test at diagnosis because it will not pick up cancer cells until the cancer has metastasized to another organ. So my next question was: "Are you telling me that my CTC was '0' when I did have cancer and it is '0' now and you are sure that I do not have cancer?" She replied, "Yes, Jenny, you do not have cancer. Eat cupcakes, exercise, and take a multivitamin. Go enjoy your life."

I paused and thought to myself, wow, I hope she is right, because if she is wrong, I could be in really big trouble. I was educated enough to know that a cancer cell does not jump from one area of the body to another area. It travels through the blood stream. I was stunned to hear her explain that the standard practice in the U.S. is to monitor lab results while a tumor can be growing large enough to be seen on a PET scan or that CTCs increase in a concentration high enough in the blood to be detected by the approved U.S. test. I walked out and never went back. That was the end of oncologist #2 for me.

The data available states that a tumor has to be about 0.5cm to 1 cm in size before it is visible on a PET scan. But what I found most surprising is that most cells in a tumor are not cancerous. I learned at a conference of the International Organization of Integrative Cancer Physicians that doctors take repetitive tissue samples – multiple biopsy sites – of a tumor because cancer cells might be found in just one or two of the samples. Less than one percent of a tumor is cancerous cells.[1]

One of the leading cancer researchers is Max Wicha, M.D., professor of oncology and director of the University of Michigan Comprehensive Cancer Center. He says standard cancer treatments can make things worse because when chemotherapy and radiation kill tumor cells, the dying cells send out inflammatory molecules that can summon *cancer stem cells*.[2] These stem cells are like the wildcard in a deck of cards. They can respond to the dying cells and essentially say, "Oh, we hear you are dying and we can help you out by making ourselves into more malignant cells like you, if you want." In that way, cancer cells can spread through the body after chemo and radiation.

The average oncologist never says one word about cancer stem cells to patients, much less treat for them.

So how do we encourage cancer stem cells not to turn into more malignant cells? It turns out a number of natural substances do just that, including cruciferous vegetables and curcumin, the spice that gives Indian food its deep yellow color.

I began to network with patients, family members, and physicians. I put together a two hour PowerPoint presentation, "Know Your Enemy and Win," and began speaking to groups. Through word of mouth, newly diagnosed patients would get my phone number. Each ring of the phone was a commitment of about three hours of education and time. Quite a few people were passionate about really healing their body and not excited to run down for surgical removal of body parts, cytotoxic chemotherapy, and radiation. It was so encouraging to be helping people. At the same time, others would choose to strictly follow traditional treatment. I would be heartbroken to receive reports of nausea, hair loss, and other side effects of harsh treatment protocols. I knew that I needed a better way to get this information out. The outline of a book was begun.

During that time, with my improving CTC counts, I must confess that I became a little complacent and stopped taking many of the things that were in my personalized protocol. I would indulge in a dessert and an occasional glass of wine with dinner. I was confident I could manage the remaining cancer cells because I had the lab reports to prove it. My mistake was that I underestimated the veracity of these cells to reproduce. After a 2 year hiatus, I decided to send my blood back to R.G.C.C. in Greece for a CTC count check. I was disappointed to learn that it was up slightly to 3.3 from my 2.9. Today I am back to managing and giving my full attention to those CTCs. I have my eye on the goal of getting that number to zero. I understand now how important it is for any person who has had cancer to never let their guard down.

As time marches on, I have found my phone rings often with calls from newly diagnosed cancer patients looking for answers to very serious questions. I received one such call in December of 2012 from a woman named Angela. She asked if I was aware of any natural alternatives to the hormone blocker, Tamoxifen.

Angela was 47-years-old, just like me when she was diagnosed with breast cancer. Her life was full and active. She was a busy single mom raising two teenagers. She had a demanding career in medical case management and was in her third season of triathlon participation.

I found that she had a very hard time saying that she had "cancer." She told me she was an avid hiker, once hiking 1600-plus miles along the Continental Divide testing equipment, the elements, and her endurance. She was a certified personal trainer and owner/operator of a sports training business for many years. She participated in multi-sports and adventure racing. She downed a green drink every day to make up for any short falls in her busy lifestyle and ate what she understood to be a healthy diet. People sought her out for health and fitness advice. She felt that her cancer diagnosis was the ultimate insult for someone who prided herself in "health and fitness."

I share Angela's history because it helps to understand that cancer can touch even the lives of those who are considered as 'healthy and fit." Also, many of the calls that I receive are coming from people in their 20s, 30s, and 40s – people we would think are too young to get cancer.

Angela explained that in May, 2012 she was feeling run down and went to see her doctor. She also went for a regular 3D mammogram and breast ultrasound to evaluate a lump in her breast that they had been "watching" since 2008 because she had a history of fibrocystic breasts. This time, the radiologist wanted more samples. This time, the diagnosis turned out to be positive for invasive lobular carcinoma in her left breast.

Angel's surgeon told her that it wasn't anything she did, it was just bad luck. She was urged not to put off surgery too long and was welcomed to "the club" with a pink bag full of brochures on breast cancer treatments, wigs, and such.

A few days later, Angela received the news that the latest

pathology report indicated infiltrating ductile carcinoma in her other breast. So she had two primary cancers, one in each breast. Her surgeon now felt that a bilateral mastectomy was the best solution. Like most people at the start of a medical crisis, Angela looked to the authority of the white coat to help her make up her mind – certainly the doctor would know best. Angela was told that removing all of her breast tissue would take care of 90 percent of any future risk. She was also told that she would "have a greater chance of dying on the freeway on the way to work than from breast cancer."

Angela will tell you that the post-surgical recovery from a bilateral mastectomy is an experience for which no one can prepare themselves. Angela's surgeon reported the good news that she had clean margins, meaning they thought they got it all. However, they did find a micro-metastasis in a lymph node that they said did not require treatment with chemotherapy. Her "Breast Cancer Recurrence Score" was 4, indicating an average distant recurrence of 5 percent.[3] With this score, she was not a candidate for chemotherapy or radiation as the benefits from chemo did not outweigh the damaging effects that it would have on her health. Her oncologist suggested that she should take Tamoxifen to suppress the estrogen hormones which fed her estrogen positive cancer. He explained that she should take the drug for just the next 5 years because after 5 years the benefits no longer outweigh the side effects. When he sensed her reluctance to take drug, he told her, "If you were stranded on a dessert island, the only thing you would want is your Tamoxifen, a bottle of water, and your boyfriend." His assurances seemed very compelling.

Yet Angela's research side kicked in and she began looking for herself into the side effects of Tamoxifen – hot flashes, fatigue, depression, deep vein thrombosis, pulmonary emboli, and additional cancers. She learned that it did not kill cancer cells; it only attempted to put any cell that is estrogen receptor positive in "remission" by blocking the estrogen receptor sites on cancer cells. The warning label states this drug is a known carcinogen. It didn't make sense to her to take a substance that caused cancer.

She was beginning to understand that the treatment was not the same thing as a cure. She was learning that the treatment of symptoms was to be followed by more treatment of more symptoms. She felt guilty that she had temporarily given up her power and submitted to radical surgery. She was realizing that her lifestyle, dietary choices, etc., played a primary role in the development of cancer. Most of all, she was feeling empowered and motivated to make changes and restore her health.

But friends and family were not happy to hear that she was not buying into the full standard plan of care for post-surgical management. Feelings of guilt and doubt began to creep in.

Angela's unopened prescription bottle was still on her night stand when she met with her breast surgeon one more time to discuss her concerns. The surgeon told her about another patient with similar ideas and concerns, a bad patient who was not following doctors' orders. This patient was even speaking on wellness and was eating kale chips, power berries, and other "nasty tasting" things. The surgeon held out a business card with my name on it. Angela was pretty convinced she did not want to be a "good girl" and take the Tamoxifen so she grabbed that business card. When Angela made that first call to me, she said it was an answered prayer.

I applauded her for her research to search for less toxic supportive therapies. I explained to her that it would be nice to have confirmation that she was cancer free. She made the same trek to Dr. Ray Hammon at the Integrative & Functional Health Center as I had made. She learned about the "Greek test" and her subsequent test result of 4.2 circulating tumor cells per 7.5 cc of blood. She now knew why her doctors wanted her to take Tamoxifen and come in for regular cancer check-ups; she was not cancer free at all.

The "Greek test" gave Angela a personalized list of the most effective chemotherapy drugs and natural substances that would be effective against her specific cancer. In the cancer arena, some call this the beginning of personalized cancer treatment.

Angela began a program to detox her body and rebuild her immune system. She radically changed her diet, eliminating processed foods and sugar. She bought a juicer and shopped for organic produce.

Both Angela and I were told that our cancers had been developing 7 to 10 years prior to our initial diagnoses. We learned that our high carbohydrate diets were feeding our cancers. Those carbohydrates break down to sugar and cancer loves sugar. The fox was in the hen house wreaking havoc and we had no idea.

Seven months later, Angela received a call from Dr. Hammon regarding a follow up CTC test from Greece to monitor the effectiveness of her new lifestyle changes and treatment protocol. Her circulating tumor cell count went down from 4.2/7.5 cc of blood to 2.0/7.5 cc of blood. This great news provided her the confidence in the dietary and lifestyle changes that she made since early February 2013, and it encourages me to continue on the course too. Even better, her count is 1.0/7.5 cc of blood as of early 2014. Angela is working to get that number to zero. And she is doing this without the use of Tamoxifen. She has the motivation and the desire to stand up to cancer. If she sticks with the program, I would expect that she will not be like so many others who experience a cancer recurrence.

During the writing of this book, I have interviewed and worked with so many incredible clinicians. I wish that I had found them sooner.

I invite you to visit my website at www.CancerFreeAreYouSure. com to contact me.

I often think about the pillow that my breast surgeon has in her office. It reads: *"Yes, they are fake, my real ones tried to kill me."* The sad truth is that even if the breasts are gone, they may still be trying to kill you.

Cancer can be detected early. And there is a lot you can do to prevent it. It is my wish that you will be empowered by the information shared in these pages. Being healthy is your birthright.

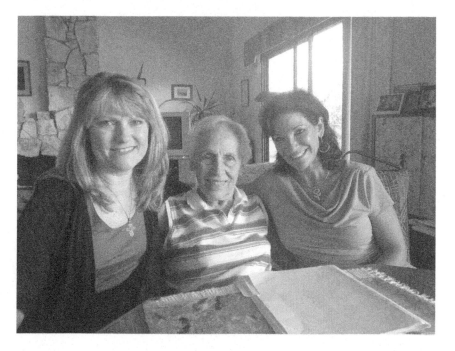

Jenny Hrbacek, Charlotte Gerson of the Gerson Institute, and Angela Lavespere – September 2013

Footnotes

1   Diehn M, Cho RW, Clarke MF. Therapeutic Implications of the Cancer Stem Cell Hypothesis. *Semin Radiat Oncol*. 2009 April; 19(2):78-86.
2   Wicha MS, Liu S, and Dontu G. Cancer Stem Cells: An Old Idea – A Paradigm Shift. *Cancer Res*. 2006; 66:(4). February 15, 2006.
3   Paik S, Shak S, et al. A multigene assay to predict recurrence of tamoxifen-treated, node-negative breast cancer. *NEJM*. 2004 Dec 30; 351(27):2817-2826.

Chapter 3

What Is Cancer?

For me, like most people, cancer was something that I simply hoped that I would never get. I really never considered myself at risk and if I was, I certainly did not want to know it. Unfortunately, widespread cancer became a reality in the 20th century when death rates started to escalate.

When the term "cancer" is mentioned, the natural reaction of most people is a feeling of trepidation. And for some reason, possibly fear or denial, I have found that most people are not really interested in learning about it either. However, the old saying "out of sight – out of mind" does not work with cancer. You can't hide from it or make it go away by ignoring it. Today almost one out of every two individuals will be diagnosed with the disease at some point in their lifetime.

I had no desire to investigate it. My first response to the disease was to follow anyone who would help me make it go away. I tried to quickly deal with the life changing diagnosis. I recall the moment when my surgeon told me that my diagnosis was not a death sentence. With that said, I got caught up in the regimented path of procedures and appointments. It was comforting that someone was taking care of me. And during these months, I went along with the program, heaved a huge sigh of relief when my surgeries were over, and started to get back into my regular routine again. All without too much thought of what was going on in my body.

My first clue that the treatment I had received was not a sure deal was picked up through conversations at cancer support groups and in physician waiting rooms. I heard many patients' personal stories and learned that many were seeking treatment for second and third recurrences. They described their course of treatment as the same one that I had just received. I quickly realized that I could be standing in their shoes someday and that there were thousands of other people on this same path, a path that relied on a bit of luck and gave no assurances.

My work began with tons of research. I can honestly say that learning about cancer is not recreational reading, but I realized my life was on the line. Ultimately, it was my responsibility for how my health would be restored. That final responsibility was not something I could outsource to anyone in a white coat, as attractive as that might have seemed at the time. To do that would be a bit like pulling the covers over my head and pretending it would go away. For far too many people, it does not go away.

Along my journey I found numerous books on cancer prevention and various treatment modalities, but no comprehensive book on early cancer detection. The primary focus of this book is not about prevention and treatment, but about *true early detection*, the type of detection that can discover cancer before the effects become devastating.

It was important for me to understand the components of this systemic disease so I could delve into the methods of detection. I also found it difficult to define cancer in just a few words, so instead, I decided to tell you about its various names, characteristics, relationships, and how it acts in the body. I urge you to read this carefully so that you can become a robust advocate for your health. I invite you to take a step up and face this reality with me.

Cancer

"Cancer" by one definition is uncontrolled cell growth. It is generally given a name according to the area in the body where the tumor first appears – colon cancer, lung cancer, breast cancer, etc.

Genes normally tell cells when to start and stop replicating themselves. But when those genes mutate – usually as we get older because of the stresses of nutritional deficiencies and environmental factors – the replication process can go haywire. In cancer, cells lose their ability to stop replicating and die as they should.

The result can be a benign tumor, generally meaning it does not sprout arteries to fuel its growth and it lacks the ability to invade neighboring tissue (metastasize). Benign tumors are usually encapsulated by fibrous connective tissue.

A malignant tumor is a cellular over-growth that builds a blood supply system that pulls nutrients away from nearby healthy tissue. It interferes with the body's normal functions, and can spread its cells via the blood vessels or lymphatic system to other parts of the body – this is known as metastasis.

Cancer has many unique characteristics. Understanding differences between a healthy cell and a cancer cell gives you with a foundation that can be used to combat and identify these cells. For instance, when you learn that your daily glass of orange juice, or that vitamin fortified breakfast bar, or that weekly Saturday morning donut contains an extraordinary amount of sugar that provides fuel for cancer growth, you come to understand why you may want to make a better food selection. Your lifestyle, including daily diet and activity choices, are huge factors in cancer progression and cancer suppression.

Knowing the characteristics of a cancer cell is the first step to formulating a plan to eradicate cancer cells from the body:

Healthy Cells	Cancer Cells
Predetermined life span. Healthy cells are programmed to die at the end of their life cycle. For example, red blood cells live about 120 days.	Unlimited life span resulting in continued growth and overgrowth.
Reproduce to replace a damaged or dead cell.	Uncontrolled growth that involves errors in DNA replication.
Aerobic (utilize oxygen to create energy).	Anaerobic (do not utilize oxygen as its primary source of energy). Use fermentation, a metabolic process converting sugar to create energy (ATP).
Thrive in a pH neutral environment.	Prefer an acidic environment.

Need a nutrient dense environment – vitamins, minerals, enzymes, amino acids, etc.	Thrive on sugar and have increased numbers of insulin receptors. Are believed to have up to 15 times the sugar receptors as healthy cells. Prefer fructose more than glucose for cell proliferation. Rob nutrients from healthy cells.
Stay in their area of operation (i.e., kidney cells stay in the kidney – you would not find a kidney cell in the liver).	Have the ability to move around the body and invade other tissues (ie., breast cancer often metastasizes to the lung).
Have checks and balances in place to prevent them from growing in unregulated fashion.	Grow faster than most of their healthy neighboring cells, because they are unregulated.
Have a regulated blood supply.	Have an unregulated ability to create new blood supply. Create claw like tentacles that invade and disrupt normal cell activity known as angiogenesis.
Are robust.	Are more vulnerable than healthy cells; this is why radiation and chemotherapy are used.
Work in unison with the immune system.	Evade detection from the immune system due to a protective protein coating around each cell.

A typical tumor has billions of cancerous cells that contain genetic mutations. These cells are unregulated and their sole function is that of reproduction and growth. They have lost sight of a limited lifespan and attempt to grow indefinitely; if left unchecked, they will eventually choke the life out of the host. Professor Thomas Seyfried tells us cancer is primarily a metabolic disease, not a genetic one:

> Regardless of cell type or tissue origin, the vast majority of cancer cells share a singular problem involving abnormal energy metabolism. . . . the gene defects in cancer cells can arise following damage to respiration. . . . many of the current cancer treatments exacerbate tumor cell energy metabolism, thus allowing the disease to progress and eventually become unmanageable.[1]

> Cancer growth and progression can be managed following a whole body transition from fermentable metabolites, primarily glucose and glutamine, to respiratory metabolites, primarily ketone bodies [diet]. As each individual is a unique metabolic entity, personalization of metabolic therapy as a broad-based cancer treatment strategy will require fine-tuning to match the therapy to an individual's unique physiology.[2]

Cancerous cells should not be able to take root and coalesce in a healthy person who is truly "cancer free." Our bodies have an immune system that should destroy these cancerous or defective cells. So when you hear someone say, "Doesn't everyone have cancer cells?" The answer is yes, but that's not the whole story. In a non-cancer patient, the immune system's natural killer cells recognize cancer cells as foreign to the body and destroy them before they have time to reproduce and grow into a tumor. A lab should not be able to detect, harvest, and grow cancer cells from a healthy person.

When the immune system falters or is overburdened, it stops doing the job it was naturally designed to do and cancer cells are allowed to flourish, unseen by the immune system. Also, there are many conditions in the body that fuel cancer cell growth, especially high blood sugar levels and chronic inflammation.

The original tumor does not have to be life threatening if caught early. It is the delayed detection and spread of the cancer that makes the disease fatal.

The Different Types of Cancer

Cancers are classified according to the kind of fluid or tissue from which they originate. There are five main categories:

Carcinoma

A carcinoma is a cancer found in body tissue known as epithelial tissue which covers or lines surfaces of organs, glands, or body structures. For example, a glandular cancer could be a breast carcinoma. Carcinomas account for the majority of all cancer cases.

Sarcoma

A sarcoma is a malignant tumor growing from connective tissues, such as cartilage, fat, muscle, tendons, and bones. The most common sarcoma is a tumor on the bone.

Lymphoma

Lymphoma refers to a cancer that originates in the nodes or glands of the lymphatic system. Lymphomas are classified into two categories: Hodgkin's lymphoma and non-Hodgkin's lymphoma.

Leukemia

Leukemia is known as a blood cancer. In leukemia the bone marrow does not produce normal red blood cells, white blood cells, and platelets.

Myeloma

Myeloma is a tumor involving the bone. Multiple myeloma refers to multiple tumors in the bone.

Two Categories of Cancer Cells

There are two different categories of cancer cells that can be identified in the blood. They are circulating stem cells (CSCs) and circulating tumor cells (CTCs).[3]

Circulating stem cells are from the primary tumor and contain the DNA necessary to begin producing more tumor cells. These stem cells can remain dormant for many years or can awaken and start producing at any time. This explains how a primary breast cancer that was removed and treated can reappear months or years later in the liver or bone. If the tumor cells stayed intact in the primary tumor, there would be no problem. The tumor could be surgically removed and that would be the end of the story. Unfortunately, some of the cancerous cells are released and swept away in the blood or lymphatic system. They have now become circulating *tumor* cells (CTCs).

Dr. Ray Hammon of the Integrative & Functional Health Center reports that a patient he had been following presented with a recurrence of cancer from a tumor, which had been treated more than 34 years earlier. The diagnosis was able to be confirmed at the autopsy via lab testing because the hospital still had his original pathology slides available.

Another way to explain this process is to think of a CSC as the "Space Ship Enterprise" or mother ship. The mother ship is big and strong and capable of maintaining life. The ship can rotate quietly in orbit, just as a cancer stem cell can quietly circulate in the body. If you can remember your days of watching the Star Trek movies, visualize the large bay doors opening on the side of the mother ship and smaller shuttle crafts shooting out into space. The same thing can happen with stem cells left in the blood stream. They can turn on and start "shooting out" or producing off-spring or CTCs. Without the patient even being aware, the cancer is growing again and looking for new tissue in which to embed.

Unfortunately, these circulating cells are not detectable on scans, and the lab tests approved for standard use in the United States are only for metastatic breast, prostate, and colon cancer, and thus not a good tool for early detection. Precious time is wasted and the mother ship's shuttle craft are still out there, looking to land somewhere. Patients are left with a high probability of developing metastatic cancer.

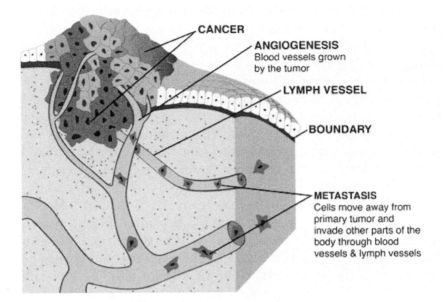

The process of cancer metastasis.

Remember, CTCs are off-spring from the primary tumor and contain cancerous DNA. This is why a lung cancer patient who has been pronounced "cancer free" may be re-diagnosed with cancer in the bone years later. That new tumor will be biopsied and lab reports will confirm that the cancer is a recurrence of the original lung cancer from years earlier.

As you read on, I will share information on how and where you can get a CTC count or other sensitive testing that will allow you to intervene in the progression and growth of possible cancer cells. Some labs can measure substances in the blood indicating cancer cells are present. Other labs can identify conditions in the body that could lead to cancer or promote its growth. All of these can sound the alarm for action, many years before cancer can be a life threatening problem.

The Sugar - Lactic Acid Connection

Cancer cells metabolize sugar for energy and when they do, they produce a substance called lactic acid.

Otto Warburg, Ph.D., documented decades ago that lactic acid levels increase in the blood if you have cancer because of a process that has become known as the "Warburg Effect."

Dr. Warburg was one of the first cancer researchers. He was awarded the Nobel Prize in 1931 for his work with cancer cell metabolism and its use of sugar fermentation for energy. He found that when cells are deprived of oxygen for a sufficient period of time, cancer developed. He said cancer cells exhibit a high rate of glycolysis – converting sugar for energy – even in the presence of oxygen (aerobic glycolysis).[4] It has since become well documented that cancer cells display high rates of glycolysis whether they were well-oxygenated or not.[5]

Life is an intensive exertion of energy to operate muscles, remove wastes, make new cells, heal wounds, and fuel the brain. Oxygen has a powerful attraction for the body's workhorses – electrons. Cells use oxygen to turn food into fuel, an *aerobic* (with oxygen) process. But cancer cells thrive in an *anaerobic* (without oxygen) environment, meaning they do not utilize oxygen as their primary source of energy. They use sugar – glucose and fructose. Dr. Warburg found cells become cancerous with only about one-third less oxygen transmission to the cell.

If you have ever worked out too hard in the gym and you feel your muscles "burning," that is lactic acid buildup at work – the muscles are fermenting glucose for energy.

A mechanism of concern with a cancer patient is that lactic acid travels to the liver where it is then converted back to glucose – the cancer cells are cleverly participating in the production of their own fuel source. This merry-go-round of lactic acid and glucose is one reason cancer cells continue to grow in end stage cancer patients even though the patient is too sick to eat. Doctors call this process gluconeogenesis.[6]

A diet high in sugar and carbohydrates creates a bountiful buffet for cancer. That is why there is an old saying amongst cancer researchers: sugar feeds cancer. Healthy cells pretty much use fats for energy, but cancer cells primarily use sugar.

The Metabolic Connection

Thomas Seyfried, Ph.D., is a biochemical geneticist and one of today's leading pioneer academic researchers promoting how to treat cancer nutritionally. He is well versed in the Warburg Effect and published an extremely well-researched book in 2012 that entices the oncology field to revisit Warburg and rethink how we view cancer:

We're not going to make major advances in the management of cancer until it becomes recognized as a metabolic disease. But in order to do that, you have to present a massive counterargument against the gene theory of cancer.

. . . if you transplant the nucleus of a cancer cell into a normal cell, you don't get cancer cells. You can actually get normal tissues and sometimes a whole normal organism from the nucleus of a cancer cell. Now, if the tumors are being driven by driver genes – all these kinds of mutations and things that we hear about – how is it possible that all of this is changed when you place this cancer nucleus into the cytoplasm of a cell with normal mitochondria?

The gene theory cannot address this. It clearly argues strongly against the concept that genes are driving this process.[7]

Seyfried argues convincingly that the traditional view of cancer as a genetic disease has been largely responsible for the failure to develop effective therapies and preventive strategies. The origin of disease, he says is malfunction of the mitochondrial energy metabolism.

You could say that mitochondria are to human cells what the engine is to the automobile. Mitochondria are energy factories inside each of our 80 trillion or more cells. Seyfried says that all cancer cells, regardless of their origin, have defective energy metabolism – dysfunctional mitochondria (car engines).

Seyfried's research documents the benefits of reduced caloric intake and a ketogenic diet as an alternate fuel source for a cell's respiratory function. Simply put, a ketogenic diet is high fat, moderate protein, and low carbohydrate. It has no sugars or starchy vegetables and grains that quickly turn into sugar in the body. Pastured eggs, butter and cream, coconut and olive oil, nuts, grass-fed meats, vegetables, and some fruit are high on the shopping list for ketogenic diets. It is a high-fat diet and it is the opposite of what the USDA food pyramid has been preaching; in fact, fat is not even on the current graphic, the one that looks like a round dinner plate.

The diet gets its name from ketones, substances made when the body breaks down fat for energy. The diet produces a high level of ketone bodies in the blood and low, stable blood sugar levels. It is a first line therapy for treating epilepsy and is being increasingly considered for the treatment of many neurological diseases and injuries, including Parkinson's, Alzheimer's, stroke, traumatic brain injuries, and cancer.[8,9]

Seyfried says that by restricting sugar and providing fat for fuel, we can dramatically reduce the rate of growth of cancer. Tumor cells cannot use ketone bodies because of their respiratory insufficiency. But as he points out, few medical professionals are trained in the diet or understand how to tell patients to implement this approach.

There is a section in the Cancer – Beat It, Don't Feed It chapter on the ketogenic diet.

The pH Connection

This simple sentence is why diet is so important: A diet high in processed foods is acid producing and most cancer patients are acidic.

An acidic body is toxic to cells because they struggle to get enough oxygen. Healthy cells need oxygen; cancerous cells don't. So, going back to the Warburg Effect, what causes cells to be deprived of oxygen? An acidic pH has a lot to do with it.

According to Dr. Robert Young, creator of *The pH Miracle for Weight Loss*, cancer is the result of toxic acidic waste products that are not properly eliminated through the four channels of elimination: urination, perspiration, respiration, and defecation. Dr. Young says:

All cancerous conditions are the expulsion of acids from the blood and then the tissues, organs and glands and are essentially the same character evolving from the same cause, namely systemic acidosis – a crisis of toxemia.

Cancer is not a noun, but an adjective expressing the process of cellular transformation. Sugar is the waste product. In fact, that's why a banana gets sweeter and sweeter as it ferments. So sugar cravings are the body's signal that the body needs more sustainable energy.[10]

I wondered why cancer patients with significant tumors often appeared swollen and puffy. We now know that the body will produce fluid in an attempt to neutralize the acidity produced by the cancer cells. The body is still trying to survive even in end stage situations.

You simply are not going to have good health if your pH is out of whack. That's why I strongly feel that any plan of action to assist the body to rid itself of cancer must include a diet and lifestyle that promotes a natural pH balance.

The Collagen Connection

Research done by the late Nobel Laureate, Linus Pauling, Ph.D., and Matthias Rath, M.D., suggests a collagen connection to cancer. Collagen is the fibrous, elastic connective tissue that holds our bodies together. It makes up much of our tendons, ligaments, joints, muscles, skin, hair, and other tissues.

Dr. Matthias Rath explains in his book, *Cellular Health Series: Cancer,* that cancer cells, viruses, and other microorganisms produce protein digesting enzymes that can destroy collagen and allow the cancer cells to move through the body and invade healthy tissues. This is part of the process of metastasis. He says that by providing the body with ample vitamin C, lysine, and proline, which are the building blocks that support strong collagen production, aggressive disease can be controlled.[11]

The Nerve Connection

Holistic practitioners say it is important to get to the root of disease, not just treat symptoms. For the purpose of this discussion, the symptom is a tumor and the root is the nerves. We know that for proper body function, the spinal column must be free of interference. With paralysis, for example, it is easy to understand that there is a disruption in the nerves of the spinal column. But what if small compressions of this important body system interfere with the body's ability to heal? A 2010 study showed the direct response between a chiropractic adjustment and body's immune fighting ability.[12] The report concluded that after a spinal adjustment, IgG and IgM antibody levels were increased for the two hour period studied. IgG and IgM are immunoglobulin antibodies produced by the body's immune system in response to foreign substances such as bacteria, viruses, fungi, or cancer cells. These antibodies attach to the foreign substances, causing them to be destroyed or neutralized.

The Hormone Connection

The largest drop in breast cancer we have seen in the last 50 years came when women stopped using synthetic hormones. In 2003, the Women's Health Initiative Study showed a 24 percent increase risk of breast cancer for women using synthetic hormone replacement therapy – estrogen plus progestin. The British Million Women Study and the French E3N Study also showed increased risk. Millions of women stopped using synthetic hormones. Breast cancer rates dropped.[13]

When we are not taking synthetic hormones to block pregnancy or dampen the effects of menopause, we are still awash in synthetic hormones. One source, for example is bisphenol A (BPA), an artificial estrogenic compound widely used in cash register receipts, plastics for food containers, and children's toys. Exposure of normal and cancerous human breast cells to low levels of BPA leads to altered expression of hundreds of genes including many involved in hormone-receptor-mediated processes.[14] About two thirds of all breast cancer tumors are hormone sensitive, which means they grow in response to excess estrogen.

Other sources of synthetic hormones and estrogen mimickers include meat and dairy, and compounds in personal care products.

We know that connective tissue around organs forms a structural biological barrier to the spread of cancer. What controls connective tissue function? Thyroid hormone. By some estimates, at least 70 percent of us are hypothyroid, meaning we don't have enough thyroid hormone to keep our cells working optimally.

The human reproductive organs are particularly prone to cancer. Statistics tell us 1 in 6 men will get a diagnosis of prostate cancer in their lifetime, 1 in 8 women will get a diagnosis of breast cancer, and a woman's risk of getting invasive ovarian cancer is about 1 in 72.[15] All of these cancers are hormonally driven.

We usually think of the sex hormones when we say "hormone," but our body uses many different kinds of hormones as messengers. Melatonin is often called the anti-cancer or antiaging hormone. Melatonin is produced in response to darkness; production peaks between 2 AM and 3 AM. The body does most of its repair work at night – we replace about a half billon cells every night while we sleep. That energy intensive process produces a lot of spare electrons, what are called free radicals. This hormone is an extremely potent antioxidant. It mops up those excess free radicals so they don't attack healthy cells. Studies have found that people who work night shifts are at increased risk for cancer, and that women with breast cancer and men with prostate cancer tend to have lower levels of melatonin than those without the disease. Melatonin is a naturally produced cytotoxin, which can induce tumor cell death (apoptosis).[16]

The Enzyme and Antibody Connection

Cancer cells make systemic changes throughout the whole body. Many of these changes are through the production of enzymes and antibodies that can be measured in the blood or urine. These components are measurable, but often over looked.

Nagalase

Nagalase (alpha-N-acetylgalactosaminidase) is an enzyme that is detectable in the blood when cancer is present. Cancerous cells or malignant cells secrete this enzyme. Nagalase suppresses the macrophages, fighter cells in the immune system. Too much nagalase and the fighter cells never get the message to go into action and attack cancer cells. Nagalase is a tool cancer cells cleverly use to ensure their own survival by allowing their continued growth to go unchecked.

More information on nagalase testing is provided in he Nagalase Test chapter.

ENOX2

Surface proteins called ENOX2 are also produced only by cancer cells – healthy cells don't make ENOX2 proteins. Cancer cells shed them into the blood stream where we can look for them. Finding them early means we can detect cancer while it is still localized and potentially curable. These proteins have molecular signatures that are used to identify the source of the cancer.

Testing for the ENOX2 protein is discussed in the ONCOLblot Labs: ENOX2 Protein Test chapter.

Thymidine Kinase (TK1)

Thymidine Kinase (TK1) is another enzyme that can be measured when cancer cells are present. Its presence in the blood serum is closely correlated to tumor development and progression. TK1 has been used in Europe for many years to monitor cancer cell proliferation/division and prognosis. Monitoring TK1 levels has been found to be quite useful for monitoring therapeutic success or failure.

Testing for TK1 levels is discussed in the RedDrop Test chapter and CA Profile Plus© chapter.

Phosphohexose Isomerase (PHI) and Carcinoembryonic Antigen (CEA)

Phosphohexose isomerase (PHI) is an enzyme implicated in the spread of cancer, and carcinoembryonic antigen (CEA) is an antigen that is present in the blood of many persons with cancer.

Refer to the CA Profile Plus Test chapter for more information on tests for these substances.

The Microbe and Fungus Connection

There is a large body of evidence to link cancer with microbes and fungus. One school of thought says microbes are a causative factor in cancer; another school of thought says they take up residence in sick cancerous cells only because a weakened body invites them.

The debate goes back to the 18th century when Louis Pasteur (1822-1895), convincingly proposed that germs caused disease. But two of his contemporaries, Claude Bernard (1813-1878) and Antoine Béchamp (1816-1908) convincingly argued that the inner terrain was more important because bacteria could not invade a healthy host and create disease on their own. It was only when the body – the inner terrain – was run down that germs would find a hospitable enough environment to set up housekeeping and do further damage to the body. The argument basically goes like this: bacteria are scavengers of nature. Flies, maggots, and rats do not cause garbage but rather feed on it. It is a debate that still continues today.

In any event, germs and fungus are part of cancer and need to be addressed and eliminated from the body for healing to take place.

Microbes or parasites come in many forms and studies show that they are prevalent in cancer patients. The human body provides a perfect environment for their reproduction as well as a food source. Tapeworms, round worms, flukes, yeast, mold, bacteria, and viruses all produce toxic waste, invade tissues, destroy cells, and steal nutrients from the body.

It is important to note that cancer cells have one big thing in common with fungus, yeast, and microbes. They all feed on sugar and Americans have a huge appetite for sugar. Athletes' foot, nail fungus, vaginal irritation, constipation, itchy scalp, and skin rashes are all examples of probable fungal infections. These common occurrences have produced a prosperous industry dedicated to providing pharmaceuticals to address all of our fungus and yeast flare-ups.

Microbes and fungus excrete waste by-products called mycotoxins that are carcinogenic, acidic, and weaken the immune system. It is also known that fungus and microbes develop a sac to provide a shield to protect them from the immune system. Cancer cells do the same type of thing by producing a protein that makes it hard for the immune system to recognize, penetrate, and destroy them.

Dr. Raphael d'Angelo, M.D., of the ParaWellness Research Program, specializes in parasite testing. He says a cancer patient's recovery will plateau and not continue until all parasitic problems are uncovered:

> What we think is happening is that the parasites create tissue inflammation and destruction which bogs down the immune system and provides fuel for cancer growth and invasion by yeast. The yeast feed on the dying tissue and they secrete more toxins that further destroy tissue keeping the cycle going. By eliminating the parasites and the yeast the immune system is freed up to do its job of attacking and resolving the cancer.[17]

It is interesting to note that plants have built in properties that protect them from fungi. Simply eating more living fruits and vegetables can transfer that protection to us. For example, coconut oil's medium-chain fatty acids exhibit antibacterial, antiviral, antifungal, and antiprotozoal properties.[18]

Many commonly eaten foods are contaminated with fungi and their by-product, mycotoxins. Peanuts, cashews, wheat, barley, cereal, corn, and alcohol have all been shown to be contaminated with fungal mycotoxins. In fact, it has been found that the reaction so many schoolchildren have to peanuts is an allergy to aflatoxin, a natural toxin produced by certain strains of the mold that grow on peanuts stored in warm, humid silos. The highest risk of aflatoxin contamination comes from corn, peanuts, and cottonseed. Aflatoxin is a potent carcinogen, known to cause liver cancer in laboratory animals.[19] We now know that mycotoxins are carcinogenic.[20]

Diet modifications and natural antifungals like oil of oregano and grape seed extract can be helpful in the battle against fungus. Often the problem requires prescriptive drugs like Diflucan, Nystatin, and Lamisil.

Use careful consideration before consuming multiple rounds of antibiotics because most antibiotics are made from fungi. Use antibiotics only when necessary and be sure to replace the good bacteria that they kill in your gut after finishing your medication.

Among the many books and websites I've researched that go into depth on the fungus and cancer connection, Doug A. Kaufmann really made the light bulb go on for me when he addressed this topic in his handbook, *The Germ that Causes Cancer*, where he presents his research implicating fungi, and what role their harmful by-products – mycotoxins – play in the cause of cancer.[21]

Dr. Pasteur's rival, Dr. Antoine Béchamp, told us a healthy inner terrain is the key to prevention and treatment of all diseases. He taught that germs thrive in unhealthy environments and not in healthy ones. Lifestyle elements such as wholesome nutrition, environmental and hygienic cleanliness, he said, were ignored in favor of "heroic" medical interventions that turned a profit for industry – and that was 150 years ago!

The smallest unit of life, Béchamp said, is not the cell, but microzyma found inside the cell. Normally, microzyma function harmoniously, but when the inner terrain shifts to favor disease, the microzyma change form into malevolent bacteria, fungi, and viruses. Then the microzyma themselves give off toxic byproducts, further contributing to a weakened terrain.[22]

Béchamp's work lives on in physicians and researchers who think mainstream medicine is on the wrong track today because germs are first and foremost symptoms. As Dr. Bernard Jensen and Mark Anderson, for example, said in their 1990 book *Empty Harvest*:

> The germ theory is still believed to be the central cause of disease because around it exists a colossal supportive infrastructure of commercial interests that built multi-billion-dollar industries based upon this theory. To the scientific satisfaction of many in the health field, it has long been disproven as the primary cause of disease. Germs are, rather, an effect of disease.[23]

Dr. Alan Cantwell (born 1934) investigated the phenomenon of cancer and bacteria for more than 30 years. In his research, he showed that "cancer microbes" were present in cancerous tissue and in the blood of cancer patients. He said one of the greatest tragedies of modern medicine was its refusal to recognize the cancer microbe – the hidden killer in cancer, AIDS, and other immune diseases.[24]

I reached the conclusion that when you have cancer, relieving the body of microbes and fungus is a proactive step that the body needs us to take, because at this point the immune system is too overwhelmed to do it on its own.

One final note: Some bacteria are good. Healthy adults carry several pounds of bacteria in their digestive tract and bowel. That amount of bacteria outnumbers the cells in our bodies by 10 to 1. Gut flora has a big job, including helping us to digest food, produce vitamins, and keep the immune system strong. However, most chemotherapy drugs can sterilize the colon, which dramatically stimulates cancer growth and invasion.[25] Many patients on a chemo regimen are also given antibiotics which kill "friendly" bacteria in the gut.[26]

The Insulin Connection

Recent studies link obesity with the incidence and mortality of a number of cancers.

Insulin resistance – sometimes called a metabolic syndrome – is when the insulin hormone is no longer able to efficiently remove blood sugar out of the blood stream. Eating a lot of sugar causes so many triggers over time for so much insulin that the mechanism becomes sluggish; cells do not bind with insulin, so glucose does not get into the cells very well. The pancreas is called upon to excrete more insulin but it cannot maintain a high insulin output indefinitely. Then insulin levels begin to go down and blood sugar levels go up. When the blood sugar rise is severe enough, diabetes is diagnosed and the door to cancer appears to swing open.

To quote Dr. Edward L. Giovannucci of the Harvard School of Public Health:

Insulin may signal cells to increase rapidly in number through a variety of mechanisms. Insulin could directly signal growth, or it could do this by increasing the levels of other potent growth factors (insulin-like growth factors [IGF]), or it could make cells more sensitive to other growth factors. Although cancer is a complex, multifactorial disease, one of the consistent characteristics of cancer cells is their ability to grow uncontrollably and to be resistant to programmed death. Thus, growth factors are critical to the initial development of cancers, as well as to their progression. A number of studies now show that individuals with higher levels of circulating IGFs are at increased risk for developing colon, premenopausal breast, and aggressive prostate cancers than are individuals with lower levels.[27]

Obese people are more likely to have higher concentrations of both insulin and glucose, a situation that may promote cancer cells to grow, multiply, and spread rapidly.

Whether the use of insulin by diabetics contributes to cancer is a debate raging among researchers right now. It makes sense to me that it does.

The Gluten Connection

Many of us crave wheat because eating it releases feel-good chemicals that have a drug-like effect on our central nervous system. That's the opioids in gluten, the protein contained in many grains, especially wheat, barley, rye, and oats.

Opiates and opioids interfere with the body's natural killer cells, also known as NK cells. These are specialized white blood cells dispatched by the immune system to kill other cells. They are part of our first line of defense against cancer and virus-infected cells.

Research shows that people with celiac disease and people with gluten sensitivities – which may be the majority of us – have a higher risk of cancer, heart disease, and death.[28]

The Inflammation Connection

Inflammation can be said to be basically one of two types:
1. The immediate healing response such as when you hit our thumb with a hammer and the skin puffs up, as your immune system sends white blood cells and other substances to start the healing process.
2. Chronic inflammation which acts as a persistent stimulus that falls below the threshold of perceived pain.

The source of the chronic stimulus might be pesticides, chemicals, heavy metals, gluten from wheat which inflames the gut, or a low-grade infection from a root canal. These persistent stimuli create a constant irritation that distorts the body's normal response.

Chronic inflammation can stimulate mutated cancer cells and enhance their survival and opportunity for metastasis:

There is a clear relationship between certain chronic in-flammatory conditions and the transformation of inflamed tissue into malignant tissue. For example, chronic gastritis (inflammation of the stomach lining) and peptic ulcers may be a causative factor in 60-90% of stomach cancers. Chronic hepatitis (inflammation of the liver) and cirrhosis of the liver are believed to be responsible for about 80% of liver cancers. Colorectal cancer is 10 times more likely to occur in patients with chronic inflammatory diseases of the colon, such as ul-cerative colitis and Crohn's disease.[29]

The Genetic Connection

Most cancers do not occur because you inherited a "cancer-causing" gene from your parents. Most cancers are caused by DNA changes that happen during your life because you have been exposed to radiation, environmental toxins, significant environmental stresses, or eat a diet that left you depleted of what a body needs to maintain a robust immune system. That is why the older we get, the more susceptible we are to cancer.

Hereditary mutations, those that are passed on from a parent to a child, account for only about 5 to 10 percent of all cancers.

Acquired mutations account for at least 90 percent of all cancers. They are DNA changes that start in one cell of the body and are found only in the offspring of that particular cell. According to the American Cancer Society:

It is important to realize that mutations in our cells happen all the time. Usually, the cell detects the change and repairs it. If it can't be repaired, the cell will get a signal telling it to die in a process called apoptosis. But if the cell doesn't die and the mutation is not repaired, it may lead to a person developing cancer. This is more likely if the mutation affects a gene involved with cell division or a gene that normally causes a defective cell to die.[30]

There are two main types of genes that play a role in cancer: oncogenes and tumor suppressor genes.

Oncogenes are a mutation of a "good" gene that would control cell division properly. When oncogenes are present, cell division goes haywire. Cells have the potential to be turned on when they are not supposed to be, allowing cells to start the process of uncontrolled growth which can lead to cancer.

Tumor suppressor genes normally work to slow down cell division, repair DNA mistakes, or tell cells when to die (apoptosis or programmed cell death). When tumor suppressor genes don't work properly, cells can grow out of control, which can lead to cancer.

Most cancer causing mutations that involve oncogenes and tumor suppressor genes are acquired, not inherited.

The Energy Connection

Our trillions of cells communicate with tiny electrical signals. We see the body's electricity at work when we have an EKG to measure heart function, or when someone is hooked up to a brain monitor in a hospital to measure ionic current flows within the neurons of the brain. Remember all those TV shows where the monitor "flatlines"? The person is pronounced dead because their brain is no longer producing voltage.

Voltage is key to life. If you have a lot of it, that's good. If you have not so much, hello disease.

Going back to Warburg, cancer is a failure of the mitochondria – the power factories inside each of our cells. If you have cancer, your mitochondria are not producing enough energy to do their job well.

"Think of a flashlight battery that doesn't have enough juice left to put out a bright light," Dr. Garry Gordon of Arizona said. "That's mitochondrial malfunction. And likewise, the Earth itself is not putting out as much juice as it used to and that affects our bodies."

Human beings evolved with the Earth's protective magnetic field. We need it as much as we need food, water, air, and sunlight. The Earth's pulsed electromagnetic frequencies, PEMF, are of great importance to internal regulation of every organism on the planet, including us.

Prolonged weakening of the Earth's magnetic field is associated with weakening of the immune system.[31] When the familiar pull of gravity is no longer present, muscles atrophy, bones lose their density, blood pressure shifts, and our ability to balance deteriorates.[32]

"The earth's magnetic field has been dropping substantially over the last 165 years," Dr. Gordon explained. "I think we are all experiencing a power failure – think of an electricity brown-out in the Northeast – because the earth's magnetic field has dropped so much."

So, if we are not getting our cellular batteries sufficiently charged from Mother Earth, can we add energy in much the same way we add supplements to our diet because the soil in which our food is grown is not as nutritious as it was centuries ago? Dr. Gordon adamantly says, "Yes."

Everything that Otto Warburg said was bad about cancer is reversed with PEMF. Pulsed electromagnetic frequency machines act as a 'whole-body battery charger' by recharging each of the cells in the body. When your cells are sick, they lose energy. Healthy cells run at about minus 70 mV. Cancer starts when you get down to minus 30 mV. Cancer cells typically have a voltage of minus 20 mV and are in fermentation, meaning they need ten times more energy from the environment. A PEMF device builds up energy within your cells; PEMF oxygenates and alkalizes the cells. All metabolic processes are driven by this cellular charge: ATP production, oxygen, nutrient absorption, waste removal, defense, and reproduction.

Dr. Gordon points to the work of Dr. William Pawluk, one of the top experts in the U.S. today on the study of PEMF:

By regenerating the cells in our bodies, we can help our cells become and stay healthy with pulsed electromagnetic fields. The earth creates magnetic fields, without which life would not be possible. Science teaches that everything is energy. All energy is electromagnetic in nature. All atoms, chemicals, and cells produce electromagnetic fields. Science has proven that our bodies actually project their own magnetic fields and our 70 trillion cells in the body communicate via electromagnetic frequencies. Disruption of electromagnetic energy in cells causes impaired cell metabolism. This is the final common pathway of disease. If cells are not healthy, the body is not healthy.[33]

It takes an electromagnetic field to support the body's regenerative efforts.

Electrons are an overlooked key nutrient, Dr. Gordon explained. "The phenomenon of electrons from one atom being shared with another atom is essential for construction of life," he said. "Modern living has created an electron-deficient environment that is creating electron-deficient bodies. Electron deficiency is another way of saying something is acidic."

And cancer, of course, thrives in an acidic environment.

The Lifestyle Connection

Smoking, obesity, alcohol, lack of exercise, and consumption of a high sugar processed food diet are just a few of the items connected to an increased risk of cancer. Americans have tremendous opportunities and a bounty of daily choices that could promote good health and the strong immune system that is needed to fight and prevent cancer.

Unfortunately, better lifestyle changes seem to be some of the hardest to accomplish. It is not uncommon to see a lung cancer patient smoking or an obese person eating a slice of cheesecake. It seems for most people, the only successful motivation is crisis – like getting a diagnosis of cancer or diabetes – and then it comes down to how strong a will to live they put forth. Personal motivation is the key to making change and I encourage you to find yours.

A diagnosis of cancer was the motivator for me; however, I can sadly say that it does not have the same effect on everyone today. We have been conditioned to depend on the so-called "easy fix" by relying on a drug or medical procedures to take care of our problems.

The Stress Connection

Cancer and stress have been shown to go hand in hand and stress is a known risk factor for cancer. The body responds to physical, mental, or emotional pressure by releasing stress hormones, namely epinephrine and norepinephrine. These hormones increase blood pressure, heart rate, and blood sugar levels. Research has shown that people who experience intense and long-term (i.e., chronic) stress can have digestive problems, fertility problems, urinary problems, and a weakened immune system. They also have been shown to suffer from viral infections, the common cold, headaches, depression, anxiety, sleep problems, and cancer.

In a 2013 study, researchers at Ohio State University linked the activation of a stress gene in immune-system cells to the spread of breast cancer to other parts of the body.[34] The gene, called ATF3, may be the crucial link between stress and cancer – enabling cancer to metastasize and lead to death. Researchers already know that the ATF3 gene is activated in response to stressful conditions in all types of cells. Under normal circumstances, triggering ATF3 protects the body from harm by causing normal cells to commit suicide if there is a stressful condition; however in a cancerous situation, the tumor cells communicate with the immune cells and cause malfunction.

The doctors with whom I have spoken have noted that their patients who process and handle stress effectively have better outcomes, and in my interviews with cancer patients, I noted that all of them had experienced a major emotional or physical trauma prior to their diagnosis. Stress is a major component of the cancer process and must be addressed. It can often be managed with exercise, counseling, support group involvement, forgiveness, learning to let go, and loving yourself.

When Cancer Was Rare and Food Was Natural

In the 1930s, Weston A. Price, D.D.S., embarked on a novel expedition to investigate the causes of physical degeneration in people. It was a unique window in time. The world was still small enough that he readily found isolated populations who had little or no contact with "modern" civilization, and yet technological advances allowed him to document his findings with photographs that spoke volumes.

He traveled to hundreds of places in 14 countries, from Switzerland to Alaska, from Africa to South Sea Islanders. He found overall excellent health in the groups of people who were eating their indigenous foods. However, where traders established trading posts, they brought with them sacks of sugar and white flour, canned goods, pasteurized milk, and refined vegetable oils. Soon after, signs of degeneration became evident. Dr. Price found that dental cavities, arthritis, and low immunity to tuberculosis became rampant. Dr. Price also found that good health could be restored when the modernized foods were removed from the diet.

He found that across the world, people ate different diets. The Eskimo, for example, ate a lot of animal protein and fat but rarely vegetables, and in some parts of Africa, protein perhaps came from bugs, not animals. But all healthy populations had diets that contained at least four times the minerals as the American diet of his day and 10 times the amount of fat soluble vitamins (A, D, E, K).

Today, Americans have not been taught how to eat well. I have found that most people don't actually know they are eating poorly. They make decisions with their taste buds, not nutritional intelligence. The food is addictive to boot. Nutrition advice from the government and associations is grossly colored by corporate lobbyists. For example, the American Heart Association for decades promoted trans fats, despite studies showing they were killing people; the FDA is now finally poised to ban them. Most doctors have precious little education in nutrition. So it is up to you to educate yourself.

It is absolutely necessary to limit processed foods. That includes foods with new-fangled vegetable oils, artificial preservatives, pesticides, and chemicals. Avoid genetically modified organisms (GMOs) which are found primarily in soybeans, sugar beets, canola, cottonseed oil, and corn. Use only natural sweeteners like stevia or raw honey in limited quantities. Don't be fooled into believing that natural sweeteners are ok. They still raise blood sugar levels and provide fuel for cancer. Cut out the cookies and cake, the vanilla coffee lattés and bagels, the sodas and sport drinks (especially the diet versions). Avoid animal foods that have been treated with hormones and antibiotics. Avoid plastic food containers. Eat your food in as close to its natural state as possible. If you can't pronounce the ingredients on the label, don't buy it. Use real, organic butter. Buy grass fed meats. Get friendly with farmers markets and vegetable co-ops. If you play golf, bring your own unsweetened ice tea in a thermos; don't buy the sugared teas and fruit juices in bottles and cans. When you go out to eat, bring your own salad dressing; simple olive oil and balsamic vinegar in a glass container works. Ask for the gluten free menu. Stop buying "diet" foods and beverages. Set a goal of eating 50 percent of your food raw. Restrict alcohol use and manage your weight.

Use non-fluoride toothpaste; fluoride has been implicated as a carcinogen. Consider a reverse osmosis filter for your drinking water. Do not put air fresheners in your car or buy scented laundry detergents and fabric softener sheets; you are just adding carcinogens to your environment. Look into smart meters your electric company may have installed on your house; their radiation emissions are classified as a 2B (possible) carcinogen. Have mercury fillings and root canals assessed by a biological dentist. Read the fine print on your prescriptions for side effects and consider their safety. Limit antibiotic use. Don't smoke. When in doubt, err on the side of what appears to be safest for your body and your environment. Exercise regularly. Let go of anger and forgive others. Find some joy in every day and use laughter as a medicine.

A Final Word on Cancer

I am hopeful that after reading the information presented in this chapter on what cancer is, you will not think of cancer as a just a "TUMOR" to be cut out or bombed out of existence with chemo, but as a complex systemic issue that has your body asking for help on many fronts.

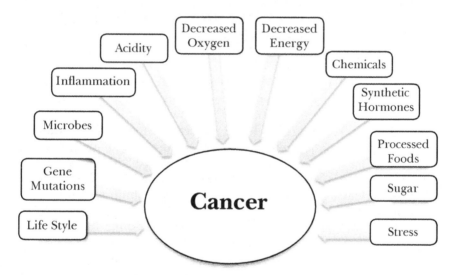

Factors contributing to cancer development.

Everything is permissible, but not everything is beneficial.

1 Corinthians 10:23

Footnotes

1   Seyfried T. *Cancer As a Metabolic Disease: On the Origin, Management, and Prevention of Cancer.* Wiley; 1 edition, 2012.

2   Seyfried T, Flores R, et al. Cancer as a metabolic disease: implications for novel therapeutics. Published by Oxford University Press. *Carcinogenesis.* vol. 00 no. 00 p.1 of 13, 2014.

3   DeVita Jr V, Lawrence TS, Rosenberg SA. *Cancer: Principles & Practice of Oncology: Primer of the Molecular Biology of Cancer.* Philadelphia, PA: Lippincott Williams & Wilkins; 1 Pap/Psc edition 2011.

4   Warburg O. The Metabolism of Tumours: *Investigations from the Kaiser Wilhelm Institute for Biology.* Translated by Dickens F. Constable & Co Ltd., 1930, 56 (out of print). Ref: *Hoppe-Seyler's Zeitschr Physiol Chem.* 1910; 66:305.

5   Lu H, Forbes RA, Verma A. Hypoxia-inducible factor 1 activation by aerobic glycolysis implicates the Warburg effect in carcinogenesis. *J Biol Chem.* 2002; 277:23111-23115.

6   Garrett RH, Grisham CM. *Biochemistry.* Boston: Cengage Learning; 5th edition, 2012.

7   Seyfried T. *Cancer as a Metabolic Disease: On the Origin, Management, and Prevention of Cancer.* Wiley, 2012

8   Schmidt M, Pfetzer N, et al. Effects of a ketogenic diet on the quality of life in 16 patients with advanced cancer: A pilot trial. *Nutrition & Metabolism.* 2011; 8:54.

9   Seyfried T, Marsh J, et al. Is the restricted ketogenic diet a viable alternative to the standard of care for managing malignant brain cancer? *Epilepsy Research.* 2012 July; 100(3):310-326.

10 pH Miracle Living website. Retrieved January 12, 2015 at: www. phmiracleliving.com/t-cancer-intro.aspxwww.phmiracleliving. com/t-cancer-intro.aspx.

11 Rath M. *Cellular Health Series: Cancer.* MR Publishing Inc., CA, 2002, p18-20.

12 Teodorczyk-Injeyan JA, McGregor M, et al. Interleukin 2-regulated in vitro antibody production following a single spinal manipulative treatment in normal subjects. *Chiropractic & Osteopathy.* 2010 Sept 2; 18:26.

13 Chlebowski RT, Kuller LH, et al. Breast cancer after use of estrogen plus progestin in postmenopausal women. *NEJM.* 2009; 360:573-587.

14 Breast Cancer Fund. Bisphenol A (BPA). Retrieved January 14, 2015 at: www.breastcancerfund.org/clear-science/radiation-chemicals-and-breast-cancer/bisphenol-a.html.

14 American Cancer Society. What is Ovarian Cancer? Updated 4-22-13. Retrieved July 20, 2014 at: www.cancer.org/cancer/ovariancancer/overviewguide/ovarian-cancer-overview-key-statistics.

16 Lynch, EM. Melatonin and Cancer Treatment. *Life Extension Magazine.* January 2004.

17 d' Angelo R. Parasites and Cancer-the Connection. Paper retrieved January 3, 2015 at: www.parawellnessresearch.com/articles.html#parasitecancer.

18 Fife B. *The Coconut Oil Miracle.* Avery, 2004, pages 66-82.

19 Cornell University, College of Agriculture and Life Sciences Website. Aflatoxins: Occurrence and Health Risks. Retrieved January 14, 2015 at: www.ansci.cornell.edu/plants/toxicagents/aflatoxin/aflatoxin.html.

20 Peraica M, Radic B, et al. Toxic effects of mycotoxins in humans. *Bull World Health Organ.* 1999; 77(9):754-766.

21 Kaufman DA, Holland D, et al. *The Germ That Causes Cancer.* Media Triton, Inc., USA, 2005.

22 Béchamp A. *The Blood and Its Third Element.* Re-edited by Review Press, 2002.

23 Jensen B, Anderson M. *Empty Harvest: Understanding the Link Between Our Food, Our Immunity and Our Planet.* Avery, 1990.

24 Cantwell A. *The Cancer Microbe.* Aries Rising Press, 1990.

25 Iida N, Dzutsev A, et al. Commensal bacteria control cancer response to therapy by modulating the tumor microenvironment. *Science.* 2013 Nov 22; 342(6161):967-970.

26 Iida N, Dzutsev A, et al. Commensal bacteria control cancer response to therapy by modulating the tumor microenvironment. *Science.* 2013 Nov 22; 342(6161):967-970.

27 Giovannucci EL. Obesity, Insulin Resistance, and Cancer Risk. *New York Presbyterian Hospital Newsletter.* Spring 2005, Issue 5.

28 Braly J, Hoggan R. *Dangerous Grains.* Avery, 2002

29 Tortora GJ, Derrickson B. *Essentials of Anatomy and Physiology.* Wiley. 9th edition. 2013.

30 American Cancer Society. Oncogenes, Tumor Suppressor Genes, and Cancer. Retrived March 4, 2014 at: www.cancer.org/acs/groups/cid/documents/webcontent/002550-pdf.pdf.

31 Roman A, Tombarkiewicz B. Prolonged weakening of the geomagnetic field affect the immune system of rats. Department of Brain Biochemistry, Institute of Pharmacology, Polish Academy of Sciences. *Bioelectromagnetics.* 2009 Jan 30; (1):21-22.

32 Cuomo C, Pflum M, Sterns O. What Happens to Your Body in Space. *ABC News*. Feb 8, 2008. Retrieved March 5, 2014 at: http://abcnews.go.com/GMA/story?id=4261638&page=1.

33 Pawluk W, Granza D. 101 Great Ways to Improve Health. Self Improvement Online, Inc. 2007.

34 Wolford CC, McConoughey SJ, et al. Transcription factor ATF3 links host adaptive response to breast cancer metastasis. *J Clin Invest*. 2013; 123(7):2893-2906; DOI: 10.1172/JCI64410.

Chapter 4

Statistics – Misconceptions of Reality

I spent a great deal of time questioning the statistical information that I had been given during treatment and examining how medical statistic misconceptions had affected the choices I had made. We as medical consumers, often in a stressful situation, want to trust that the information we receive concerning important medical decisions is absolutely factual, complete, and reliable.

Today, countless Americans trust the statistics when making life and death decisions and many others are walking around with a false sense of security after treatment having been told their PET scan is clean and they are cancer free. They do not fully understand the side effects of treatments and that they are prime candidates for a disease recurrence.

The cancer statistics they are given and rely upon are difficult to understand because of the way that they are calculated and gathered. Statistics are manipulated to imply that patients who are counted as "cured" never experience cancer again and live a long life.

This chapter is not meant to criticize, but to shed light on the truth and help you navigate your way through a very confusing trail of information.

The 5 Year Statistic

You need to know that cancer survival rates are the first big manipulation you are likely to encounter. Survival rates are measured just 5 years out. They describe the percentage of people who are alive 5 years after a cancer diagnosis, excluding those who die from other diseases.[1] If a patient dies 5 years and one day after diagnosis, that patient is still counted in the 5 year survival statistic. If the patient dies of a treatment-induced side effect like pneumonia, due to a compromised immune system caused by the chemotherapy, the death most likely is not counted as a cancer death in the statistics; it would be reported as a death from pneumonia.

For example, take cancer patients treated with radiation therapy who later die from a radiation-induced stroke: a study of head and neck cancer patients who received radiation therapy found that stroke rates over their lifetimes were five times greater than expected. The average time between radiation treatment and stroke was 10.9 years, and the increased risk of stroke persisted for 15 years after radiation therapy.[2]

The cancer industry's manipulations disguise the fact that the toxic therapies used to eradicate cancer can themselves cause premature death. The death rate for cancer has barely changed since 1950.[3]

Reputable people have been speaking up for a long time about the cancer industry's poor outcomes. Dr. John Bailer, who spent 20 years on the staff of the National Cancer Institute and was editor of its journal, took the industry to task in 1985. Speaking at the Annual Meeting of the American Association for the Advancement of Science, he said:

> My overall assessment is that the national cancer program must be judged a qualified failure. The 5 year cancer survival statistics of the American Cancer Society are very misleading. They now count things that are not cancer, and, because we are able to diagnose at an earlier stage of the disease, patients falsely appear to live longer. Our whole cancer research in the past 20 years has been a failure. More people over 30 are dying from cancer than ever before. More women with mild or benign diseases are being included in statistics and reported as being "cured." When government officials point to survival figures and say they are winning the war against cancer they are using those survival rates improperly.[4]

Linus Pauling, two-time Nobel Prize winner, was even more blunt the following year:

> Everyone should know that most cancer research is largely a fraud and that the major cancer research organizations are derelict in their duties to the people who support them.[5]

It simply is not true that we are winning the war on cancer. What we have is an effective way of manipulating data to sell harsh and toxic treatments that are profitable for those who make a diagnosis.

Meanwhile, cancer is striking earlier than ever before. It is not uncommon to see patients in their thirties with cancer. This was not the case 50 years ago. Cancer is now the second highest cause of death in American children, second only to accidents.[6]

Early clinical diagnosis also has a lot to do with the statistical manipulation. If the cancer is caught earlier, patients appear to be living longer. They reach the 5 year survival date and are therefore counted amongst the survivors even though they later succumb to the disease. It is basically just a matter of moving the goal post.

The 5 year survival rate should be meaningless to you. What you want and should insist on is a treatment that will heal the body of cancer to the point that you live a normal lifespan, and do not die a premature death from cancer. You want to die of something else – preferably from old age.

Manipulating "Prevention" for Revenue

It is important to realize that the good intentions of physicians and the media to promote the value of cancer screening does not in any way equate to cancer prevention. Looking for a lump is not the same as working to prevent the lump. In some circles, cancer screening is described as "tolling for business." If you have a lump, great – bring on the biopsies, and sign 'em up for the very profitable surgery/chemo/radiation.

We need to be leery of marketing campaigns advertising cancer screening and treatment under the guise of "being helpful" or increasing "awareness." Where is the prevention factor? Where is the prevention campaign? Could it be that there are no revenues produced from prevention campaigns? But wait, couldn't a small portion of the billions of dollars raised for the cure be allocated for this? If it is, it is hard to see.

If you don't have a lump or a high PSA number or something else indicative of cancer, you typically are sent home with nothing – not even a pamphlet – about how to prevent cancer.

One good resource is the 2010 President's Cancer Panel report which has a surprisingly candid discussion of the environmental causes of cancer. At the very least, oncologists could be handing out copies of the executive summary to advise people to avoid known environmental carcinogens. Additionally, many of the medical screening methods used today are ineffective or downright harmful. As the President's Cancer Panel report said:

> The use of radiation-emitting medical tests is growing rapidly. Efforts are needed to eliminate unnecessary testing . . . No mechanism currently exists to enable individuals to estimate their personal cumulative radiation exposure, which would help patients and physicians weigh the benefits and potential harm of contemplated imaging and nuclear medicine tests.[7]

It is well established that exposure to ionizing radiation can result in mutations or other genetic damage that cause cells to turn cancerous. In other words, medical devices that use radiation to screen or treat can cause cancer.

A 2010 study by researchers at the U.S. Department of Energy's Lawrence Berkeley National Laboratory showed how radiation exposure can alter the environment surrounding human breast cells so that future cells are more likely to become cancerous.[8] "By getting normal cells to prematurely age and stop dividing, the radiation exposure created space for epigenetically altered cells that would otherwise have been filled by normal cells," said Paul Yaswen, a cell biologist and breast cancer research specialist with Berkeley Lab's Life Sciences Division.[9] In other words, radiation promoted the growth of pre-cancerous cells by making the environment surrounding the cells more hospitable to their continued growth.

When the U.S. Preventive Services Task Force in recent years issued new guidelines calling for less screening with mammograms and PSA tests, their goal was to reduce the significant harm from overtreatment. The move was met with howls of protest from various groups who promote annual screenings. Yet these tests are far from perfect.

In the U.S., the risk of having a false-positive test within 10 mammograms ranges from 58 to percent to 77 percent.[10,11] A number of studies have concluded that mammography's benefits fall far short of the advertising.

A major study reported in the *British Medical Journal* in 2014 concluded that the rationale for screening by mammography should be urgently reassessed by policy makers.[12] As Gina Kolata reported in the *New York Times*:

> One of the largest and most meticulous studies of mammography ever done, involving 90,000 women and lasting a quarter-century, has added powerful new doubts about the value of the screening test for women of any age.
>
> It found that the death rates from breast cancer and from all causes were the same in women who got mammograms and those who did not. And the screening had harms: One in five cancers found with mammography and treated was not a threat to the woman's health and did not need treatment such as chemotherapy, surgery or radiation.[13]

Many cancers grow slowly, or not at all, and do not require treatment. In fact, they may be best left alone.

Studies find that mammography detects lesions in women that are inherently benign, but are termed "pre-cancerous" and treated preemptively at both financial and emotional cost to women.

A 2012 study that looked at three decades of screening in the United States concluded:

> Our study raises serious questions about the value of screening mammography. It clarifies that the benefit of mortality reduction is probably smaller, and the harm of overdiagnosis probably larger, than has been previously recognized. And although no one can say with certainty which women have cancers that are overdiagnosed, there is certainty about what happens to them: they undergo surgery, radiation therapy, hormonal therapy for 5 years or more, chemotherapy, or (usually) a combination of these treatments for abnormalities that otherwise would not have caused illness.[14]

Annual mammography does not result in a reduction in breast cancer specific mortality for women aged 40-59 beyond that of physical examination alone or usual care in the community. The data suggest that the value of mammography screening should be reassessed.[15]

In addition, a study of 1.8 million Norwegian women published in 2014 found much the same results – screening has a limited effect on the occurrence of serious and aggressive cancer cases, and causes significant overtreatment of conditions best left alone.[16]

In January 2013, the Swiss Medical Board conducted a global review of mammography screening studies and recommended that no new systematic mammography screening programs be introduced and that a time limit be placed on existing programs:

It is easy to promote mammography screening if the majority of women believe that it prevents or reduces the risk of getting breast cancer and saves many lives through early detection of aggressive tumors. We would be in favor of mammography screening if these beliefs were valid. Unfortunately, they are not, and we believe that women need to be told so. From an ethical perspective, a public health program that does not clearly produce more benefits than harms is hard to justify.[17]

A modern thermogram, which does not deliver an annual dose of radiation, has proven to be a better tool for early detection because it can see tumor formation perhaps 10 years before a mammogram can pinpoint it. However, radiologists and business interests are not aligned with thermography machines – the makers of thermography machines do not sit on the boards of the American Cancer Society and Susan G. Komen. Thus the mainstream breast cancer groups say nothing positive about thermography. The industry is still invested in the old, ineffective status quo despite overwhelming scientific evidence that change is needed.

Colonoscopy is another commonly recommended cancer screening. People assume colonoscopies save lives because it makes sense that removing pre-cancerous polyps should reduce the incidence of cancer. But actually strong evidence for that has been lacking. According to the National Cancer Institute: "Because there are no RCTs [random controlled trials] of colonoscopy, evidence of benefit is indirect."[18]

Evidence finally came in 2014. A Yale Cancer Center study concluded that an estimated half a million cancers were prevented by colorectal cancer screening in the U.S. from 1976 to 2009.[19]

Arguments about effectiveness aside, one thing had never been in doubt about colonoscopy screenings – they are revenue generators. As the *New York Times* put it in a 2013 series on the high cost of American health care:

> Colonoscopies . . . are the most expensive screening test that healthy Americans routinely undergo. They are often prescribed and performed more frequently than medical guidelines recommend. The high price paid for colonoscopies mostly results not from top-notch patient care, according to interviews with health care experts and economists, but from business plans seeking to maximize revenue; haggling between hospitals and insurers that have no relation to the actual costs of performing the procedure; and lobbying, marketing and turf battles among specialists that increase patient fees.[20]

Money often incentivizes motivations other than really good health care, and puts the emphasis on revenue-generating procedures rather than prevention. Efforts to look for cancer are not the same as efforts to prevent cancer.

The BRCA1 and BRCA2 genetic testing is an example of money dominating outcomes. If you are a carrier of the BRCA genes, you are perhaps more prone to develop cancer. The full test costs roughly $3,000 and is not always covered by insurance. A positive result will put a woman into a panic and often comes with the recommendation to remove the breasts, uterus, and/ or ovaries. Those surgeries, and the reconstructive surgery that follows, are good revenue generators.

Doctors typically do not focus on the other side of the story – of all the cases of breast cancer, the patients with a positive BRCA test are in the low single digits, about 5 percent. And, only about half the women with the BRCA1 gene mutation eventually develop breast cancer, and 11 to 17 percent of women with the BRCA2 mutation will develop ovarian cancer.[21]

Why don't all people with the BRCA mutation go on to develop cancer? This is the science of epigenetics – what causes some genes to express and other genes not to express. We inherit two copies of each gene, one gene from our mother, one from our father. Usually, we inherit at least one good gene and that one keeps us healthy. But when we inactivate the good gene through smoking, environmental chemicals, stress, and a number of other factors still not completely understood, the "bad" gene can take over. Our genes are not our destiny. How we influence our genes is worthy of developing large educational and prevention programs from the government and the various cancer organizations.

Very often, the BRCA test is simply used to get women into the operating room. What doctors could be doing is giving people a choice by explaining the statistics and explaining what we know about how to affect genetic expression in favor of the "good" genes expressing.

What of the other 95 percent or more of patients with breast cancer who have no genetic mutation? What caused their cancer? Most point the finger of blame primarily at environmental and emotional factors. Yet the medical establishment has not made it a priority to educate the public about non-drug and non-surgical interventions.

For example, there is a wealth of research – some 5,000 peer-reviewed studies – on curcumin, the active principal in the herb turmeric. This is the spice that gives Indian food its yellow color. Curcumin is an anti-inflammatory, anti-oxidant, anti-microbial, and anti-carcinogenic herb that has been shown to reverse the tendency for bad genes to express. Research shows that curcumin promotes apoptosis (cancer cell death), scavenges reactive oxidative species (ROS), and reduces the inflammatory cancer microenvironment.[22] Curcumin is not toxic, it is affordable, and you can find it in any grocery store. Did my doctors mention curcumin to me? Did they ever suggest it would be a good thing to add to my diet in terms of preventing a recurrence of cancer?

Nope, not a word during my conventional treatment. I first heard about it a year later when I met Dr. Hammon and Dr. Oliveras.

There is an urgent need to give patients information about validated interventions that can target cancer's multiple causative factors before they take hold. Curcumin is one of the most compelling interventions.

Manipulating Drug Research

Drug companies, the FDA, the media, and many doctors use a numerical shell game to cleverly promote the limited benefits of many of the pharmaceuticals. By presenting only lucrative patented treatments and expensive insurance-approved tests, patients are rarely given all of the information available so that they can make a fully informed decision. Also, a very important factor left out of the statistics is the harmful and possibly deadly side effects of many of the recommended treatments.

Tamoxifen, the breast cancer treatment drug, is a classic case. It is classified by the World Health Organization and the American Cancer Society as a human carcinogen. Yet it is prescribed for cancer prevention.

In September 2000, *The Lancet* reported a study which showed that women who had taken Tamoxifen and subsequently developed endometrial cancers had biologically aggressive endometrial cancers and therefore had a poor prognosis. Also, Tamoxifen users were more likely to develop malignant mixed mesodermal tumors and sarcomas of the endometrium, and had significantly reduced cancer-specific 3-year survival rates.[23]

According to a 2008 study, the treatment of breast cancer with Tamoxifen results in an increased risk of uterine cancer and higher chances of dying from it.[24]

It is a rare day that an oncologist takes the time to walk a breast cancer patient through the pros and cons of the research on the drugs used – they just use them. Oncologists often do not tell cancer patients when they are being subjected to one-size-fits-all therapy. For example, researchers found that women with early-stage breast cancer who were HER2 negative derived absolutely no benefit from taking the commonly used anthracycline drugs in their chemotherapy.[25] Anthracycline is a type of antibiotic that comes from certain types of streptomyces bacteria. However, approximately 80 percent of breast cancers are HER2 negative; thus only 1 out of 5 women with breast cancer can benefit from these drugs that have considerable toxicity associated with their use. In another study, seven percent of patients treated with Adriamycin®, an anthracycline drug, developed congestive heart failure.[26] This is a serious side effect; the heart is a much needed organ.

Chemotherapy drugs are toxic. It is a long-standing reality that oncologists hope the chemo will kill the cancer faster than it kills the patient. Why are we using drugs with serious side effects when the benefits are questionable at best?

Please understand the statistics that patients are betting their lives on are compiled by companies that stand to make a lucrative profit from selling their wares. These companies are able to choose the sample group that make up the studies as well as decide what data is included into the final report. Drug companies do not have to report all their studies, so the ones that didn't look good just go in the trash can – the FDA and the public never see those. Details of clinical trials published in medical journals are too often written by authors with financial ties to the companies whose drugs they are writing about. As the *New York Times* reported:

> For years, researchers have talked about the problem of publication bias, or selectively publishing results of trials. Concern about such bias gathered force in the 1990s and early 2000s, when researchers documented how, time and again, positive results were published while negative ones were not. Taken together, studies have shown that results of only about half of clinical trials make their way into medical journals.

> . . . [GlaxoSmithKline in 2012] pleaded guilty to criminal charges and agreed to pay $3 billion in fines after the United States Justice Department accused the company, based in London, of failing to report safety data about its diabetes drug Avandia, and of publishing misleading information about Paxil, the antidepressant, in a medical journal.[27]

Manipulating Standard of Care for Profit

Did you know that the drug companies are the only ones allowed to make health claims on their products? The U.S. law says that only drugs can make claims to cure, prevent, or treat a disease.[28]

The FDA has taken draconian steps to suppress information about foods that reduce disease risk. In 2005, for example, the FDA banned information about cherries' health benefits from appearing on websites and product labels – tart cherries have the ability to reduce the risk of colon cancer because of the anthocyanins and cyanidin contained in the cherry. Also, cherry juice helps to eliminate gout and reduce inflammation and pain in arthritis. According to the FDA, when cherry companies disseminated this peer-reviewed scientific information, the cherries became "unapproved new drugs" and were subject to seizure.[29]

Just the year before, researchers from Johns Hopkins Hospital reported that phytocompounds in tart cherries suppress pain caused by inflammation about as well as the drug Indocin® (indomethacin). Indocin is a powerful nonsteroidal anti-inflammatory drug (NSAID) that can cause many side effects.[30]

God, or nature if you prefer, created natural tools for us like B17 (laetrile) and vitamin C. These are not part of the American "Standard of Care," even though thousands of cancer patients have stepped out of the box and have chosen to use these substances with great success.

Conventional medicine presents its options for treating cancer confidently and offers little room for debate or flexibility. When you dig deeper and look at survival rates, it seems strange that patients and physicians are placing their confidence in protocols that offer such poor outcomes. Every day, patients and their families are led into making decisions that will affect their lives based on the data they are given. In oncology where success is measured in months and not years, this seems criminal. This reductionist and fear-based approach puts patients at a huge disadvantage when making decisions. The pharmaceuticals, surgeries, and radiation are not simple solutions and have major – sometimes deadly – side effects.

During my cancer journey, I was offered only the options of surgery, chemotherapy, and radiation. In fact, they were presented as an everyday activity like sitting down to a plate of milk and cookies. It is shocking – the ease at which these protocols are arranged. Get the diagnosis on Wednesday, and be scheduled for surgery or chemo the following Monday. Sign here, get this lab work. Within a matter of days, you are in the system. A very profitable system that may, or may not, do more than put a bandage on your problem. We spend more time shopping for a car than we do considering our options after a cancer diagnosis.

How many cancer patients read the drug inserts on the chemotherapy drugs being dripped into their veins? You should ask to read those inserts before consenting to the first chemo session. You need to understand that the side effects and warnings that are in small print can and often do occur. Organ damage, pain, and nausea top the list. Remember, you have time to do your homework. *There is no need to be scheduled for treatment within days of the diagnosis.* That is more about salesmanship than what it best for you.

Understanding Risk

Oncologists frequently express the benefits of chemotherapy in terms of "relative risk" rather than giving a straight assessment of the likely impact on overall survival of the individual patient. Some of the commonly used terms are: relative risk reduction, *absolute risk* reduction, and absolute survival benefit, and the number needed to treat, abbreviated as (NNT). The whole statistic thing can get very confusing. But hang in here – this is vitally important to your ability to make an objective choice about treatment.

Remember the trouble with mammography screenings? Well, saving a life is great, yes. But at what price to hundreds of others who had benign anomalies, benign tumors, or cancerous tumors that would have spontaneously regressed or never presented a threat in a woman's lifetime? And what of the expense and emotional trauma all those over-diagnosed and over-treated women endure? How many cancers are caused by the annual dose of carcinogenic radiation to which this old technology exposes them?

Relative risk is a statistical means of expressing the benefit of receiving a medical intervention in a way that, while technically accurate, has the effect of making the intervention look considerably more beneficial than it truly is. If receiving a treatment causes a patient's risk to drop from 4 percent to 2%, this can be expressed as a decrease in relative risk reduction of 50 percent. On face value that sounds good. But another, equally valid way of expressing this is to say that it offers a 2% reduction in absolute risk, which is less likely to convince patients to take the treatment.

If a patient has a 98% probability of surviving 10 years without chemotherapy and has a 99% chance with chemotherapy, the statistics would be reported as:

- Absolute survival benefit = 1%.
- Relative risk reduction = 50%.

It is unlikely that many patients would opt for chemotherapy because of the 1 percent absolute survival benefit. If the patient is given only the relative risk reduction statistic of 50 percent, along with a recommendation from their oncologist to take the therapy, would most likely agree and begin the protocol.

In any study where you want to exaggerate the benefits, use this concept of relative risk. Then minimize the side effects by reporting them in terms of absolute risk.

Many people would choose a drug that improves their chances of killing cancer cells by 50 percent rather than a drug that eliminates cancer in one out of 100 people. Both of these statistics are describing the same drug. They are just two different ways of looking at the same statistic. That is why it is of utmost importance that as a patient and chief decision maker, you understand relative benefit in contrast to absolute benefit.

In 2011, the Cochrane Collaboration looked at randomized trials comparing the number of women who died of breast cancer who participated in mammography screening and those who did not participate. The Cochrane Collaboration is not in the business of selling mammograms or treating cancer, so they make no effort to paint a brighter picture of mammography than the research actually shows. Researchers laid out their findings in terms of absolute risk:

As the effect [screening to reduce mortality] was lowest in the adequately randomised trials, a reasonable estimate is a 15% reduction corresponding to an absolute risk reduction of 0.05%. Screening led to 30% overdiagnosis and overtreatment, or an absolute risk increase of 0.5%. This means that for every 2000 women invited for screening throughout 10 years, one will have her life prolonged and 10 healthy women, who would not have been diagnosed if there had not been screening, will be treated unnecessarily. Furthermore, more than 200 women will experience important psychological distress for many months because of false positive findings. It is thus not clear whether screening does more good than harm.[31]

In the award-winning video, *Healing Cancer From Inside Out*, director Mike Anderson provides an example of how drug companies come up with percentages that their drugs benefit certain patient populations:

For example, 100 people are enrolled in a clinical trial of a new . . . drug. Out of 100 people [they] expect two people to get [breast] cancer, but during the trial, after all 100 people were put on the drug, only one person got breast cancer, meaning the reduction in breast cancer was 1 person in 100, or 1%. This is called the absolute benefit. This is not good news for the drug company because 1 in 100 could happen by chance. But remember, 2 people were expected to get breast cancer, but only 1 person got it – and 1 divided by 2 equals ½ or a 50% reduction. Through the magic of number manipulation this drug can all of a sudden reduce your chances of getting breast cancer by 50%. This is called the relative benefit. It magically turns the 1% absolute benefit into a 50% relative benefit . . . not to mention the side effects in all 100 people who took the drug for one person to benefit. Everyone suffered harm but only one person may have been helped by it and that could have happened purely by chance.[32]

Drug advertisements boast about their latest "breakthrough" treatment. Pharmaceutical companies and cancer treatment centers advertise the relative risk to deceptively raise cure rates. Many media reports are not researched news reports, but regurgitated press releases – marketing tools making the treatments appear more beneficial than they actually are. These reports present a study's findings in relative risk terms rather than absolute risk reduction.

So the bottom line? Find out the "Absolute Survivor Benefit." Ask your doctor: out of 100 people, how many benefitted from this treatment? Insist on clarification about how much time this treatment will buy you – is it days, months, or years? And if just days or months, what will your quality of life be like during that time? Will the toxicity of the treatment be worth it? If your doctor won't tell you this information, look it up. Beware of what you read online from organizations who take sponsorship money from the pharmaceutical industry.

And most of all, remember that orthodox medicine does not have proven cures for cancer. "Effective" does not mean cure; it just means temporary tumor shrinkage.

"Then you will know the truth and the truth will set you free."

– John 8:32 (KJV)

Footnotes

1   American Society of Clinical Oncology. Understanding Statistics Used to Guide Prognosis and Evaluate Treatment. Updated 02/2013. Retrieved April 19, 2013 at: www.cancer.net/all-about-cancer/newly-diagnosed/understanding-statistics-used-guide-prognosis-and-evaluate-treatment.

2   Dorresteijn LD, Kappelle AC, et al. Increased risk of ischemic stroke after radiotherapy on the neck in patients younger than 60 years. *J Clin Oncol.* 2002 Jan 1; 20(1):282-288.

3   Kolata G. Forty Years' War: Advances prove elusive in the drive to cure cancer. *New York Times.* April 24, 2009.

4   Overell B. *Animal Research Takes Lives: Humans and Animals Both Suffer.* The N-Z Anti-Vivisection Society, Inc. 1993; p 132.

5   *Outrage* magazine. Oct/Nov 1986.
6   American Cancer Society. Cancer In Children. September 2013.
    Retrieved October 1, 2015 at: www.cancer.org/acs/groups/cid/
    documents/webcontent/002287-pdf.pdf.
7   President's Cancer Panel. Reducing Environmental Cancer
    Risk-What We can do Now. 2008-2009 Annual Report of the
    President's Cancer Panel. Released May, 2010. Retrieved
    December 30, 2014 at: http://deainfo.nci.nih.gov/advisory/pcp/
    annualReports/pcp08-09rpt/PCP_Report_08-09_508.pdf.
8   Yaswen, P; Mukhopadhyay, P; Costes, S. Promotion of variant
    human mammary epithelial cell outgrowth by ionizing radiation:
    an agent-based model supported by in vitro studies. *Breast Cancer
    Research*. February, 2010; 12:R11.
9   Lawrence Berkeley National Laboratory. Press release: Study
    Raises New Concerns About Radiation and Breast Cancer. May
    13, 2010.
10 Euler-Cheplin M, Kuchiki M, Vejborg I. Increased risk of
    breast cancer in women with false-positive test: The role of
    misclassification. *Cancer Epidemiology*. 2014 Oct; 38(5):619-622.
11 Cohen, R. Mammography false alarms linked with later tumor
    risk. Reuters. August 22, 2014.
12 Miller A, Wall C, et al. Twenty five year follow-up for breast
    cancer incidence and mortality of the Canadian National Breast
    Screening Study: randomised screening trial. *BMJ*. February 11,
    2014; 348:g366. doi: 10.1136/bmj.g366.
13 Kolata G. Vast Study Casts Doubts on Value of Mammograms.
    New York Times, February 11, 2014.
14 Bleyer A, Welch HG. Effect of three decades of screening
    mammography on breast-cancer incidence. *NJEM*. 2012;
    367(21):1998-2005.
15 Miller A, Wall C, et al. Twenty five year follow-up for breast
    cancer incidence and mortality of the Canadian National Breast
    Screening Study: randomised screening trial. *BMJ*. February 11,
    2014; 348:g366. doi: 10.1136/bmj.g366.
16 Lousdal ML, Kristiansen IS, et al. Trends in breast cancer stage
    distribution before, during and after introduction of a screening
    programme in Norway. *Eur J Public Health*. 2014 Dec; 24(6):1017-
    1022.
17 Biller-Andorno N, Jüni P. Abolishing mammography screening
    programs? A view from the Swiss Medical Board. *NEJM*. 2014
    May 22; 370:1965-1967.

18 National Cancer Institute. Colorectal Cancer Screening PDQ. Retrieved January 13, 2015 at: www.cancer.gov/cancertopics/pdq/ screening/colorectal/HealthProfessional/page3.

19 NCI News. Yale study estimates that screening has prevented half a million colorectal cancers. Retrieved January 19, 2015 at: www.cancer.gov/newscenter/cancerresearchnews/2014/ YaleEstimateScreeningColorectalCancerPrevention.

20 Rosenthal E. The $2.7 Trillion Medical Bill-Colonoscopies Explain Why U.S. Leads the World in Health Expenditures. *New York Times*. June 1, 2013.

21 National Cancer Institute Fact sheet. BRCA1 and BRCA2: Cancer Risk and Genetic Testing. Retrieved January 18, 2015 at: www. cancer.gov/cancertopics/factsheet/Risk/BRCA.

22 Park W, Amin AR, et al. New perspectives of curcumin in cancer prevention. *Cancer Prev Res* (Phila). 2013 May; 6(5):387-400.

23 Bergman L, Beelen MLR, et al. Risk and prognosis of endometrial cancer after tamoxifen for breast cancer. *Lancet*. 2000; 356:881-887.

24 Lavie O, Barnett-Griness O, et al. The risk of developing uterine sarcoma after tamoxifen use. *International Journal of Gynecological Cancer*. 2008 March/April; 18(2,);352-356.

25 Gennari A, Sormani MP, et al. HER2 status and efficacy of adjuvant anthracyclines in early breast cancer: a pooled analysis of randomized trials. *J Natl Cancer Inst*. 2008 Jan 2; 100(1):14-20.

26 Swain SM, Whaley FS, Ewe MS. Congestive heart failure in patients treated with doxorubicin: a retrospective analysis of three trials. *Cancer*. 2003 Jun 1; 97(11):2869-2879.

27 Thomas K. Breaking the Seal on Drug Research. *New York Times*. June 29, 2013.

28 FDA-Food-Structure/Function Claims. Retrieved October 15, 2013 at: www.fda.gov/Food/IngredientsPackagingLabeling/ LabelingNutrition/ucm2006881.htm Page updated 08/21/2013.

29 FDA press release October 24, 2005. FDA Warns Companies to Stop Marketing Fruit Products with Unproven Disease Treatment and Prevention Claims. Retrieved at www.fda.gov/NewsEvents/ Newsroom/PressAnnouncements/2005/ucm108503.htm.

30 Tall JM, Seeram NP, et al. Tart cherry anthocyanins suppress inflammation-induced pain behavior in rat. *Behav Brain Res*. 2004 Aug 12; 153(1):181-188.

31 Gøtzsche PC, Nielsen M. Screening for breast cancer with mammography. Cochrane Breast Cancer Group. January 19, 2011.

32 *Healing Cancer From Inside Out*. Directed by Mike Anderson. 2008. DVD.

Chapter 5

Conventional Treatments –
The Wait, Watch, and Wonder Program

As a newly diagnosed cancer patient, it often seems that your world is turned upside down in an instant. The diagnosis is usually followed by strong recommendations from the healthcare system to immediately – within a week or two – begin an aggressive treatment program that typically involves surgery, chemotherapy, and radiation in different combinations. It is so easy to get swept up by the system, and give up your right to take a step back and further examine the additional treatment options. In a situation where you are fearful and overwhelmed, your first thought probably is not to question what you are told by medical "authorities." But it should be; I wish I had.

You do have time to examine the proposed conventional treatments you will be pressured to undergo.

In the United States, we use about three times more chemotherapy than other nations do. We spend about five times more on chemotherapy. Yet our cancer survival rates are not appreciably different.[1] We have more cancer among us today than in 1971 when the "war on cancer" was begun.

A lot of the standardized care we are doing is simply not working. Overall cancer rates are not coming down. Even the elite in our society do not fare better than the average citizen.

The Status Quo

When Senator Ted Kennedy was diagnosed with brain cancer in 2008, he had access to the absolute, best care available. Yet he did not live longer than the average patient with his kind of cancer. According to *New York Times* reporters Gina Kolata and Dr. Lawrence K. Altman:

> [Kennedy] became one of the millions whose fate was not much changed by the cancer war. Despite billions that have been spent, the death rate from most cancers barely budged.

Mr. Kennedy's cancer, a glioblastoma, kills almost everyone
who gets it, usually in a little over a year. Although he got
the most aggressive treatment, Mr. Kennedy lived just 15
months after his diagnosis – just about the median survival
for patients with his type of tumor who got the radiation and
chemotherapy regimen that has become the standard of care.

As has happened with most cancers in the nation's 40-year war
on cancer, progress on glioblastomas has been incremental.
With these deadly brain cancers in particular, the disease
remains poorly understood.[2]

The American Cancer Society, the largest private financier
of cancer research, has spent more than $3.4 billion on research
grants since 1946. The National Cancer Institute receives roughly
$5 billion each year. If both public and private investments are
to be accounted for, estimates put the U.S. spending on cancer
research at about *$16 billion each year*.[3] Where is the cure? Kolata
tells us:

> One major impediment, scientists agree, is the grant
> system itself. It has become a sort of jobs program, a way
> to keep research laboratories going year after year with the
> understanding that the focus will be on small projects unlikely
> to take significant steps toward curing cancer.

> "These grants are not silly, but they are only likely to produce
> incremental progress," said Dr. Robert C. Young, chancellor
> at Fox Chase Cancer Center in Philadelphia and chairman of
> the Board of Scientific Advisors, an independent group that
> makes recommendations to the cancer institute.

> Dr. Otis W. Brawley, chief medical officer at the American
> Cancer Society, said the whole cancer research effort
> remained too cautious.

> "The problem in science is that the way you get ahead is
> by staying within narrow parameters and doing what other
> people are doing," Dr. Brawley said. "No one wants to fund
> wild new ideas."[4]

Researchers have jobs, but the rest of us are waiting for "the cure."

Drug Research Still Leads the Way

We are relentlessly bombarded with drug advertising on television, and that has trained us to expect a cure from the pharmaceutical industry. But it isn't happening. The headlines tell the story:

- 2013 – The U.S. wastes an estimated $6 billion annually on popular white blood cell boosting drugs that have no medical benefits for most cancer patients using them.[5]
- 2012 – Chemotherapy can make cancers more resistant to treatment and even encourage them to grow because chemotherapy causes healthy cells to release a protein that actually feeds cancer cells and causes them to thrive and proliferate.[6]
- 2011 – The FDA declared the blockbuster pharmaceutical Avastin no longer be prescribed for the treatment of breast cancer, claiming that the drug has proven to be neither safe nor effective in treating the disease.[7]
- 2011 – $100,000 cancer drugs are ineffective – "The latest expensive treatment is Dendreon's Provenge cancer vaccine. It costs $93,000 for each patient that uses it, no matter whether it works or not. In fact, there is no way to tell whether it worked in an individual patient, because it doesn't shrink tumors or slow progression of the disease in any measurable way . . ."[8]

And a 2013 paper, authored by Dr. Hagop Kantarjian, Professor of Medicine and Chair of the Leukemia Department at MD Anderson, and signed by 120 leukemia specialists, shows that the costs of leukemia drugs are actually harming patients – call this one a case of "financial toxicity."[9]

Many people involved in the cancer field, like Harmala Gupta, founder-president of CanSupport in New Delhi, note that that money and politics got in the way of winning the war on cancer:

Institutions like the NIH and the NCI [are] turning over the fruits of basic research to private collaborators who in turn dictate the terms on which they will be made available to the public . . . By ceding ground to pharmaceutical lobbies, America has significantly nullified the huge research advantage that the NIH gave it. As a result, Americans not only have a poorer health status than Europeans, but also pay a much higher price for their drugs than Europeans do.[10]

Most pharmaceutical drugs are designed to work on one target (such as a gene, a protein, or a cellular receptor) or one physiologic pathway (such as inflammation, glucose metabolism, or immune modulation). However, cancer is driven by hundreds, perhaps thousands of targets and pathways. Cancer is a complex disease. It seems highly unlikely that a drug can deliver a "cure" for most cancers. We have been waiting 50 years or more for the silver bullet that has never come.

With all of the money raised for cancer research, cancer is still killing better than ever before. People are suffering and are being run through tests and treatments like a national cattle call. The truth is that there is no liability on the medical industry's part for prescribing conventional, NCCN backed cancer treatments.

Marketing Versus Reality

Despite the paltry victories, the U.S. cancer industry has done a fantastic job at marketing its wares. People see the Susan G. Komen races and the American Cancer Society's ads implying that if you give a little more money, the cure is right around the corner. Most people do not research or read beyond the pamphlet their doctor may have given them until they are well into treatment or after.

The cancer industry's public relations machine keeps the public thinking that results for cancer treatment are getting better all the time. The system works well for the research grant recipients and the pharmaceutical industry's shareholders, but it doesn't work nearly as well for most patients.

According to Dr. Guy B. Faguet, author of *An Anatomy of Failure: A Blueprint for Future Years*, chemotherapy is just 2% effective in late stage cancers after a 5 year period. He asserts that chemotherapy drugs have shown benefits in treating a few types of cancers, including acute lymphocytic leukemia and choriocarcinom in children, but beyond that, chemo has a disappointing track-record. Chemotherapy, he says, is largely ineffective in dealing with advanced cancers or malignancies.

Many other doctors agree. Robert C. Atkins, M.D., author of *Dr. Atkins' New Diet Revolution*, judged the American cancer industry's approach as dismal for patients:

> My studies have proved conclusively that untreated cancer victims live up to four times longer than treated individuals. If one has cancer and opts to do nothing at all, he will live longer and feel better than if he undergoes radiation, chemotherapy or surgery. Then, why is this still the gold standard for treatment?

While 67 percent of newly diagnosed cancer patients are expected to survive, that only means they are alive 5 years after their diagnosis; fewer than a fifth of patients with cancers of the lung, pancreas, liver or esophagus are expected to live that long. And if the disease has metastasized – about 90 percent of those cancer patients will die of their disease.[11]

When I was diagnosed, I did not know that the standard of care for cancer had such a bad track record. I had been a big believer in its effectiveness. After all, it is what the experts say we should do.

I did not fully understand the impact of indiscriminately killing both cancerous and healthy cells with chemotherapy and radiation. I did not understand the full impact of a weakened body trying to detox toxic drug treatments. I did not understand the importance of a healthy immune system. No one mentioned any of that as I was scheduled for surgery and chemo shortly after my diagnosis.

The Same Old War on Cancer

I have firsthand experience from my diagnosis and journey through the halls of Houston's best hospitals. I watched as information on alternative, less expensive, less toxic, and less invasive treatments was suppressed and even laughed at by those in the oncology business. Remember, I was told to eat cupcakes after my initial treatment.

The American Medical Association (AMA), National Cancer Institute (NCI), and American Cancer Society (ACS) regulate the protocols that are the gold standard for all official cancer treatments in the U.S. Expensive drugs, invasive surgeries, and radiation are the primary components on the menu and all I was offered. It is hard to resist the sales pitch when you are scared and you have been taught that doctors have all the answers. You find yourself literally putting your life in the hands of persons or institutions unknown to you.

Physicians, like most people, don't feel comfortable discussing things that they know very little about. Unfortunately, our accredited medical schools do not offer courses on homeopathy and the wide array of natural therapies. Several physicians interviewed said that not only did they not learn about natural therapies, but they only had one class on nutrition while in medical school.

In 2010, only 27 percent of the 105 medical schools in the U.S. met the minimum 25 required nutritional hours set by the National Academy of Sciences.[12]

Our medical schools receive funding from pharmaceutical companies and the pharmaceutical representatives are responsible for educating doctors on the drug therapies. Deep-pocketed pharmaceutical companies sponsor destination medical conferences and events. Physicians need continuing education hours for their license renewals and gladly attend these events. Did you know that some physicians receive research grants, perks, and gifts as well as monetary payment for enrolling a patient in a research study?

Realize that cancer is big money and big business. Don't let money and the insurance companies dictate your treatment. Keep in mind deductibles and co-pays. This money might be better spent on a healing therapy or on an early diagnostic test. Know that there are many options. Cancer is much easier and less expensive to deal with when it is caught early.

Unlike other kinds of doctors, cancer doctors are allowed to profit from the sale of drugs. Whereas doctors in other specialties simply write prescriptions, oncologists can make a significant part of their income by buying chemotherapy drugs wholesale and selling them to patients at a marked up prices – you don't go to a pharmacy and buy your chemo; the doctor has it.[13] That sets the stage for the sale of drugs and therapies that may be very expensive with little hope of success.

Also, keep in mind physicians have to deal with HMOs, insurance companies, and government agencies looking over their shoulders and more doctors have become fearful of the legal ramifications of not going "with the flow." To step outside the box and recommend any treatments that are not blessed as being part of the standard of care – rules for treatment devised by state licensing boards and medical societies – can put doctors' licenses at grave risk.

So the old system changes very slowly. Cancer Treatment Centers of America, a relative newcomer, is helping to bring meaningful change with the addition of organic food and holistic practitioners.

Here are key things to know about the three commonly used modalities to treat cancer:

Surgery

Surgery is the oldest form of cancer treatment. It plays a role in diagnosing cancer and finding out how far it has spread, a process called *staging*. Surgery can play a useful role by reducing the tumor burden – debulking the mass – and leaving the patient with less cancer to treat by other means.

Surgery weakens immunity and places great systemic stress on the patient. Also, we know that cancer is not a localized disease; it is part of a systemic health problem. Surgical removal of the known tumor seems to make everyone feel better, but the elephant is still in the room.

Surgeons routinely tell cancer patients, "I got it all," but many studies have shown that some cancer cells are left behind in 25 to 60 percent of patients, allowing malignant growths to recur. I had significant surgery to remove my cancer only to find plenty of cancer cells still circulating in my blood.

Research has shown that a tumor as small as 1-2 mm has blood perfusion, thus giving cancer cells access to the blood supply and the rest of the body. The hope is that even with clean surgical margins, no cancer cells have been released into the blood stream. After the successful removal of a tumor, the patient is usually told they have "no evidence of disease (NED)."

What the patient is not told is that it is not safe to assume surgery makes them cancer free. They are not told they can confirm that diagnosis with one of the tests listed in this book. Instead, they are encouraged with the news that the surgeon got most of the tumor or all of the tumor and the pathology report indicated clean margins. That means that they could not see any cancer cells in the tissue that was removed from the area surrounding the tumor.

Surgery is not the curative treatment that is thought to be; in fact, cutting into a tumor can spread cancer cells into the patient's bloodstream. Biopsies can be problematic too. During a biopsy, a needle is inserted directly into the tumor leaving behind an open pathway for cancer cells to escape into the body.[14] This practice is tragic, in my opinion.

Mastectomies have become a standard procedure that subjects women to a futile, mutilating surgery. Furthermore, I have found no evidence that mastectomies affect survival. Susan Moss says in her book, *Keep Your Breasts*, that if patients knew this, they would likely refuse surgery. She healed herself of breast and uterine cancer using natural therapies.

Chemotherapy

The cornerstone of a conventional treatment plan is chemotherapy, usually a "cocktail" of aggressive chemical cellular toxins. Chemo drugs kill both cancerous and healthy cells alike, and wreak havoc on the body's immune system and organs. Dosages are set by NCCN standards and a low-dose option such as insulin potentiated therapy (see Treatment Options and Complementary Therapies chapter) is not offered.

In the event your doctor does not give you the package inserts from your chemo drugs so you can read the side effects for yourself, I'll list a few of them:

- Nausea and vomiting.
- Alopecia (hair loss).
- Liver toxicity.

- Kidney toxicity.
- Cardiac toxicity (reducing heart function).
- Fatigue.
- Hearing loss and damage.
- Bone marrow suppression.
- Immune suppression.
- Neutropenia (low white blood cell count).
- Thrombocytopenia (low blood platelet count, clotting problems).
- Anemia (low red blood cell count).
- Inflammation to mucous membranes (ulcers).
- Loss of appetite.
- Peripheral neuropathy.
- Vision damage.
- Skin and nail damage.
- Cognitive problems (memory).
- Loss of libido (sex drive).
- Infertility.
- Diarrhea and constipation.

Chemo sessions are often spaced several weeks apart because the patient must have time to recover from the harsh effects of the treatment. Particularly, the white blood cell count needs to recover to keep the patient from dying of infection, and the red blood cell count needs to recover to carry oxygen throughout the body. Blood cells are made in the bone marrow, and bone marrow cells are rapidly dividing cells – the kind of cells most susceptible to being killed by chemotherapy drugs. As the chemo kills the bone marrow cells, the body cannot rapidly make a generous supply of blood cells.

Some cancer cells will survive the pharmaceutical onslaught. During recovery time, those surviving cells keep growing and getting stronger.

Months or years later, these stronger cells can start reproducing and the result is a stronger cancer that is resistant to chemotherapy. How does that happen? At least a couple of ways.

The p53 gene is part of the body's machinery to prevent cancer in the first place. It was one of the first tumor suppressor genes ever discovered. It is on the lookout for cell damage and dispatches proteins to activate repair systems when DNA is damaged and initiates cell death (apoptosis) if the damage is irreparable. Cell death is a good thing because you want cancer cells to die. But when the p53 gene becomes mutated – part of its gene sequence is lost or deleted – it cannot manufacture the proper proteins. Most cancer patients have p53 protein mutations.

It has been unclear whether p53 mutations made tumors easier or harder to treat – you find examples of both arguments in the medical literature. In any event, there is substantial agreement that a mutated p53 gene makes you resistant to chemotherapy.[15,16,17] Chemotherapeutic drugs cause DNA damage. The p53 gene senses that and sends out proteins whose first mission is to try to repair damaged cells. In some cases, that effort is successful. However, cells live after their DNA has been damaged by chemotherapeutic agents and in this way, they become resistant to chemotherapy. Cancer cells damaged by chemo can develop in time into a recurrence of cancer.[18]

We know today that 90 percent of cancer patients with metastatic breast, prostate, lung or colon cancers develop resistance to chemotherapy.

What is missing in the literature is emphasis on finding out why the p53 gene goes bad as we get older, and what we can do to encourage our tumor suppressor genes to stay healthy.

In 2012, scientists led by the Fred Hutchinson Cancer Research Center reported that DNA-damaging cancer treatment coaxes fibroblasts to crank out a protein called WNT16B within the tumor's microenvironment. This protein is taken up by nearby cancer cells, causing them to grow, invade, and resist subsequent therapy.[19] In other words, chemotherapy damages the DNA of healthy, non-cancerous cells, causing them to produce molecules that in turn produce more cancer cells.

Then there is the problem of the cancer stem cells. About a decade ago, Max Wicha, M.D., professor of oncology and director of the University of Michigan Comprehensive Cancer Center, told us that standard cancer treatments can actually make things worse because they can activate cancer stem cells. He found that when tumor cells die from chemotherapy and radiation, they give off inflammatory signals that "wake up" these stem cells. These cells can act like a wildcard and reproduce themselves as malignant cells, remaining dormant for years, then triggering a recurrence of cancer.[20]

Just about every doctor would agree that cancer is fundamentally a failure of the immune system. We all have cancer cells in us. If our immune system is working well, it cleans out those errant cells every day, long before they have a chance to take root and form a tumor.

Chemotherapy, unfortunately, does not strengthen the patient's immune system; chemotherapy actually weakens it. Cells are most vulnerable to chemotherapy's killing effects of when the chemo hits them as the cells are dividing. So rapidly dividing cells like your hair follicles, bone marrow, and your gut lining, are most likely to die after a chemo session. Add to that list the rapidly dividing immune system killer-cells which deal with fungi, bacteria, viruses, and damaged cells.

Bill Henderson, author, radio talk show host, and cancer coach, puts it this way:

> Conventional cancer treatment (surgery, chemotherapy and radiation) destroys your immune system. Oncologists pay little attention to rebuilding it or changing your lifestyle. This is why patients with cancer treated with conventional treatment seem to get better, only to have the cancer recur in a few months or years in a more aggressive form. Additionally, the cancer that returns is usually resistant to the previous chemotherapeutic agents used. The weaker cancer cells have been killed off by the treatment and the stronger ones survive, only to reproduce themselves. Eventually, all are strong and treatment resistant.[21]

We are still waiting for the cancer industry to integrate less toxic approaches to treatment, such as including therapeutic levels of vitamin C into the standard of care since we know it kills cancer cells without killing healthy cells or prompting drug resistance. We are also still waiting for healing the immune system to become part of the standard of care.

Radiation

Radiation is perhaps the most toxic of the three regulation-issue cancer treatments. Like chemotherapy, it damages normal, healthy cells in the process of killing cancer cells. Radiotherapy is a powerful carcinogen; it causes secondary cancers in many patients exposed to it. Using radiation is the equivalent of burning the cancer cells to death in an effort to cripple cancer cells' ability to replicate.

But cancer is a systemic disease, so burning a small section of the body does not make much sense. Radiation can reduce the tumor size, but the side effects are significant and harmful. Healthy cells are killed along with the cancerous cells.

Depending on the part of your body being treated, you may experience:

- Skin dryness, itching, peeling, or blistering.
- Fatigue.
- Diarrhea.
- Hair loss in the treatment area.
- Nausea and vomiting.
- Sexual changes.
- Swelling.
- Trouble swallowing.
- Urinary and bladder changes.

Most of these side effects go away within two months after radiation therapy is finished. Late side effects may first occur six or more months after radiation therapy is over. They vary by the part of your body that was treated and the dose of radiation you received. Late side effects may include:

- Infertility.
- Joint problems.
- Brittle, broken bones.
- Lymphedema.
- Necrosis.
- Secondary cancer.

"For many survivors, the cost of the cure of their cancer has been late, life-threatening effects of therapy," said Dr. Lois B. Travis, director of the Rubin Center for Cancer Survivorship at the University of Rochester Medical Center. "We recognized that secondary malignant neoplasms and cardiovascular disease are among the most serious adverse effects experienced by the growing number of survivors worldwide."[22]

Patients who receive radiation to a part of their body where lymph nodes were removed are at high risk to develop lymphedema – an accumulation of fluid near the site of surgery or radiation. This comes as a result of burning or removing lymph nodes which are part of a vast network of vessels running through the entire body. Lymphedema is a painful condition that produces swelling in the limbs, fingers, or toes, a feeling of tightness, heaviness, or a tingling sensation, and thickening of the skin. Data reports that upwards of 70 percent of patients will experience lymphedema after a modified radical mastectomy (removal of breast and axillary lymph nodes) with regional nodal radiation.[23]

Radiation can produce scaring and reduce the blood flow to the treated area leaving patients at risk for infection and delayed healing. This problem can become chronic and debilitating and can require lifelong management.

Recently, I was talking to a breast cancer patient who had undergone radiation. She was reporting chest soreness and pain. Her oncologist told her radiation can cause her ribs to fracture easily. I asked her if anyone had warned her about this possible side effect. She said no, it must have been in that tiny print on the forms that she was told to sign.

Additionally, the National Cancer Institute reports on their website that radiation therapy can cause new cancers many years after the completion of finished treatment.[24]

Radiation adds to the list of health problems.

Terms Commonly Used in Conventional Treatment

Remission

Let's define remission. According to the American Cancer Society, there are two different types of remission:

1. When a treatment completely gets rid of all tumors that could be measured or seen on a test, it's called a complete response or complete remission. (It's important to note the use of the words "could be measured.")
2. A partial response or partial remission means the cancer partly responded to treatment, but still did not go away. A partial response is most often defined as at least a 50% reduction in measurable tumor.[25]

Wow, I thought that remission meant the patient was successfully treated and is cancer free for the time being. Unfortunately, most people have a distorted and incorrect understanding of remission. What we now know is that the patient may still have microscopic cancer cells, but they are not clumped together in large enough numbers to be seen on a scan. They have just quieted down for a time or could not be measured by the test outlined by the cancer and insurance industries in the United States.

No Evidence of Disease

"No Evidence of Disease" or NED is a term that is used when the oncologist can't detect cancer. NED is used more now than the word "remission." I guess that it is the best that they have to offer. However, what is really wanted by the patient is a cure.

Survivor

Last, but not least, is the big "S" word, "survivor." What does that really mean? Basically, it means that you have lived 5 years beyond your diagnosis – so far.

Alternative Approaches Pushed Aside

On April 24, 2013, the FDA and FBI raided the Camelot Cancer Care Center in Tulsa, Oklahoma, for treating cancer patients with B17, also known as amygdalin and laetrile. The FDA did not send Camelot a "cease and desist" letter prior to the unannounced raid. The search warrant was specific for B17. As this is written months later, the government's case is still ongoing. To date, one employee has pleaded guilty to misdemeanor interfering with federal agents, but other than that, no charges have been filed. Bank accounts have been frozen; patient records and office equipment remain seized.

Camelot is yet another piece of collateral damage in a long running war against B-17. The history is long so let us briefly relate just one chapter from this travesty because cancer patients need to know what they are up against.

Word about the success of cancer treatments using laetrile began to spread in the 1950s. In 1972 Sloan Kettering commissioned Dr. Kanematsu Sugiura, one of the most respected cancer research scientists, to conduct tests over a 5 year period to determine the effectiveness of laetrile in cancer treatment. His repeated tests yielded consistent results:

*   Laetrile inhibited the growth of tumors.
*   It stopped the spreading (metastasizing) of cancer in mice 77 percent of the time.
*   It relieved pain.
*   It acted as a cancer preventative.
*   It improved general health.

At the conclusion of the trials in 1977, Sloan Kettering released a press statement that said: ". . . laetrile was found to possess neither preventative, nor tumor-regressent, nor anti-metastatic, nor curative anticancer activity."

Dr. Sugiura was fired, and so too was Ralph Moss, head of public relations at Sloan Kettering who protested the cover up and blew the whistle in a press conference on November 18, 1977.

Although technically not a vitamin, vitamin B17 was the name given to amygdalin by bio-chemist Dr. Ernst Krebs in 1952. It has been used for more than 50 years by cancer treatment centers outside the U.S. because it works. It still is not FDA-approved.

B17 is present in many foods and most fruit seeds including apples, cherries, nectarines, pears, and plums. Edward Griffin's 2010 edition of his book, *World Without Cancer - The Story of Vitamin B17*, cites case after case of its beneficial use. Griffin contends that the medical establishment has waged war against

B17, not because the science convinces us we should do so, but because politics demands we do so based upon the economic power of those who dominate the medical establishment. B17, he writes, ". . . is not widely available to the public because it cannot be patented, and therefore is not commercially attractive to the pharmaceutical industry."

You can find stories from people occasionally saying that B17 did not work for them; many more saying it did work. If the voices from the grave could talk, we would hear the countless testimonials that conventional cancer treatment did not save them. Note: We would also hear from some 60,000 voices from the grave that the FDA-approved Vioxx for arthritis caused their deaths. Or consider this: a study released in 2013 found more people are dying in the U.S. from FDA-approved prescription drugs than from heroin and cocaine combined.

People often find out about B17 after conventional oncology has basically told them they are going to die. So who is protecting whom?

Pioneers in healing cancer naturally such as Harry Hoxsey, Dr. Royal Raymond Rife, and Dr. Max Gerson presented patient records documenting the success of their treatments, yet the evidence of their work has been dismissed or suppressed.

One has to question why the organizations we believe are working to help us, are giving us such limited options to treat cancer. If surgery, chemotherapy, and radiation fail, patients are sent home to die, with no mention of other proven therapies. Shouldn't the profession that we trust with our lives have a responsibility to give us all the options, not just the financially profitable ones?

Cancer is a wily beast. We need to be open to therapies other than just those provided by the pharmaceutical industry. The FDA gets half its budget funded by drug companies, but that should not mean chemical assaults are the only approach we take in treating cancer.

I toured several cancer clinics in Tijuana, Mexico and was able to speak with many of the doctors, staff, and patients. Like most people, I thought that a person must have to be desperate to go to one of these clinics on the other side of the U.S. border.

After my firsthand experience, I completely changed my opinion. I learned that many of these doctors have purposefully left the U.S. and set up clinics just 15 minutes into Mexico. These doctors have a deep compassion and desire to help their patients heal of cancer and refuse to be limited to the age-old trio of surgery/radiation/chemo. I found they were using many protocols that are not allowed or accepted as cancer treatments in the U.S. such as B17, intravenous infusions of vitamin C, immune therapies, diet, insulin potentiation therapy (IPT), energy medicine, and detoxification. These clinics report that they are healing approximately 40 percent of the "terminal" patients that show up on their door step.

An eye opening book that gave me a new perspective is Daniel Haley's *Politics in Healing: The Suppression and Manipulation of American Medicine*. In the book he explains why we don't have effective non-toxic cancer cures and how the status quo prevents new ideas from entering medical research and practice. Here you can read about cancer cures which were and still are being relentlessly suppressed by the FDA and the AMA.

It Is Time to Stop the War

We have twice as much breast cancer as we did when the National Cancer Act was signed in 1971, kicking off the "war on cancer." That sounds like a failed agenda.

At the time, curing cancer looked like an easy task. It had taken America just a decade to successfully land a man on the moon. Surely, in less time, we could find a cure for cancer. Heck, we sequenced the entire human genome just 18 years from the time the idea was born. But curing cancer focused on treatment, not causes or prevention, and we have not made much progress with that approach. We still don't have the "cure"; we only have "hope" for a cure and endless requests for more money.

"It's time to admit that our efforts have often targeted the wrong enemies and used the wrong weapons," said Devra Davis, Ph.D., M.P.H., ecological epidemiologist, and world specialist on patterns of cancer in space and time. The National Cancer Institute tells us that two-thirds of all cancers have environmental causes. That, she says, ought to make research into what causes cancer a high priority, but it does not:

The war on cancer remains focused on commercially fueled efforts to develop drugs and technologies that can find and treat the disease – to the tune of more than $100 billion a year in the United States alone. Meanwhile, the struggle basically ignores most of the things known to cause cancer, such as tobacco, radiation, sunlight, benzene, asbestos, solvents, and some drugs and hormones. Even now, modern cancer-causing agents such as gasoline exhaust, pesticides and other air pollutants are simply deemed the inevitable price of progress.

They're not. Scientists understand that most cancer is not born but made . . . Of the nearly 80,000 chemicals regularly bought and sold today, according to the National Academy of Sciences, fewer than 10 percent have been tested for their capacity to cause cancer or do other damage . . . No matter how much our efforts to treat cancer may advance, the best way to reduce cancer's toll is to keep people from getting it.[26]

Statistics tell us that in 2013, more than 1.6 million Americans were diagnosed with cancer and nearly 600,000 died from it.[27] That is about equal to the death toll from 9/11 happening every two days.

Yet the cancer industry spends very little of its multi-billion dollar resources on effective prevention strategies, such as dietary awareness, environmental toxins awareness, and immune system enhancements.

Dr. Kathleen T. Ruddy, a breast cancer surgeon in New Jersey, formed the Breast Health and Healing Foundation to focus public attention on the urgent obligation to discover the causes of breast cancer. Her question gets right to the point for women like me who have experienced breast cancer:

At least 30% of breast cancer is deemed preventable using known and proven risk reduction strategies. Yet less than 1% of all research funding is used toward this goal. If 30% of breast cancer is preventable, shouldn't we spend that portion of our research dollars trying to do so?[28]

It is preferable to prevent cancer rather than treat it. Isolated cancer cells are not threatening because they have no built-in support mechanisms. Kudos to the healthy immune system which sweeps out those cells every day, just as we take out the household trash every night. But when the immune system is overwhelmed and those isolated cancer cells coalesce and take root, they build their own fortresses inside our bodies. They connect to the bloodstream and build their own highways – a network of blood vessels for ready access to food. Cancer cells are first at the feeding trough, robbing us of nutrition our immune system needs to wipe them out. And cancer cells can travel through the bloodstream to other areas of our body. This is why cancer is a systemic disease.

Recognize that when you receive a cancer diagnosis, you are about to be sold something – a course of treatment. It really isn't much different than entering the marketplace to buy, say, cookware for your kitchen. You can buy Teflon-coated pans, or aluminum, or stainless steel, or glass, or several other options. The salespeople who sell the Teflon-coated pans will talk a great story about the non-stick, easy clean-up features. But they won't tell you the EPA has identified a cancer-causing chemical used in the production of Teflon. The aluminum pans do not come with warnings about the health hazards of aluminum leeching into your food. You can choose glass and stainless, but you have to ignore the salespeople pushing toxic non-stick and aluminum.

Likewise, when it comes to cancer treatments, there are options, and there is something to know about those options before you make your choice. Take time to educate yourself about the choices – look before you leap, as they say. Don't fall for the ploy that you absolutely must have surgery or start chemo within a few days of getting a cancer diagnosis. You owe it to yourself to do some homework. Your life is at stake.

Traditional cancer treatments are just that – treatments, not cures. After completion, patients begin the process for which I call the: "The Wait, Watch, and Wonder Program."

Don't Wait, Watch, & Wonder

The Wait, Watch, and Wonder program is what is offered to most cancer patients after completing their prescribed course of treatment. The patient is released to WAIT until the next oncology check-up, where the doctor will WATCH their lab and test results. All the while, the patient will WONDER if their cancer will come back.

Stop wondering, "Am I really cancer free?" If you have already undergone treatment, choose one or more of the tests I talk about in this book to confirm a "cancer free" or "survivor" status.

Don't be an obedient patient and partake of this watch and see approach. Don't let cancer grow large enough to be seen on a mammogram or PET scan, or via a biopsy. Detect it now. Treat it now. Detox and support your body with the nutrients that it requires. It is easier to reverse and the treatments can be less toxic when cancer is in its earlier stages.

And one final note: Never lose faith in the body's own healing abilities. The body can reverse a cancer on its own – spontaneous remission it is called – and doctors see it happen often. Sometimes the body does it and we only know it happened because tests showed that the cancer "went away." Sometimes we don't even know the body did it. Sometimes we can reverse a diagnosed cancer by giving the body tools to fight it – great nutrition, detoxification, and avoidance of carcinogens.

Get off of the revolving door of the cancer industry and take control. Take your health back.

Footnotes

1   Faguet G. The *War on Cancer: An Anatomy of Failure, a Blueprint for the Future*. Springer. 2006.

2   Kolata G, Altman LK. Forty Years' War-Weighing Hope and Reality in Kennedy's Cancer Battle. *New York Times*. August 28, 2009.

3   Leaf C. *The Truth in Small Doses*. Atria Books. 2013.

4   Kolata G. Forty Years' War-Grant System Leads Cancer Researchers to Play It Safe. *New York Times*. June 28, 2009.

5   Nebraska City News website. Study confirms drug given routinely during cancer treatment ineffective for most, costs $6 billion. March 21, 2013. Retrieved January 19, 2015 at: www. ncnewspress.com/article/20130321/NEWS/130329988.

6   Bates C. Chemotherapy "can make cancers more resistant to treatment and even encourage them to grow." *Daily Mail*. August 6, 2012.

7   FDA News Release November 18, 2011. FDA Commissioner Announces Avastin Decision. Retrieved January 3, 2015 at: www.fda.gov/NewsEvents/Newsroom/PressAnnouncements/ucm280536.htm.

8   Langreth R. $100,000 Cancer Drugs, Ineffective $50,000 Back Operations, Unnecessary MRI Scans Will Bankrupt America: A Forbes Conversation. *Forbes*. February 9, 2011.

9   Kantarjian H. Price of drugs for chronic myeloid leukemia (CML), reflection of the unsustainable cancer drug prices: perspective of CML Experts. *Blood*. April 25, 2013.

10 Gupta H. Money first, ethics second. *The Hindu*. April 6, 2013.

11 Leaf C. Why we are losing the war on cancer (and how to win it). *Fortune*. 2004 Mar 22; 149(6):76-82, 84-6, 88 passim.

12 Adams KM, et al. Nutrition education in U.S. medical schools: latest update of a national survey. *Acad Med*. 2010 Sep; 85(9):1537-1542.

13 Ellis R. Cancer docs profit from chemotherapy drugs-situation begs the ethical question: Are they overprescribing? NBC Nightly News. September 21, 2006.

14 Baum M. Does Surgery desseminate or accelerate cancer? *Lancet*. 1996 Jan 27; 347(8996):260.

15 Reles A, Wen WH, et al. Correlation of p53 mutations with resistance to platinum-based chemotherapy and shortened survival in ovarian cancer. *Clin Cancer Res*. 2001 Oct; 7(10):2984-2997.

16 Soussi T. p53 mutations and resistance to chemotherapy: A stab in the back for p73. *Cancer Cell*. 2003 Apr; 3(4):303-305.

17 Breen L, Heenan M, et al. Investigation of the role of p53 in chemotherapy resistance of lung cancer cell lines. *Anticancer Research*. 2007 May-Jun; 27(3A):1361-1364.

18 Moreno CS, Matyunina L, Dickerson EB, et al. Evidence that p53-mediated cell-cycle-arrest inhibits chemotherapeutic treatment of ovarian carcinomas. *PLoS ONE*. May 2007; 2(5):e441.

19 Sun Y, Campisi J, et al. Treatment-induced damage to the tumor microenvironment promotes prostate cancer therapy resistance through WNT16B. *Nature Medicine*. August 2012; 18:1359-1368.

20 Wicha MS, Liu S, Dontu G. Cancer stem cells: an old idea – a paradigm shift. *Cancer Res*. 2006 Feb 15; 66(4):1883-1890; discussion 1895-1896.

21   Henderson B, Garcia CM. *Cancer-Free: Your Guide to Gentle, Non-toxic Healing.* Fourth Edition, Booklocker.com, Inc., 2011, p 89.

22   Survival at a Cost: Common Cancer Treatment Carries Huge Risks. *ABC News.* March 7, 2012.

23   Shah C, Vicini FA. Breast cancer related arm lymphedema: incidence rates, diagnostic techniques, optimal management and risk reduction strategies. *J Radiat Oncol Biol Phys.* 2011; 81:907-914. Also, see more at: www.cancernetwork.com/cancer-complications/lymphedema-separating-fact-fiction/page/0/2#sthash.6tn5ARX1.dpuf

24   National Cancer Institute Fact Sheet: Radiation Therapy for Cancer. Retrieved January 3, 2015 from: www.cancer.gov/cancertopics/factsheet/Therapy/radiation.

25   American Cancer Society. When Cancer Doesn't Go Away. Retrieved January 3, 2015 from: www.cancer.org/treatment/survivorshipduringandaftertreatment/when-cancer-doesnt-go-away

26   Davis D. Off Target in the War on Cancer. *Washington Post.* November 4, 2007.

27   National Cancer Institute. SEER Stat Fact Sheets: All Cancer Sites. Retrieved January 3, 2015 from: http://seer.cancer.gov/statfacts/html/all.html

28   Ruddy KT. Setting The Agenda For The PURE CURE. Ruddy's blog. November 21, 2011. Retrieved January 3, 2015 from: http://breastcancerbydrruddy.com/?p=3338

Chapter 6

Treatment Options and Complementary Therapies

Now that conventional cancer treatments have been reviewed, I feel that this book would not be complete without discussing some of the other approaches available today. Surgery, chemotherapy, and radiation are blunt, invasive instruments; there are other effective and more elegant ways to defeat cancer. It is essential that all options be considered and I hope that someday they will be included in the standard of care.

The following material was supplied by Best Answer for Cancer Foundation, a 501(c)3 based in Austin, Texas.

Insulin Potentiation Therapy (IPT) – A Powerful Target, Low Dose Approach to Chemotherapy

Insulin potentiation therapy (IPT) is a time-proven and powerful method of treating cancer. It has been in use since 1946. It is often called "a kinder, gentler approach."

IPT, also called insulin potentiation targeted low dose (IPTLD), uses traditional chemotherapy drugs, but is very different than conventional chemotherapy.

IPTLD is able to selectively target chemo drugs directly to cancer cells, largely bypassing healthy cells. Because of this, patients undergoing IPTLD experience far fewer side effects; their quality of life is higher. Whereas most people undergoing conventional chemotherapy can be instantly recognized by their bald heads, for example, most IPTLD patients do not lose their hair.

IPTLD uses about one-tenth the chemotherapy drug dosages used in conventional oncology.

IPTLD is also different because most physicians who make use of IPTLD realize that chemotherapy, even at reduced dosages, is not the only tool available. They make use of complementary therapies to eliminate cancer and rebuild the immune system.

IPTLD physicians also typically make use of chemosensitivity tests to determine which drugs and complementary therapies will be most effective, and which would not be. This process of selection and elimination spares patients unnecessary exposure to the effects and costs of a regime that would have little opportunity for a good outcome.

The Insulin Advantage

Each of our trillions of cells has a membrane, an outer skin, that protects it from toxins. Conventional chemotherapy needs to flood the body with drugs to force penetration through that membrane.

IPTLD, on the other hand, recognizes that the membrane of cancer cells is built differently than healthy cells. Cancer cells use sugar as their primary fuel; healthy cells use fat as their primary fuel. The membrane of cancer cells is built to give them plenty of access to glucose moving through the bloodstream.

Cancer cells love glucose. The faster they get glucose, the faster they can grow and spread. PET scans (positron emission tomography) find cancer by looking at the cellular uptake of sugar. A radioactive tracer is mixed with glucose (sugar water) and injected into a vein. The cancer cells take up the radioactive agent as they take in the sugar. The resulting three-dimensional images of tracer concentration within the body are then constructed by computer analysis to reveal a mass, the tumor.

This need for glucose – sugar – also creates a vulnerability, however, and IPT uses that vulnerability to full advantage.

Insulin is the same natural hormone we hear about in diabetes, and it is what actually "escorts" glucose into cells. In medical parlance, we say cancer cells are equipped with more insulin receptors, upwards of 16 times more than healthy cells. Insulin can't work to pump glucose into a cell unless it can find an insulin receptor to work through so cancer cells have a lot of them. Glucose is so important to cancer cells that they have the ability to secrete their own insulin to ensure their supply of fuel.

What if we pair a small dose of chemo drugs with insulin and glucose, in much the same way a PET scan pairs sugar with a tracer? The cancer cells take in the chemotherapy drugs in their effort to get at the sugar. Think of it as a Trojan horse effect.

When a doctor administers IPT, the first thing he or she does is to carefully lower the patient's blood sugar level with insulin. As the blood sugar drops, the patient's healthy cells rely on fat metabolism, but the patient's cancer cells become seriously compromised. The cancer cells sense the threat to their survival and open wide their cell walls (insulin receptors) to get at whatever sugar they can find in the blood stream's diminishing supply. When the blood sugar level has dropped enough – what is called the "therapeutic moment" – the doctor will administer a low dose of chemotherapy followed by glucose. Then the patient's blood sugar level is brought back up to normal.

"Potentiation" means "to make more effective." Because insulin and glucose target the delivery of the drugs, IPT uses about 90 percent less chemotherapy compared to conventional oncology. This means that patients continue to thrive, maintain their lifestyle, and be vital while the cancer is eradicated.

Insulin helps us in another way. Chemo is most effective when it connects with a cancer cell as it is dividing because cells are most vulnerable when they expend energy to divide. Insulin prompts cancer cells to divide. Thus, insulin helps us deliver chemo to more cells at a more vulnerable moment in their life cycle.

The cells that turn over the fastest in the human body – the ones most likely to be dividing at any one time – include those in the intestine, bone marrow, the mouth, and hair follicles. Without insulin, the conventional large dose of chemotherapy forces itself through the membrane of any cancer cells that happen to be dividing, plus the other rapidly dividing cells in the body. That is why the side effects with conventional chemo cause people to go bald, produce nausea, lower red and white blood cell counts, and often lead to mouth and stomach ulcers and organ failure. By using insulin to target the drugs to the cancer cells, the healthy cells are largely spared.

Conventional use of chemotherapy comes down to whether we can kill the cancer without killing the patient.

To summarize the process that takes place with IPT:

*   Insulin allows us to differentiate the cancer cells from the normal cells.
*   Insulin targets the drugs to the cancer cells, largely by-passing healthy cells.
*   Cancer cells take up larger amounts of chemotherapy medications than they ordinarily would without the use of insulin.
*   Just as insulin facilitates the entry of chemo drugs into the cell, it facilitates the release of metabolic toxins out of the cell so it assists with detoxification.
*   Insulin prompts cancer cells to divide, a process during which they are much more sensitive to the toxic effects of the drugs. The result is a level of cancer cell death and growth control comparable to or even better than standard chemotherapy.
*   The lower dose means there are far fewer side effects. Patients do not experience the severe side effects that lead to the debilitating loss of hope and lowered quality of life.
*   The lower dose does not break down the immune system's ability to protect against other infections common to the traditional chemotherapy protocols.
*   The lower dose means IPT treatments can be used as long as they are needed without the concern of long-term toxicity to healthy cells and tissues.
*   IPT gives us the ability to aggressively pursue immune therapy while simultaneously using chemotherapy, a combined treatment which is usually not possible with the standard high-dose chemotherapy approach.

IPT has been reported to work especially well for breast, prostate, lung, colon, stomach cancers, lymphoma, and melanoma. There are also reports of IPT bringing responses and remissions to patients with pancreatic, ovarian, renal cell cancers, blood, bone, cervical, esophageal, lip, mouth, neck, small intestines, testicular, throat, thyroid, uterine and vaginal cancers.

Chemosensitivity Tests

There are dozens of chemotherapy drugs and hundreds of possible combinations available. Conventional one-size-fits-all treatments provide average outcomes, with the majority of patients failing to show long-term improvement from these protocols. Cancer is an individual disease, and protocols need to be customized for best outcomes. Which drug combinations will work best for you, and which would not work while exposing you to toxic side effects? It is of great value to be able to determine the effectiveness of chemotherapies in the individual patient prior to starting the treatment.

A chemosensitivity test uses blood and/or tissue to determine a personalized treatment protocol. A patient's individual sample is tested against various chemotherapy drugs in a laboratory to determine which best target a patient's unique cancer, and which complementary therapies will be effective.

For example, some breast cancers have a receptor on the surface of the cancer cells called HER 2, and some do not. If your breast cancer has these receptors, Herceptin® may be helpful; if not, it definitely will not be helpful. The side effects of this drug can lead to serious heart problems, including heart failure, so it is in a patient's best interest to know if it is worth the risk of including this drug in their protocol.

There are robust discussions at this time as to whether it is best to test blood or tissue, and much progress will be made in the years to come. Today, chemosensitivity testing provides real-time information about the sensitivities of a patient's tumor, even at different times during therapy, and the tests correlate with treatment success.[1,2] Chemosensitivity testing is an essential component in the use of IPTLD. (More details in the Cancer Testing – An Overview chapter.)

What It Is Like to Receive IPTLD

The patient is seated in the physician's office, usually in a comfortable lounge chair. Medical staff will insert an IV into a vein or port. The patient will be given a dose of insulin based on their body weight, enough to take the blood glucose level down to about 35-45 mg/dL.

At this level patients start to feel "fuzzy" or lightheaded. They may also feel weak, hungry, and flushed. The insulin dose is adjusted to keep them in this state for 5-6 minutes. This is enough time to cause the cancer cells to open their insulin receptors (glucose flood gates).

Think of the lowering of the blood sugar as you might think of holding your breath. You know you can do it for maybe 2-3 minutes, but much longer than that and you will die. If it were possible to completely deprive cancer cells of glucose, they would die within a matter of minutes. Unfortunately to keep you alive, we cannot do that, but IPTLD can decrease the amount of glucose by about 70 percent. This is enough of a decrease to cause cancer cells to go into "emergency mode" and make them more vulnerable to chemotherapy drugs.

At the therapeutic moment, the chemotherapy drugs are delivered, followed immediately by an intravenous infusion of glucose. Anti-inflammatories, anti-fungal, anti-bacterial, anti-viral, and liver support substances are also often administered at this time.

Clinical experience with the IPTLD protocol has demonstrated that the therapeutic moment comes approximately 25 to 30 minutes after insulin is given. A session of IPT lasts about two hours.

On days when IPTLD is not administered, patients may undergo a number of complementary therapies.

Each person is treated on a case-by-case basis, but generally doctors advise between 14 and 25 IPT sessions combined with complementary therapies and lifestyle changes.

Technically Speaking

Insulin plays an important role in the mechanisms of malignancy. Fractionated low-dose chemotherapy utilizes insulin as a biologic response modifier to target cancer cells and not the immune system or vital body organs. IPT manipulates the mechanisms of malignancy to therapeutic advantage by employing exogenous insulin to enhance anticancer drug cytotoxicity and safety.

It is well recognized that the cell-cycle phase-specific anticancer drugs work best on cells in S-phase of the growth cycle. Because of the much richer distribution of insulin and IGF-I receptors on cancer cell membranes versus normal somatic cells, drug potentiating effects will predominate in the cancer cells with a relative sparing of normal tissues.

Insulin has been found to increase the cell-killing effects of the chemotherapy drug methotrexate in a population of human breast cancer cells in tissue culture by a factor of up to 10,000.[3] In a study of three cases where IPT was used in the treatment of metastatic tumors following failure of standard chemotherapy, the findings were:

Remission for 15, 21 and 8 months, respectively. The first patient was lost to follow up after June 2008 and the other two are in remission until now, receiving maintenance treatment. Their quality of life improved rapidly after the first 2-3 courses and gave the patients the opportunity to restore their normal work activity after 2-3 months from the beginning of treatment. The third patient was additionally treated with LHRH agonist.

Treatment was very well tolerated, the only complaints being weakness and sleepiness during the first day. Lab examinations showed no significant toxicity. In our 3 patients we observed insignificant increase of liver function tests in the first 6 weeks, while these normalized without any additional measures during treatment.[4]

In another study of 196 patients diagnosed with a variety of neoplastic diseases:

Laboratory tests demonstrate that the dose related toxicity of chemotherapeutics can be largely mitigated when applying them in conjunction with insulin, at a fractionated dose following a dose dense regimen. . . The average number of IPT treatments received amongst patients who completed the initial six was thirteen treatments total . . . Patients easily tolerated IPT . . . Only two of the one hundred forty-eight patients with initially low Hb level needed blood transfusion while in active treatment . . .

Upon follow-up, eighty-eight of 108 patients (81%) with advanced metastatic disease reported a subjectively significant improvement in their quality of life.[5]

IPT is an empirically derived innovation for which good scientific evidence exists to affirm its formulation. Being consistent with the natural biology of the cancer cell, the operational mechanisms of IPT make it an ideal candidate for cancer treatment.

Since most diseased cells have an excess of insulin receptors, IPTLD can be used to treat conditions as diverse as arthritis, herpes, hepatitis C, and AIDS, as well as cardiovascular, respiratory (including pneumonia), neurological and intestinal disorders.

IPTLD is an off-label use of chemotherapy and other medications and insulin; off-label use of drugs is common practice throughout the world.

Complementary Therapies

Most conventional cancer treatment focuses on only controlling cancer growth. While that is obviously essential, it is just part of the treatment necessary for what is a complex, systemic disease. Long term control of cancer takes a comprehensive approach. The cancer must be eliminated or brought under control, and the patient's compromised immune system function must be optimized. The goal of complementary cancer therapies is to:

- Provide more effective and targeted cancer treatments that leave surrounding healthy tissue unharmed.
- Utilize other cancer-killing agents and thereby decrease dependency upon chemo drugs.
- Help the body detoxify.
- Provide nutrition to a depleted body.
- Nurture and strengthen the immune system.

Here are some common complementary cancer therapies used by the International Organization of Integrative Cancer Physicians (IOICP):

High-dose Vitamin C

Intravenous, high-dose vitamin C treatments have proven to be highly effective at killing cancer cells. Unlike chemotherapy drugs, vitamin C does not have significant toxicity associated with its use, and patients do not develop a resistance to it. Vitamin C therapy also helps tamp down infections which are common to the makeup of people with cancer.

Poly-MVA®

Lipoic acid is uniquely bound to Palladium (LAPd), and combined with minerals, vitamins, and amino acids. Many doctors like to use it because it provides so many benefits and has no side effects. It is highly selective for malignant tissue. It influences oxygen, water, and electrical inputs to the malignancy. It reduces tumor size, supports the liver in removing spent chemo agents from the body, invigorates normal cells, and helps to repair any damage invasive cancers may have left behind. Its enzymatic complex of polynucleotide reductase assists in correcting malfunctional nucleic acids in the DNA of genes. In June of 2008, Poly-MVA submitted and was approved for an IND (Investigational New Drug) application. It is believed that this study will lead to the use of Poly-MVA in more integrative and supportive approaches for various types of degenerative disease conditions (see the Nutrients – Critical Components chapter for more information on Poly-MVA).

UV Therapy

Ultraviolet Therapy is a time-honored medical procedure where a portion of a patient's blood is withdrawn, exposed to sanitizing ultraviolet light, and then reintroduced to the patient's body. Some of its effects are:

- Improved circulation and oxygenation of tissues.
- Anti-inflammatory effects.
- Stimulation of the immune system.
- Increased tolerance of the body to chemotherapy and radiation.
- Cardiovascular protection.
- Powerful anti-infection properties.

Hyperbaric Oxygen Therapy (HBOT)

In a hyperbaric chamber, pure oxygen is delivered under pressure, which has the effect of dissolving oxygen into the plasma – delivering as much as 10 times more oxygen as the bloodstream normally delivers and reaching further into the tissues. That provides fuel for healing and re-growth. Oxygen is also the enemy of cancer which prefers an oxygen-free environment.

Epigenetics and Gene Therapy

These include methods to reprogram the cancer cell to accept a "death" switch. Cancer cells have a birth switch and a life switch, but no death switch.

Enzymatic Therapy

Embryologist Dr. John Beard proposed in 1906 that pancreatic proteolytic digestive enzymes represent the body's main defense against cancer, and that enzyme therapy would be useful as a treatment for all types of cancer. Today, Dr. Nicholas Gonzales in New York has done the most to document the success of enzymes in creating cases of exceptional survival and in many cases evidence of tumor reduction. Enzymes are natural proteins that stimulate and accelerate many biological reactions in the body. Certain enzymes break down the protective coating of cancer cells making them more susceptible for white blood cells to identify and attack them.

IV Chelation

Toxic chemicals and heavy metals promote cancer and po-tentiate other carcinogens. EDTA is a highly effective way to eliminate excessive heavy metals that serve as cancer's shield and lower the metals content from tissues and organs. Heavy metals include: aluminum, barium, cadmium, mercury, nickel, plati-num, thallium, tungsten, uranium, creatinine, cobalt and lead, among many others. In addition to heavy metals, EDTA also re-moves excessive free iron, which promotes cancer by catalyzing free radical pathology. Most cancer cells have a strong affinity for iron. Removal of excessive iron is a vital factor of many anticancer therapies. When heavy metals are contained in the body, they cause a number of symptoms, not the least of which is they assist in cancer's growth and provide a nice home for cancer cells.

Oncothermia and Hyperthermia

Oncothermia utilizes heat as a means of therapy, a fundamental practice that has been in use for centuries. Heat can cause considerable damage to living cells, hence the body can only survive for a short time in temperatures in excess of 42°C. However, the destructive force of heat, when applied skillfully, can help to treat cancer. Malignant tumors can be controlled or even recede as a result of targeted oncothermia.

IPT/HT

Chemo drugs are not the only substances that can be combined with insulin to make for a more effective delivery. When IPT was first used, it was a combination of antibiotics with insulin. Homeopathic formulas can be delivered more effectively with insulin. Custom made homeopathic medicines are designed to reach deeply into the body to release and remove toxins, and stimulate the natural repair and regrowth process. In IPT/HT, natural homeopathic medications are used in place of chemotherapy drugs. Whereas drugs force the body to do something that it is not naturally doing, homeopathic remedies always work with nature to stimulate natural healing processes and have no side effects.

Ozone Therapy

Ozone therapy is a unique form of therapy that both heals and detoxifies at the same time. Cancer cells can thrive and grow only in an oxygen-poor environment. With more oxygen in tumors, they behave less aggressively and with less metastases. Ozone modulates the immune system, increases oxygen delivery to the tissues and cells, kills bacteria and viruses, and increases cellular energy production.

Vaccines

Tumor cells churn out defensive molecules that repel or destroy T cells, the white blood cells that make up part of the immune system and help the body fight diseases. For example, much research is being done on developing vaccines to prompt dendritic cells to stimulate immune cells and direct them to act against specific cancers. Dendritic cells are also part of the immune system; they interact with T cells to initiate and shape the adaptive immune response. Dendritic cell vaccines must be individually formulated from each patient's blood. Immune stimulating vaccines are in use in many other countries, but have not been widely accepted in the U.S.

Mushroom Extracts

These have traditionally used to boost immune system vitality. They are used to support the body's production of endogenous antioxidant enzymes, including superoxide dismutase (SOD), catalase, and glutathione, which, in turn, support the body's natural immune defenses against free radical damage. A mushroom extract supplement can be used to stimulate natural killer cells, thus limiting tumor growth. Some extracts have antiviral, antibacterial, and antifungal properties.

Fermented Soy

In his book, *What Your Doctor May Not Tell You About Breast Cancer*, Dr. John R. Lee, M.D., specifically recommends only fermented soy products to reap the benefits of soy phytochemicals. According to the National Cancer Institute of the National Institutes of Health, soy isoflavones have been shown to reduce tumor cell proliferation and induce tumor cell apoptosis, as well as regulate hormone balance and reduce the risks of breast cancer, heart disease, and osteoporosis. The Haelan 951 product is the choice of integrative cancer physicians because the product is sugar free, made with non-genetically modified (non-GMO) beans, and provides a high quality form of predigested soy proteins for cancer patients experiencing cachexia, anorexia, protein calorie malnutrition, the toxic side effects of chemotherapy, and undesirable hormonal imbalances that promote faster tumor growth.

"Myers' Cocktail"

An intravenous vitamin and mineral protocol developed in

the 1970s by Dr. John Myers at Johns Hopkins University. Dr. Myers pioneered the use of intravenous vitamins and minerals in the treatment of a wide variety of medical conditions, including cancer. Doctors often customize the "cocktail" for each patient; the formula typically includes vitamin C, the B vitamins, magnesium, and calcium. A "Myers' cocktail" is used to coax nutrients directly into the cells, by-passing the digestive system, because many cancer patients have compromised digestive systems and are nutrient deficient.

Emotional and Spiritual Support
There is a well-founded school of thought that cancer often follows a traumatic incident in life, or is an outgrowth of repressed emotional baggage. Bernie Siegel, M.D., for one, has written much about cancer's connections to our emotions. Encouraging patients to clear emotional traumas can result in better survival rates.

Biological Dentistry
Although conventional medicine largely disconnects itself from the mouth, integrative cancer physicians recognize that chronic infections from root canals and cavitations, and mercury exposure from fillings, are detrimental to the immune system. Initiators of cancer can include heavy metals in the oral cavity as they influence organs connected to meridians. Removing metal and infections from the mouth is an important step to boost the immune system's ability to identify and kill cancer cells.

Mind-body Medicine
There are numerous approaches to mind-body medicine. Yoga, tai chi, relaxation-visualization, affirmations, breathing exercises, forgiveness of others, as well as gratitude and prayer are common applications that help make for healing on a deeper level.

Why Doesn't My Regular Oncologist Use IPTLD?
IPTLD uses only about 10 to 15 percent of the amount of pharmaceutical drugs used in conventional chemotherapy. Understandably, the pharmaceutical industry has been slow to

encourage doctors to use less of their product. Medical associations and schools dependent upon pharmaceutical funding have not been motivated to embrace it.

According to the American Cancer Society:

Despite individual reports, there are no published scientific studies available showing that IPT is safe or effective in treating cancer in humans. IPT may have serious side effects.[6]

Medical literature and clinical experience show quite the opposite. The Best Answer for Cancer Foundation maintains a list of studies and papers on IPT.

Insulin potentiation therapy was developed by a family of physicians – the doctors Donato Perez Garcia. Over the last 25 years they and other doctors have collaborated to provide a sound scientific basis for the therapy, and getting documentation of this published in the scientific medical literature. Their common goal has always been, and remains, to get IPTLD properly studied in the United States so greater numbers of physicians and patients in the United States will use it.

The side effect of using insulin is the occurrence of hypoglycemia, or low blood sugar. Patients are closely monitored by professionals and provided appropriate amount of glucose intravenously to offset the insulin. Patients will feel hungry, and it would not be unusual to experience mild and temporary symptoms of hypoglycemia, which can include fatigue, headache, or sweating.

Note that diabetic patients administer and manage their own insulin without the daily oversight of professionals.

Since chemotherapy drugs have considerable toxicity associated with their use, there is always a risk, but because IPTLD uses much lower doses than conventional chemotherapy, the risk is significantly reduced.

Patients may experience some constipation and nausea after the first two IPTLD treatments. Anemia and decreased WBC and platelet counts are unusual; rarely are decreases so severe as to require transfusions.

Shifting the Cancer Paradigm

Best Answer for Cancer Foundation is at the forefront of the emerging shift from the traditional one-size-fits-all approach to an enlightened integrative cancer treatment approach that is more personalized and more patient-centered with an emphasis on better outcomes. It is our mission to provide prevention education, awareness, options, and support to patients and physicians dealing with cancer.

IPTLD is exciting because it allows so many patients to devote full attention to their wellness, thus increasing their chances of recovery, and improving the quality and duration of their lives.

Two books the Foundation recommends about IPTLD:

* *The Kinder, Gentler Cancer Treatment: Insulin Potentiation Targeted LowDose(TM) Therapy* by Best Answer for Cancer Foundation, 2009.
* *Treating Cancer with Insulin Potentiation Therapy* by Ross A. Hauser, M.D. and Marion A. Houser, M.S., R.D., 2002.

For more about the Best Answer for Cancer Foundation and the International Organization of Integrative Cancer Physicians, see:

www.bestanswerforcancer.org
www.IOICP.com
www.IPTLD.com

Footnotes

1   Rudiger N, Stein E-L, et al. Chemosensitivity Testing of Circulating Epithelial Tumor Cells (CETC) in Vitro: Correlation to in Vivo Sensitivity and Clinical Outcome. *Journal of Cancer Therapy*. 2013 Apr; 4:597-605.
2   Lau G, Loo W, Chow L. Neoadjuvant chemotherapy for breast cancer determined by chemosensitivity assay achieves better tumor response. *Biomedicine & Pharmacotherapy*. 2007 Oct. 61(9):562-565.
3   Alabaster O, Vonderhaar B, Shafie S. Metabolic modification by insulin enhances methotrexate cytotoxicity in MCF-7 human breast cells. *Eur J Cancer Clin Oncol*. 1961. 17(11):1223-1228.

4   Damyanov C, Radoslavova M, et al. Low dose chemotherapy in combination with insulin for the treatment of metastatic tumors. Medical Center of Integrative Medicine, Sofia, Bulgaria. *Journal of BUON*. 2009. 14:711-715.

5   Damyanov C, Gerasimova D, et al. Insulin Potentiation Therapy in the treatment of malignant neoplastic diseases: a three year study. *J Cancer Sci Ther*. 2012 Apr; 4:088-091. doi:10.4172/1948-5956.1000117

6   American Cancer Society. Insulin Potentiation Therapy. Overview. Retrieved January 8, 2015 from: www.cancer.org/treatment/ treatmentsandsideeffects/complementaryandalternativemedicine/ pharmacologicalandbiologicaltreatment/insulin-potentiation-therapy.

Chapter 7

Cancer Testing – An Overview

There are many new and little known tests that can give you an early warning about cancer and dramatically reduce the chances you would find out about a cancer when it is already in stage 2, 3, or 4.

Why wait until the cancer is far enough along for you to develop signs and symptoms? What a blessing it would be to find out that you are in an early or pre-cancerous stage. I can honestly say that if I had known about the testing that I tell you about, I could have saved myself a tremendous amount of anxiety, pain, suffering, time, and money. Don't wait for a tissue biopsy or PET scan to find out that you have cancer. It takes many years for cancer cells to form a tumor large enough to be detected or cause symptoms. A 2009 study, for example, showed that most early stage ovarian tumors exist for years at a size that is a thousand times smaller than standard routine tests can detect reliably.[1]

Symptoms that Indicate the Need for Testing
The American Cancer Society reports that a *symptom* is a signal that is felt or noticed by the person who has it, but may not be easily seen by anyone else. Symptoms like fever, extreme tiredness, or weight loss are fairly common because cancer cells use up much of the body's energy supply. Some lung cancers make hormone-like substances that raise blood calcium levels which affect nerves and muscles, making the person feel weak and dizzy. Cancers of the pancreas usually do not cause symptoms until they grow large enough to press on nearby nerves or organs, causing back or belly pain.

Cancer is a group of diseases that can cause almost any sign or symptom. The signs and symptoms will depend on where the cancer is, how big it is, and how much it affects the organs or tissues. If a cancer has spread (metastasized), signs or symptoms may appear in different parts of the body.[2] Don't ignore even the smallest of symptoms. Better yet, get tested before symptoms develop.

I no longer subscribe to the philosophy that ignorance is bliss. Cancer is all too common today. Finding out sooner rather than later can make the difference between being able to live your life and pursue your dreams to the fullest, verses an event that derails your career or, in the worst case scenario, leads to an early and expensive death.

Here are a few reasons and/or symptoms that should prompt you to get an early detection test:

- Unexplained sudden weight loss.
- Fever.
- Fatigue.
- Pain.
- Yellow skin or eyes.
- Itching.
- Wounds that won't heal.
- Blood in the stool or urine.
- Diarrhea or constipation.
- Vomiting.
- Indigestion.
- Trouble swallowing.
- Pain with urination or decreased flow.
- Unusual bleeding or discharge.
- Chronic cough or hoarseness in the voice.
- Shortness of breath.
- Thickening or lump in the breast or other part of the body.
- Change in personality.
- Chronic exposure to hazardous chemicals or low-level radiation.
- History of consuming known dietary carcinogens, e.g., large amounts of artificial sweeteners, colorings, flavorings, and preservative agents.
- Chronic exposure to drinking water containing high concentrations of chlorine, fluorides, pesticides, and other potentially carcinogenic chemicals.
- History of smoking, or a non-smoker chronically exposed to "second hand smoke."
- Chronic stress.

- Depression.
- Habitual caffeine or alcohol abuser.
- History of chronic viral infections, i.e., herpes and HIV families.
- History of sun overexposure and sunburns.
- Family history of cancer.
- Past history of cancer.
- Undergoing treatment for an ongoing cancer.
- Taking medications having carcinogenic potential side effects.
- Diet that consists of a majority of processed food and cooked food.
- Early detection of cancer.
- Emotional turmoil.

Chemosensitivity Testing

Chemosensitivity testing (CST) is an emerging field with great promise for improving patient outcomes. With today's medical advancements, CST can be utilized once cancer is confirmed to determine which drugs will be most effective for you – in other words, personalized treatment.

The new buzz in the oncology industry is genomics, which is advertised as the very best in personalized treatment. We hear terms such as gene testing, genetic profiling, molecular testing, target profiling, whole cell cytometric profiling, chemosensitivity testing, and genomic testing. I will shed some light on their differences so you can decide what tests are best for you.

First, the most common way a CST is used is to shape a personalized treatment protocol. The National Cancer Institute describes a chemosensitivity assay as:

A laboratory test that measures the number of tumor cells that are killed by a cancer drug. The test is done after the tumor cells are removed from the body. A chemosensitivity assay may help in choosing the best drug or drugs for the cancer being treated.[3]

CST is a huge step in providing a personalized approach to chemotherapy. The goal is to give each patient the very best opportunity for a positive response to their drug treatment. The word "goal" is used because even through drug therapy can be effective against cancer cells, it is not a cure. There are inherent problems administering any cytotoxic drug, even if it is the best one for the patient's tested cancer cells. Side effects can be debilitating and lasting. Plus, tumors have the ability to develop drug resistance. That means patients need repeat sensitivity testing and adjustments to the treatment plan.

Drug efficacy (or response) testing has been around since the 19th century through the work of Drs. Louis Pasteur and Paul Ehrlich for determining which antimicrobial (antibiotic) would kill a certain strain of bacteria.[4]

Drug efficacy testing is routinely done today, for example, with bladder infections. Patients give a urine sample to the lab where it is tested against the various antibiotics used for urinary tract infections. The doctor then writes a prescription for the antibiotic that was shown to do the best job of knocking out that particular infection.

Likewise, doctors can use the results of a chemosensitivity test to formulate the most effective and targeted cancer treatment plan.

If CST is not done, you fall victim to the one-size-fits-all approach of conventional oncology. Standard drugs from the National Comprehensive Cancer Network (NCCN) guidelines will be prescribed; a more effective drug may remain on the shelf. CST can prevent your exposure to a drug that not only would be ineffective at fighting the cancer, but could be extremely damaging to the immune system.

Integrative oncologists have been using CST for years. It is my experience that conventional oncologists are not up to speed on them – but they should be. The one-size-fits-all testing and treatment plans are old school, a thing of the past.

Suzanne Somers interviewed many cancer doctors and wrote several books on cancer therapy after her first-hand experience with breast cancer. She said:

Now that I realize chemo sensitivity tests exist, it feels un- conscionable that chemotherapy would ever, ever be admin- istered without testing first to find out if the chemo is even compatible with the specific cancer.

If these tests could help us to take less chemo, or a better chemo for our specific cancer, why wouldn't we ALL be given these tests?[5]

Suzanne Somers is absolutely right. A personalized, targeted approach is a much better approach. There are three different primary methods of doing CST.

The first method utilizes whole cell cytometric profiling done on living tumor tissue. The tumor sample is surgically removed, and must arrive at the lab within 24 hours of collection, where the cells are exposed to different chemotherapy drugs and the best drug reactions are identified. Cell lines or genes are not evaluated. This type of test is not considered "early detection" because you must have a known tumor to get the test. Rational Therapeutics in Long Beach, California, is a leading lab offering this type of testing. Their contact information is www.rationaltherapeutics. com or 800-542-4357. Testing must be prearranged with the lab and your surgeon so that a tumor tissue sample can be acquired during surgery. Representatives at Rational Therapeutics said they frequently receive phone calls from cancer patients after their surgery has been done and it is too late to get the sample for testing. The current cost of the Rational Therapeutics CTC is $4,000 and to date, the test is not covered by insurance.

The second method uses genetic molecular expression, also called genomic, gene, or molecular testing. This test also uses tumor tissue to identify the chemo drugs that should produce the best potential treatment outcome. The goal of this type of test is to match known characteristics of a chemotherapy drug with the identified characteristics or "gene patterns" of the patient's cancer cells. In gene testing, the chemotherapy drugs are not physically tested against the patient's cancer cells as they are with whole cell cytometric profiling. Genomic testing provides a "theoretical potential" for the drug's success and other biological mechanisms of the cancer cell like drug resistances are often not considered.

There is a great deal of data addressing the relevancy of this type of gene based test. A clinical trial presented in the 2011 *Journal of Translational Medicine* involving ovarian cancer patients, for example, found that patterns of gene expression identified through molecular gene testing were compared with results of cytometric testing. This process exposes living cancer cells to chemotherapy drugs that are possible candidates for use against your cancer cells. Four different genes were included in the molecular part of the study. The four genes were selected as those which researchers believe to have the greatest likelihood of accurately predicting individual patient response to specific chemo drugs. Study results reported that for two of the genes studied, there was no significant correlation between gene expression pattern and patient response. In other words, results for these genes were found to be meaningless. For the third gene studied, there was a 75 percent correlation between expression and patient response. This means that the gene was 75 percent accurate when it came to identifying an active drug for that patient. For the fourth gene studied, the accuracy in identifying an active drug was only 25 percent. In marked contrast, the cytometric testing was found by the researchers to be 90 percent accurate in identifying active drugs for the ovarian cancer patients in this study.[6] You can see that the research is indicating that the cytometric method is superior to the genomic method; however, it is important to remember that any test that requires a tumor tissue sample is NOT early detection.

The third method falls a bit outside the National Cancer Institute's definition of CST. This is because the laboratory, Research Genetic Cancer Center (R.G.C.C.), is based outside of the United States and uses the cytometric method of CST on cancer cells they are able to extract from a *blood sample*. This changes things quite a bit because the test can be performed on cells that are extracted from a patient years *before* a tumor is found. In addition to analyzing the genetic markers on the cancer cells to determine the best drugs, Dr. Ioannis Papasotiriou of R.G.C.C. in Greece said:

> R.G.C.C. labs adds one final step not used by any other labs that we know of at this time. This final step is verification of the genetic findings. This means we actually test each patient's CTCs and CSCs independently against each chemotherapeutic agent and on the list. This ex-vivo type testing is accomplished by expanding the few CTCs and CSCs harvested from each patient by using our proprietary cell culture.

In other words, the extracted cancer cells of each individual are cultured (grown) in the laboratory where they are then brought into direct contact with the chemo drugs. During this process the cells are observed and the effectiveness of each drug is measured (AKA an ex-vivo study). R.G.C.C. is working with hundreds of integrated physicians treating cancer at its earliest stages. You can find more details on all of the tests R.G.C.C. offers in the Research Genetic Cancer Center chapter or at www.rgccusa.com.

There is one other lab that does CTC testing from a blood sample. It is Biofocus® in Germany (www.biofocus.de). The major difference between these two labs that do CST testing with cells extracted from a blood sample is:

- R.G.C.C. uses the cytometric method of testing with living cancer cells being brought into direct contact with each chemo in addition to analyzing the genomic markers.
- Biofocus uses the genomic, "theoretical potential," method. (More details in the Biofocus Tests chapter.)

It is important to know that if R.G.C.C. or Biofocus is not able to isolate any cancer cells from the blood sample they receive for the CST, the test cannot be performed. That is a very good thing because blood without extractable circulating tumor cells is what you want to have. The exception is with cancers in the brain. Due to the blood brain barrier, cancer cells are not detectable in the peripheral blood.

Just as everyone's finger prints are different, cancer cells are different too and the information obtained from this type of test can be invaluable. Unfortunately, insurance companies are resistant to pay for such testing at this time. If you have decided to take chemo and can afford CST, exercise the choice to get it.

Natural Substance Sensitivity Testing

This is a companion test to the effort to look for the most effective chemo drugs. This test looks for natural substances that will be the most effective in treatment to kill cancer cells, cancer stem cells, and boost immune system function. Therapeutic doses of vitamin C, for example, have been shown to kill cancer cells and vitamin C does not have the toxicity or the tendency for the development of drug resistance that chemo does.

There are only two labs I have identified which offer any type of testing for natural substances even though there are increasing numbers of patients who are seeking natural therapies. Many of the tested substances support the immune system while aiding in the reduction of the number of cancer cells through a process called angiogenesis or apoptosis.

Angiogenesis is the process that the body uses to signal the growth of blood vessels to a tumor to provide it with nutrition for growth. The Angiogenesis Foundation in Cambridge, Massachusetts, reports that all cancerous tumors release angiogenic growth factor proteins that stimulate blood vessel growth to tumors and that anti-angiogenic therapies literally starve the tumor of its blood supply by interfering with this process. This test identifies natural substances that are anti-angiogenic to the individual patients' tumor cells.

Apoptosis is the process of inducing cell death. However, cancer cells have lost their natural programming to die – they keep duplicating endlessly. This test identifies natural substances that cause cell death to the individual patient's tumor cells.

The following labs provide natural substance sensitivity testing:

Research Genetic Cancer Center (R.G.C.C.), Greece
The R.G.C.C. lab requires a blood sample. If circulating tumor cells are present, they are isolated for testing.

First, cell lines/genetic markers on the individual's tumor cells are used to identify effective natural substances. Second, a verification process is utilized where the living tumor cells are brought into direct contact with the natural/tested substances. R.G.C.C. is the only lab I know of that offers this extensive ex-vivo (out of body) form of testing. Every testing procedure R.G.C.C. uses is always done in triplicate and very few labs offer this level of accuracy.

The lab tests for 46-48 natural substances ranging from mistletoe and Metformin to Artecin® and Thymex®. They are adding new substances periodically. The full current list is in the Research Genetic Cancer Center chapter.

Biofocus®, Germany

The Biofocus test is done with a blood sample and the extracted tumor cells are analyzed for their genetic molecular expression. The results are predicted based on the markers on the tumor cells and known mechanism of action of the proposed natural substances.

As of this writing, the tested natural substances are:

* Quercetin.
* IP6 (Inositol-6-P).
* C-statin.
* Dammarane sapogenins.
* Acetogenin graviola.
* Haelan951 fermented soy extract.
* Curcumin.
* Ellagic acid.
* Arglabin.
* Artemisinin.
* Amygdalin B17 (laetrile).

Non-Early Detection Tests for Cancer

"Non-early" detection tests for cancer are tests that look for a cancer that usually has been around for many years and has finally gotten large enough to be detected by these tests.

PET Scan

A Positron Emission Tomography (PET) scan is non-early detection because the cancer must form a tumor large enough to absorb the radioactive glucose that is reflected on the images. We can learn a lot about the operation of a cancer cell by understanding how a PET scan works. Before a PET scan, the patient receives an intravenous infusion of radioactive glucose. Cancer cells rapidly metabolize (take in and use) sugar and synthesize (absorb) the radioactive glucose. The body is then scanned and areas of the body with cancer cells will light up on the scanned images. Cancer cells take up sugar much faster than non-cancerous cells. If the tumors are large enough, the scan can pin-point the source of the cancer and detect whether cancer is isolated to one specific area or has spread to other organs, bones, or tissues. Small tumors under 1 cm may not show up on the scans, thus the patient will be told they are fine.[7]

However, a clean or negative PET scan does not mean that you don't have cancer. Patients are not told they could have microscopic tumors and that there are steps they can take now to prevent cancer growth, such as consuming a low sugar diet. Also, the patient just received a dose of fuel for any cancer cells in their body. Most oncologists do not warn their patients about the dangers of the radioactive sugar that they are being injected with, or the carcinogenic effects of radiation.

Alternate "non-early" detection imaging techniques include computed tomography (CT) scans which use X-rays to produce detailed pictures of structures inside of the body, and magnetic resonance imaging (MRI) which uses a magnetic field and pulses of radio wave energy to produce the pictures. MRIs often provide different information about structures in the body than can be seen with an X-ray or CT scan.

Tumor Markers

Looking for tumor markers is a non-early detection kind of test because tumor markers are produced by cancer cells, and in most cases you must have a significant number of cancer cells for the tests to report as HIGH. Monitoring tumor markers has become a standard of care that oncologists use at follow-up appointments. If a patient's labs show an increase in tumor markers, the oncologist will most likely order a PET scan and/or a CT imaging test. These tests have become essential diagnostic tools that physicians use to reveal the presence and severity of cancers.

According to the National Cancer Institute:

> Tumor markers are substances that are produced by cancer or by other cells of the body in response to cancer or certain benign (noncancerous) conditions. Most tumor markers are made by normal cells as well as by cancer cells; however, they are produced at much higher levels in cancerous conditions. These substances can be found in the blood, urine, stool, tumor tissue, or other tissues or bodily fluids of some patients with cancer. Most tumor markers are proteins. However,

more recently, patterns of gene expression and changes to DNA have also begun to be used as tumor markers. Markers of the latter type are assessed in tumor tissue specifically.

Thus far, more than 20 different tumor markers have been characterized and are in clinical use. Some are associated with only one type of cancer, whereas others are associated with two or more cancer types. There is no "universal" tumor marker that can detect any type of cancer.[8]

Many cancer types have associated tumor markers that are present in the blood. These tumor makers are used to look for possible disease progression. You should be familiar with your tumor marker levels so you will be able immediately to notice a change. Many times, the patient's tumor markers are not elevated enough to register as "high" on lab report and thereby sound an alarm that there is a problem. So, it is important to know what is normal for each patient and reference that number as your personal baseline. Do not feel safe just because your number is lower than the number that is considered high on the lab report. I did not have elevated tumor markers when I was diagnosed with cancer.

By the time a patient has elevated tumor markers, the cancer may be well established. This information was a huge motivator for me to write this book to present other testing and early detection methods. I caution you against solely relying upon the customary tumor marker blood tests. These tumor marker tests are a poor, or late, indicator of disease presence and progression because the measurable markers are only released into the blood by established cancer cells.

Know too that tumor marker tests have major limitations as a diagnostic tool:

- Sometimes, noncancerous conditions can cause the levels of certain tumor markers to increase.
- Not everyone with a particular type of cancer will have a higher level of a tumor marker associated with that cancer.
- Tumor markers have not been identified for every type of cancer.

Below is a list of some of the more common specific cancer tumor markers that are currently used in the clinical setting. Some are associated with only one type of cancer, whereas others are associated with two or more cancer types. There is no "universal" tumor marker that can detect any type of cancer.

Cancer Tumor Markers	Applicable Cancer(s)
Alpha-fetoprotein (AFP)	Liver cancer and germ cell tumors
Beta-2-microglobulin (B2M)	Multiple myeloma, chronic lymphocytic leukemia, and some lymphomas
Beta-human chorionic gonadotropin (Beta-hCG)	Choriocarcinoma and testicular cancer
BCR-ABL fusion gene	Chronic myeloid leukemia
CA15-3/CA27.29	Breast cancer
CA19-9	Pancreatic cancer, gallbladder cancer, bile duct cancer, and gastric cancer
CA-125	Ovarian cancer
Calcitonin	Medullary thyroid cancer
Carcinoembryonic antigen (CEA)	Colorectal cancer and breast cancer
CD20	Non-Hodgkin lymphoma
Chromogranin A (CgA)	Neuroendocrine tumors
Cytokeratin fragments 21-1	Lung cancer
Fibrin/fibrinogen, Nuclear matrix protein 22	Bladder cancer
HE4	Ovarian cancer
Immunoglobulins	Multiple myeloma and Waldenström macroglobulinemia
Lactate dehydrogenase	Germ cell tumors
Prostate-specific antigen (PSA)	Prostate cancer
5-Protein signature (Ova1)	Ovarian cancer

Biopsy

This is a non-early detection test because a tumor large enough to be visualized must be present.

For the majority of cancers, a biopsy is the procedure used to make a definitive cancer diagnosis. It can often be done in the doctor's office with a local anesthetic.

During a biopsy, a tumor may be punctured several times with a needle to retrieve an adequate amount of tissue to be examined under a microscope by a pathologist (a doctor who specializes in interpreting laboratory tests and evaluating cells, tissues, and organs to diagnose disease). Often, doctors will recommend a biopsy after a physical examination or an imaging study, such as an X-ray, has identified a possible tumor. Based on this analysis, the pathologist determines whether the tissue removed contains tumor cells and whether this tumor is benign (noncancerous) or malignant (cancerous, meaning that it has the ability to spread to other parts of the body).

But there is a long simmering debate about the safety of biopsies.

The human body, in its wisdom, tries to contain a cancer growth inside a walled-off box we call a tumor. But in some cases, penetrating the tumor wall with a needle several times may allow cancer cells to inadvertently break away from a tumor and escape, thus spreading the cancer beyond the immediate tumor area.

Several studies have found a higher incidence of cancer after biopsies.[9,10,11]

Biopsies became routine practice in the U.S. by the 1940s and they were endorsed by both the American Cancer Society and the American Medical Association. But as cancer researcher Ralph Moss tells us, many people have strong reservations since the practice was developed:

In 1940, the first American textbook on cancer treatment contained warnings on the dangers of biopsies. "The medical literature is full of pleas for and against biopsy of all types of tumors," wrote Cushman D. Haagensen, MD, of Columbia University, NY, in 1940. Some doctors are "inquisitive but afraid of doing harm with biopsy" (Haagensen 1940). Bradley

Coley, MD, a bone surgeon at Memorial Sloan-Kettering Cancer Center (and son of the famous immunotherapy pioneer, William B. Coley, MD), wrote that "there is some doubt as to the harmlessness of needling such tumors. It may not be a wholly innocuous procedure" (Pack 1940). A survey taken at the time showed that most surgeons agreed that the excision of suspect tissue was to be condemned and avoided.[12]

Disrupting a tumor by sticking a needle into it appears to leave an opening and the opportunity for cancer cells to exit into other areas of the body. Since it is known that cancers cells attempt to move about the body, be aware that a biopsy may just help them achieve that task.

Early Detection Tests and Functional Tests

"Early detection" tests find cancer when it is in the pre-cancerous or early years of development and before it is able to produce signs and symptoms.

"Functional" tests can indicate a potential problem or condition in the body that lead to and make the body more susceptible to cancer development.

The tests range in price and vary in the data that they provide. These tests range in complexity from a simple pH test that cost only pennies per test strip to a blood test that checks for circulating tumor cells that costs about 550 euros (roughly $740 USD). And, if cells are found, more elaborate chemosensitivity and nutrient sensitivity tests can be run on the cells for around 1,350 additional euros (roughly $1,820 USD). Several of the tests are available without the assistance of a physician and some require that you have your physician order the test for you.

Each test is different and has a specific mechanism through which it can indicate a pre-cancerous or cancerous condition. Some detect substances that are present in the blood when cancer is present, and others monitor blood hormone levels that respond to cancer cells. Yet others warn you of a condition in the body that can lead to potential cancer growth. Still others can extract cancer cells from a blood sample for further examination. Other tests help your physician to develop a personalized cancer treatment program.

When you are discussing cancer detection or the monitoring of cancer with classically trained physicians, they will most likely not offer the tests discussed in this book. The conventional medical paradigm is one of treating symptoms and illness, not correcting the root cause of the health issue or strengthening the immune system.

In addition to early detection tests, there are the circulating tumor cell (CTC) tests. These tests examine the blood for tumor cells that have broken free from the tumor. During the process CTCs are extracted from the patient's blood sample. Tests of this nature can be used to screen for new cancers, monitor remaining disease that may not be visible by standard imaging methods, and for diagnosis when the primary tumor is unknown or a biopsy is not possible.

Controlling circulating tumor cells is essential to preventing cancer from metastasizing (spreading) and becoming life-threatening. If you are at risk or have been diagnosed with cancer I strongly encourage you to have your blood tested for CTCs.

The following labs offer blood testing for CTCs:

Research Genetic Cancer Center (R.G.C.C.), Greece.

This lab has a branch office in the USA, the United Kingdom, Germany, Cyprus, Hungary, and Australia.

R.G.C.C.'s "ONCOCOUNT" test is used for early detection. The lab provides a count of the number of CTCs present in the tested sample. It is important to be aware this test is not effective for brain or central nervous system tumors. R.G.C.C. reports that that by using whole blood, they are able to maintain the expression of the cancer cell, i.e., phenotype, genotype, and epigenetics.

CELLSEARCH®, United States

This lab is located in Raritan, NJ. It is a part of the Johnson & Johnson Family of Companies and is run by Janssen Diagnostics,

LLC (formerly Veridex Corporation).

It is the first and only FDA-cleared blood test for enumerating or counting circulating tumor cells (CTCs) in patients with metastatic cancers of the breast, colon, and prostate. The CELLSEARCH test has not been identified as an early detection test.

Biofocus, Germany

The Biofocus test is a CTC detection test and does NOT provide a numerical value of the cancer cells present in the tested blood sample. This test is preferably used for monitoring of patients with known cancer.

Conclusion

It is unfortunate but true that many people do more research when purchasing a camera than when purchasing a cancer treatment. They research brands of cameras, consider the number of pixels, and refer to online reviews before making the purchase. We all want to be knowledgeable consumers; however, when it comes to being a medical consumer, most of us relinquish our rights. Insist on the very best. Be informed and validate the efficacy of the treatments that you are considering or have received.

Use one of the tests discussed as a yard stick to measure the effectiveness of any cancer treatment, or to make sure that you don't have a brewing cancer problem. It is much less costly to treat cancer in its early stages than to wait for a big bad tumor to rear its ugly head.

If you have been diagnosed, please do not retreat if your insurance company or Medicare will not pay for your testing. Your life is very important and the proverbial buck stops with you, not someone in the medical establishment. Keep an open mind. If you can afford to get tested, do it. If you have chosen the chemotherapy route, beginning treatment with a personalized targeted plan of attack is much better than starting with the standard generic rounds of chemo. The upfront costs may seem high, but it is a much better approach in the long run.

You will find that the battle is not just to be cancer free, but to obtain the very best in diagnostic testing and monitoring. The goal is not just getting rid of the tumor and lowering your tumor markers, but maintaining and repairing a healthy immune system. It is about *outcomes*.

The following pages provide information on how and where you can obtain each test. Each of these labs is making great strides in the fight against cancer. I invite you to carefully examine the attributes as well as the limitations of each test.

I have personally used the tests offered by Research Genetic Cancer Center-USA, LLC for both early detection and for the formulation of treatment protocols. I used the R.G.C.C. test after PET scans told me I was "all clear." This test showed me that the number of circulating tumor cells in my body was actually increasing. I also used the R.G.C.C. test to find out which natural substances are most effective for me and to keep cancer stem cells in check.

I thank Dr. Ray Hammon of the Integrative & Functional Health Center for introducing me to this test. I attribute my health today to the work done at this state-of-the-art laboratory. With the R.G.C.C. tests you are able to intervene early and deal with the residual cancer cells.

Before the test, I was living the illusion of being cancer free. Today, I am empowered and have my eye on the target.

Express your rights as a consumer and insist on the very best testing available.

Footnotes

1   Brown P, Palmer C. The preclinical natural history of serous ovarian cancer: defining the target for early detection. *PLoS Med.* 2009 Jul; 6(7):e1000114. doi: 10.1371/journal.pmed.1000114.

2   American Cancer Society. Signs and Symptoms of Cancer: What Are Signs and Symptoms? Retrieved January 15, 2015 at: www. cancer.org/cancer/cancerbasics/signs-and-symptoms-of-cancer.

3   National Cancer Institute. NCI Dictionary of Cancer Terms. Chemosensitivity Assay. Retrieved January 18, 2015 at: www. cancer.gov/dictionary?cdrid=45990.

4   Canetti G, Froman S, et al. Mycrobacteria: laboratory methods for testing drug sensitivity and resistance. *Bull World Health Organization.* 1963; 29:565-578.

5   Somers S. *Knockout: Interviews with Doctors Who Are Curing Cancer and How to Prevent Getting It In the First Place.* Crown Publishing, 2009: 127.
6   Von Hoff DD, Clark GM, et al. Prospective clinical trial of a human tumor cloning system. *Cancer Research.* 1983; April; 43(4):1926-1931.
7   Kostakoglu L, Agress H, Goldsmith SJ. Clinical role of FDG PET in evaluation of cancer patients. *RSNA RadioGraphics.* March-April 2003; 23(2):315-340.
8   National Cancer Institute. Fact Sheet-Tumor Markers. Updated 12-07-11. Retrieved January 20, 2015 at: www.cancer.gov/cancertopics/factsheet/detection/tumor-markers.
9   Hansen NM, Ye X, et al. Manipulation of the primary breast tumor and the incidence of sentinel node metastases from invasive breast cancer. *Arch Surg.* 2004 Jun; 139(6):634-639; discussion 639-640.
10   Metcalfe MS, Bridgewater FHG, et al. Useless and dangerous-fine needle aspiration of hepatic colorectal metastases. *BMJ.* 2004; 328:507-508.
11   Loughran CF, Keeling CR. Seeding of tumour cells following breast biopsy: a literature review. *Br J Radiology.* 2011 Oct; 84(1006):869-974.
12   Moss R. Are Needle Biopsies Safe? Retrieved January 30, 2015 at http://chetday.com/needlebiopsy.htm.

Part 1

Tests to Detect Cancer:

Early Detection

(Prices for tests subject to change.)

Chapter 8

CA Profile Plus

NOTE: The original CA Profile test was updated in 2013 with the addition of the Thymidine Kinase component. It is now called the CA Profile Plus.

American Metabolic Laboratories
1818 Sheridan Street
Hollywood, FL 33020
www.americanmetaboliclaboratories.net
Phone: 954-929-4814
Email: customerservice@americanmetaboliclaboratories.net

*The following information was provided by Emil Schandl,
Ph.D., M.D., at American Metabolic Laboratories. Please
refer to their website for additional information and updates.*

TEST

Summary and Explanation

The CA Profile Plus is an early screening test for cancer. It is also an effective tool for monitoring regression or progression of disease. It was developed by Emil Schandl, Ph.D., M.D., and is available from American Metabolic Laboratories in Hollywood, Florida.

The CA Profile Plus is composed of nine tests:

HCG – Human chorionic gonadotropin, also called the pregnancy or malignancy hormone by Dr. Schandl, is an autocrine proliferating factor and is tested three different ways:

* HCG (IRMA): a highly sensitive test used to measure the intact HCG molecule in the blood.
* HCG (IMM): tests for intact and all molecular forms of HCG in the blood.

- HCG-Urine: a highly sensitive quantitative test for HCG in the urine. American Metabolic Laboratories uses an exclusive method of performing this test.

PHI – Phosphohexose Isomerase. The PHI enzyme has been called the human autocrine motility factor (AMF) and has been an implicating factor in the metastasis or spread of cancer. It regulates and channels cells into anaerobic metabolism (i.e., sugar metabolism).

TK1 – Thymidine Kinase. TK1 is a dynamic growth factor.

CEA – Carcinoembryonic Antigen. CEA is an antigen that is present in the blood of many persons with cancer.

GGTP – Gamma-glutamyltranspeptidase. GGTP is an enzyme that is present when the liver, pancreas, or the biliary system has been damaged due to therapy or disease.

TSH – Thyroid stimulating hormone. Detects high or low thyroid activity. Many cancer patients and those who are developing cancer or receiving chemotherapy are hypothyroid.

DHEA-S – Dehydroepiandrosterone sulfate. DHEA is the adrenal anti-stress, pro-immunity, longevity hormone. Most cancer patients, and those who are developing cancer, have low serum DHEA levels. This hormone is needed for T-lymphocyte production as part of the immune cellular response system against cancer, bacterial, and viral infections.

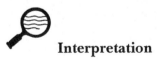 **Interpretation**

The test includes a 15 minute phone consult. Positive test results may warrant a lifestyle change through metabolic therapy. An absolute final diagnosis is done with tissue pathology.

The following are a few factors related to specific components of the test:

HCG can be elevated in an existing cancer, stress that is leading to cancer, or in a developing cancer – in some instances as many as 10-12 years before an actual tumor could be detected by any other method.

- Normal levels are less than 1.0. (0.3 mIU/mL is the lowest detectable quantity).
- GRAY ZONE, is a result of less certainty and may be 1.0 - 3.0.
- Results above 3.0 should be more seriously considered.

Remember, a positive or suggestive result does not necessarily indicate an existing cancer but perhaps a developing cancer since cancers may take 10-12 years to develop to the point of a diagnosis.

PHI can be elevated in a developing cancer, existing cancer, or an acute heart, liver, muscle disease, acute hypothyroidism or acute viral infection. Examples of these acute conditions are myocardial infarction, hepatitis, AIDS, and traumatic muscle injury. If an acute condition can be ruled out, cancer may be the cause of the elevated result and the 10-12 year cancer development clock may be ticking. This enzyme is also the autocrine motility factor (AMF) which causes cell motility (i.e. it is the malignancy factor). Normal results are less than 34.0 U/L; however, in an established malignancy a change even within normal range could be significant.

TK1 is an enzyme necessary for DNA synthesis. It is responsible for attaching a phosphate group to the nucleic acid base thymine. Its level in the blood of a cancer patient can be interpreted as a direct indication of tumor cell replication (i.e., increase or decrease of tumor size). Transient elevations have also been found in wound healing, B12 vitamin deficiency, or some viral infections, and acute stages of infection. The normal reference range is 0.6 – 6.1 U/L.

CEA test was originally developed to monitor colorectal cancers. It is actually an excellent non-organ specific cancer marker. It can be elevated in most types of cancers. Normal results are less than 3.0 ng/mL.

GGTP levels are considered normal when less than 29 in females and 35 in males.

TSH levels are normal when in the range of 0.4 – 4.0 mico IU/L.

DHEA-S levels are low or zero in most cancer patients. Normal is 35 - 430 for females and 80 - 560 for males.

HCG IRMA	May be elevated in cancer, stress-related to cancer, a developing cancer, or pregnancy. It will detect only intact hormone. It may not detect HCG-L.	Normal: Less than 1 mIU/mL; gray zone: up to 3.0 mIU/mL.
HCG IMM	May be elevated in cancer, stress-related to cancer, a developing cancer, or pregnancy. It measures intact and all other molecular forms of the hormone, including HCGL-S (HCG-like).	Normal: Less than 1mIU/mL; gray zone: up to 3.0 mIU/mL.
HCG Urine*	May be elevated in cancer, stress-related to cancer, a developing cancer, pregnancy, or the presence of HCG like substance (HCGL).	Normal: 0.0 - 1.0; gray zone 1.1 - 3.8 mIU/mL.
PHI	Elevations may warn of a developing cancer; cancer; active AIDS, acute viral disease, acute heart, liver, or muscle disease.	Normal: Less than 34 U/L; gray zone: up to 40.00 U/L.
TK1	Elevations may be interpreted as a direct indicator of tumor cell replication.	Normal: 0.6 – 6.1 U/L.
GGTP	Diseases of the liver, pancreas, and the biliary system. Also heart, lung, kidney ailments.	Normal: Females less than 29 IU/L, Males less than 35 IU/L.

TSH	Thyroid stimulating hormone, for thyroid and oxygen metabolism. This ultra sensitive method measures low or high thyroid activity.	Normal: 0.4 - 4.0 mcIU/mL.
DHEA-S	Adrenal anti-stress, immunity, and longevity hormone; low or zero in most cancer patients.	Normal: Females 35 - 430 mcg/dL, Males 80-560 mcg/dL. Results must be interpreted in reference to a person's age.
CEA	Carcinoembryonic antigen may be elevated in any malignancy.	Normal: Less than 3.0 ng/mL; gray zone is 3.1 - 5.0 ng/mL.

* Laboratory studies indicated that urinary HCG (IRMA) was negative in 99 percent of the tested subjects. This means that very little, if any, tumor generated HCG was filtered out. The urine should be tested by the IMM method, however, because tumor originated fragments can be present that the IRMA method excludes.

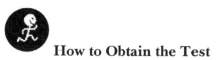

How to Obtain the Test

Call 954-929-4814 or 954-929-4895 to order and have a test kit shipped to you.

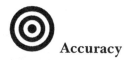

Accuracy

CA Profile reports that 89% - 97% of positive test results were confirmed by biopsy in diagnosed cancer cases.

Cost

- $576.00 for the CA Profile PLUS. (NINE tests, including TK1)
- $426.00 for the original CA Profile. (EIGHT tests, does not include the TK1)
- Credit cards are accepted.
- There is an additional fee for the blood drawing service to be paid to the laboratory that you use (typically $25 - $50).
- If you need a doctor to order your blood draw, American Metabolic Laboratories can provide this service for an additional fee of $20.
- All insurance claims are considered as "out of network" and require your own physician's prescription, which must be written by a licensed M.D. or D.O. for consideration by your insurance company.
- Medicare and Medicaid are not accepted by American Metabolic Laboratories.
- Inquire about shipping charges when ordering.
- American Metabolic Laboratories offers an additional test called the Longevity Profile Plus that includes the CA Profile Plus. This test costs is $1,065.00. See their website for details.

Process Time

Tests are run every Wednesday. Results are mailed out via USPS First Class mail on Friday of that week.

Special Instructions
For shipping domestic or international orders, no ice is required. Test kits must reach American Metabolic Laboratories within 7 – 10 days. Be sure to collect the first morning urine and transfer it to the collection vial before going to the laboratory to

have blood drawn. International orders should be shipped using Global Express.

Benefits

- The tests are designed to detect malignant neoplasms at their earliest stages, before other currently available diagnostic measures are successful. The CA Profile has been proven to be an excellent adjunct tool for early detection of malignancies when producing abnormal clinical laboratory results, even years prior to actual diagnosis by current state-of-the-art methods.
- It is valuable in monitoring the progress of cancer patients as well.
- It is able to detect brain tumors (note: some tests are not able to detect brain cancer due to limitations placed by the blood brain barrier).

Limitations

- Must have a physician's prescription if filing an insurance claim.
- The CA Profile is neither organ nor site specific.
- Does not stage cancers, however, monitoring the TK1 levels can reflect the rate of cancer growth.

Confidentiality

- Tests ordered by a personal physician for a patient will have the results mailed to the ordering physician. The doctor can authorize the release of the results directly to the patient.
- Tests ordered directly with American Metabolic Laboratories will have the result mailed directly to the person tested.

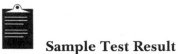

Sample Test Result

This is a sample test Longevity Profile, which includes the CA Profile, on a 60-year-old female, who had breast cancer 10 years prior. She shows elevated tumor markers, elevated coronary factors, no sex hormones, low DHEA-S.

AmericanMetabolicLaboratories.net
1818 Sheridan Street, Suite 102
Hollywood, FL 33020
Phone: 954-929-4895   Fax: 954-929-4896

Patient Name	Jane Doe	Patient I.D. Number:	19624
Address		Requisition Number:	19624,19625,19626

Phone	( )	Sex F		Age 60	
Date Drawn	11/19/12	Date Blood Received		11/21/12	
Time Drawn	9:05	Time Blood Received		11:00	
Clinical History	CA BR (SURGERY 10 YEARS AGO)				

Referring Physician: American Metabolic Laboratories
                  C. A. Schandl, M.D., Ph.D.   FCAP
     Address   1818 Sheridan Street Suite 102
                  Hollywood , FL 33020
     Phone   (954) 929-4814   Fax   (954) 929-4896   UPIN   ME 86046

Test Name	Result	Normal Ranges
CA Profile (HCG : IRMA, IMM, IMM-Urine, PHI GGTP, CEA, TSH, DHEA-S; for PLUS add TK1)		
HCG * (IRMA)	5.3▲	mIU/mL (<1.0; gray zone 1.0 - 3.0)
HCG * (IMM)	7.3▲	mIU/mL (<1.1; gray zone 1.1 - 3.0)
HCG Urine* (IMM)	2.6▲	mIU/mL (0.0 - 1.0 ; gray zone 1.1 - 3.0)
PHI *	58.9▲	U/L (0 - 34.0; gray zone 35.0 - 40.0)
GGTP	15	IU/L (F 3.0 - 28.7, M 3.3 - 35.0)
CEA	1.3	ng/mL (0.0 -3.0; gray zone 3.1 - 5.0)
DHEA-S	65.0	µg/dL (F 35.0 - 430.0, M 80.0 - 560.0, see chart)
TSH (Third Generation)	3.02	µIU/mL (0.4 - 4.0)
TK1 **		U/L (0.0 - 6.1)
PSA		ng/mL (0.0 - 4.0)
OM-MA (CA-125, Ovary)		U/mL (1.9 - 16.3)
BR-MR (CA 15-3, Breast)	31.3	U/mL (7.5 - 53.0)
GI-MA** (CA 19-9, Gastric & Pancreatic)		U/mL (0.0 - 35.0)
IGF-1	220.0	ng/mL (See attached graph for interpretation)
ESTRADIOL	< 0.0	pg/mL (See attached "Normal Values" for interpretation)
PROGESTERONE	< 0.0	ng/mL (See attached "Normal Values" for interpretation)
TOTAL TESTOSTERONE	29.2	ng/dL (See attached "Normal Values" for interpretation)
FREE TESTOSTERONE		pg/mL (See attached "Normal Values" for interpretation)
CORTISOL A.M.	12.2	µg/dL (5 - 25)
CORTISOL P.M.	5.5	µg/dL (approx. 2.5 - 12.5)
PTH	37.2	pg/mL (13.0 - 59.0)
PYRILINKS-D (DPD)		nM DPD/mM creatinine (F 3.0 - 7.4, M 2.3 - 5.4)
hsC-REACTIVE PROTEIN	0.34▲	mg/dL (0.00 - 0.30; coronary risk may exist at 0.15 and above)
HOMOCYSTEINE	7.5▲	µmol/L (5.0 - 7.0; recommended below 7.0)
Lp(a)	75.1▲	mg/dL (10.0 - 30.0), coronary risk factor
LDL (direct)	179.0▲	mg/dL (<130; 130-159 moderate/high risk, >160 high risk)

* Well documented, yet, not approved for tumor market.
** For research only: the performance characteristics
   of this product have not been established.

< less than   ▲ higher than normal value
> greater than   ▼ lower than normal value

Signature _____   Date   05/06/2014
CLIA No. 10D0918662 State of Florida Lic. No. L800010873

Note from Emil K. Schandl, Ph.D., M.D,
American Metabolic Laboratories:

I have personally designed these profiles and many years of experience have shown success as high as 97 percent. This means that if there are 100 biopsy diagnosed cancer cases, 97 may yield positive results. These observations were generated by examining some 40,000 plus patients. I can assure you these series of clinical laboratory tests are very useful for early detection of biochemical changes leading to cancer. The panels are also very productive in monitoring an individual's progress while receiving therapies, metabolic, conventional or the judicious combination of both.

A positive result is a warning sign that may warrant a complete change of lifestyle risk factors through evaluation and implementation of metabolic therapy. It is much easier to prevent cancer than to cure it.

I strongly recommend the Cancer Profile, and even more so, the Longevity Profile, on an annual basis as part of your most comprehensive health watch. In the event of abnormal cancer marker/s results, it is wise to also perform the TK1 test for additional confirmation and follow-up of those findings.

Cordially yours,

E. K. Schandl, M.S., Ph.D., M.D.(MA), FACB, CC(NRCC), SC(ASCP), LNC, Oncobiologist, Clinical and Nutritional Biochemist, Clinical Laboratory Director (States of FL, NY, CA)

Thoughts

The CA Profile Plus test can be lifesaving. Not only can it be used to monitor known disease, but it can identify pre-cancerous conditions.

The nine tests included provide a multifaceted result and each test can be used to validate the other results. For example, the CA Profile provides multiple indicators and if more than one of the nine tests results returns positive, then there is a stronger body of evidence to identify a problem.

Just as Dr. Schandl stated in his note to the reader, this test can be used as a proactive part of your annual physical exam. It can be utilized to identify a new cancer or a cancer recurrence at its earliest stages. For example, I received a phone call from a patient who was treated for breast cancer 2 1/2 years ago. She was declared as having no evidence of disease at the time. She said that her MRI and PET scan last month indicated a lesion on her chest wall, liver, and in the lymph nodes. Had she been monitoring her health status with a test such as the CA Profile, she may have been able to begin treatment long before the tumors would have been large enough to appear on the scans.

In talking with the staff at American Metabolic Laboratories, we discussed the reality that approximately 40 percent of the normal population tested had a "false" positive CA Profile©. According to national statistics 1 out of every 2.5 individuals will develop cancer in America (i.e., 40 percent of the U.S. population). Maybe these 40 percent "false" positives are the individuals who are unknowingly in the process of developing cancer?

Reference

See: www.americanmetaboliclaboratories.net/CA_Profile-The_ Original.html

Chapter 9

Cologuard®

Stool DNA Home Screening Kit

Exact Sciences Labs
Phone: 844-870-8870
www.cologuardtest.com

The following information was provided by Exact Sciences Labs.
Please refer to their website for more information and updates.

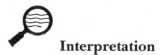

Summary and Explanation

Colorectal cancer is the third most commonly diagnosed cancer and the second leading cause of cancer deaths in men and women combined in the U.S. Unfortunately, most cases are not found early or before it has spread beyond the tissues of the colon or rectum. Cologuard was approved by the FDA in August of 2014. It requires a prescription and can be done in the privacy of your home.

This cancer screening test looks for blood in the stool and altered DNA. The wall of the colon naturally sheds cells daily; abnormal cells will be picked up by stool as it passes through. Cologuard uses advanced stool DNA technology to find altered DNA from these abnormal cells, which could be associated with cancer or pre-cancer. Cologuard is a screening test. Any positive result should be discussed with your doctor and followed by a diagnostic colonoscopy.

Interpretation

- The test result is reported as "positive" or "negative."

- Information from the DNA analysis and blood test are combined to reach the test result.
- The test is capable of detecting pre-cancerous polyps and cancer through stage 4 with 92 percent sensitivity.

How to Obtain the Test

- www.cologuard.com provides a "Find a Doctor" tab.
- The test must be ordered by prescription through a licensed clinician. If your doctor would like to know more about Cologuard, he can contact Exact Sciences at 844-870-8870.
- Cologuard is shipped directly to your home. You must use a street address; P.O. boxes are not permitted. Instructions for collecting a stool sample are included and easy to understand. The kit includes a prepaid UPS shipping label. Please note that the sample must be shipped within 24 hours of collection, and received by Exact Sciences Labs within 72 hours. They recommend shipping completed test kits Sunday through Thursday for this reason.

Accuracy

- In a 10,000 patient clinical study, Cologuard found 92% of colon cancers. It also found 69% of high-risk pre-cancers (high-grade dysplasia), those most likely to develop into cancer. Cologuard achieved a specificity of 87%.
- Both false positives and false negatives do occur. In a clinical study of Cologuard, 13% of people without cancer or pre-cancer tested positive. Any positive should be followed by a diagnostic colonoscopy. Following a negative result, patients should continue participating in a screening program at an interval and with a method appropriate for the individual patient.

- Cologuard performance when used for repeat testing has not been evaluated or established. However, the Centers for Medicare and Medicaid Services (CMS) recommend Cologuard be performed every 3 years for patients 50 and older, who do not have symptoms of colorectal cancer, and who do not have an increased risk of colorectal cancer

 Cost

Medicare covers Cologuard once every 3 years as long as you are between 50-85 years old and you are at average risk for developing colon cancer. Medicare will not cover the test if you have symptoms that your doctor thinks may be related to colon cancer, if you previously had a positive colonoscopy that found polyps or cancer, or if your doctor determines that you have a high-risk family history of colon cancer.

It is also covered by a variety of private insurers. Check with your provider to confirm coverage. Co-pays and/or deductibles may apply. If you have private insurance coverage, the Cologuard Assurance program is designed to bill your insurance company on your behalf. They do require a $50 prepayment and a signed Assignment of Benefits from you. Next, after your test is complete, they will bill and if necessary appeal to your insurance company for the remaining unpaid balance. Please note that if insurance coverage is denied, you will be responsible for the unpaid balance. The $50 can be refunded if insurance coverage is approved. The maximum out-of-pocket cost of Cologuard is $599, depending on the covered benefits of your specific insurance plan.

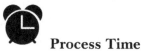 **Process Time**

Test results will be delivered to your doctor within two weeks of the lab receiving the completed test kit.

BENEFITS

Benefits

- The test can identify the presence of cancer and pre-cancerous cells.
- Available for Medicare coverage for adults 50-85 years of age who are at average risk for colon cancer.
- No special bowel preparation or dietary restrictions are required prior to taking the test.
- Done in the privacy of your home.
- Less invasive than a colonoscopy.

LIMITATIONS

Limitations

- Results should be interpreted with caution for individuals over age 75, as the rate of false positives increase with age.
- Cologuard is NOT approved for people with a "HIGH" risk of colon cancer. These may include:
  o A personal history of colon cancer, polyps, or other related cancers.
  o A family history of colon cancer.
  o A positive result for another screening method in the last six months.
  o Patients who have been diagnosed with a condition that is associated with high risk for colorectal cancer, which include but are not limited to inflammatory bowel disease (IBD), chronic ulcerative colitis (CUC), and Crohn's disease.
- Cologuard should not be used by those who have or may have blood in their stool due to actively bleeding hemorrhoids, menstruation, or other existing conditions, as this may result in a false positive.
- Cologuard is not a replacement for diagnostic colonoscopy or surveillance colonoscopy in high risk individuals.
- Cologuard may produce false positive or false negative results.

Confidentiality

Results are reported to the ordering physician and become part of the your medical record.

Thoughts

Colorectal cancer is no longer a disease of those with advanced age. We are seeing rates increase for people under the age of 50. Studies report that approximately 13 percent of people diagnosed when the cancer has spread to distant sites, will reach the 5 year survival milestone. Knowing this, it has become critical to do early screening.

This test adds the component of stool DNA analysis to the "Occult Blood Stool Test" that I described in the Colon Health Screening chapter. However, the cost is considerably higher. Consider both and decide which test is best for your circumstances.

References

References are available at: www.cologuardtest.com

Chapter 10

Colon Health Screening for Occult
Blood in Stool – Home Test Kit

Colorectal cancer is often called the "silent killer." Excluding skin cancers, colorectal cancer is the third most common cancer diagnosed in both men and women in the United States.[1]

Cancer that begins in the colon is called colon cancer. Cancer that begins in the last six inches of the large intestine (the rectum) is called rectal cancer. Cancer that begins in either of these areas is called colorectal cancer (CRC). About 75 percent of patients with CRC have no family history of the disease, so it does not appear to be primarily inherited.[2] Colorectal cancer deaths could be nearly eliminated if most people learn the basics and get tested.

TEST

Summary and Explanation

A home test kit, available at specialty drugstores or online, can be used to detect "occult" or invisible blood in the stool. Fecal occult blood can be a sign of a problem in your digestive system, such as a growth, polyp, or cancer in the colon or rectum.

If microscopic or visible blood is detected, it is important for your doctor to determine the source of the bleeding to properly diagnose and treat the problem. Blood may be seen as red or black tar-like feces and may appear in the stool because there are:

- Benign (noncancerous) or malignant (cancerous) growths or polyps of the colon.
- Hemorrhoids (swollen blood vessels near the anus and lower rectum that can rupture causing bleeding).
- Anal fissures (splits or cracks in the lining of the anal opening).

- Intestinal infections that cause inflammation.
- Ulcers.
- Possible bowel conditions such as colitis, Crohn's disease, celiac disease, or diverticular disease.
- Bacterial infections.
- Food allergies to items such as dairy and wheat.

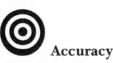 **How to Obtain the Test**

You can purchase fecal occult blood test kits at specialty pharmacies or order them online. Each test kit provides specific instructions, and most offer a toll-free number to call if you have questions. Since colon cancers may bleed from time to time, rather than continually, you will need to collect three different stool samples. The stool samples should be taken one day apart. Be sure to purchase a kit that includes at least three separate test cards.

Do not perform the test if you have one of the conditions in the bulleted list above, diarrhea, or if you are menstruating.

Interpretation

Stool samples are collected in a clean container and evaluated by detecting color changes on the test card. Some test kits instruct you to simply drop the test card into the toilet after a bowel movement. Follow instructions included in your kit.

Accuracy

A negative test result means that no blood was found in the collected stool sample during the testing period. Always continue to follow your doctor's recommendations for regular cancer screening.

Cost

Most test kits are priced at $5 - $15 per testing card.

Process Time

Usually results are read in two minutes. Follow test kit instructions.

Benefits

- Can detect the presence of unknown colon cancer so that treatment can be started earlier.
- Cost is low compared to a colonoscopy.
- Non-invasive.
- Convenient, quick, easy and can be done at home.
- No cleansing of the colon is necessary.

Limitations

- Positive results may be due to a condition other than cancer.
- Requires further testing to determine the cause of the bleeding.
- Fails to detect non-bleeding polyps.
- False positives can occur.

Confidentiality

Testing is done in the privacy of your home.

Thoughts

Many people do not want to do a colonoscopy or don't have the funds or insurance available to get one. A home fecal blood test kit provides a more affordable option. I feel that for the early detection of colorectal cancer, the fecal occult blood test should be done by everyone starting in their thirties. Regular screening can often find colorectal cancer early, when it is most likely to be curable.

When relying on colonoscopies for colon cancer testing, it is important to remember that a colonoscopy is done on the large intestine and can miss a bleeding lesion in the small intestine.

Footnotes

1 American Cancer Society. Colorectal Cancer- What Are the Key Statistics About Colorectal Cancer? 1/31/2014. Retrieved January 31, 2015 at: www.cancer.org/cancer/colonandrectumcancer/ detailedguide/colorectal-cancer-key-statistics.

2 National Cancer Institute. Genetics of Colorectal Cancer. Retrieved January 15, 2015 at: www.cancer.gov/cancertopics/pdq/ genetics/colorectal/healthprofessional.

Chapter 11

EarlyCDT – Lung Test

Oncimmune (USA) LLC
8960 Commerce Drive, Building #6
De Soto, Kansas 66018
Phone: 888-583-9030
www.oncimmune.com

The information provided on this test was obtained from Oncimmune. Please refer to their website for updates.

TEST

Summary and Explanation

The EarlyCDT® is a test that detects the presence of seven lung cancer-associated antigens in the blood. Oncimmune reports that it is effective in detecting all stages of lung cancer, including the earliest stages. Oncimmune's goal is to advance early lung cancer detection to the greatest extent possible using the autoantibody assay technology utilized in the EarlyCDT test.

The test works by evaluating a known process: When a tumor is present in the lung, it produces abnormal proteins/antigens that are not normally found in the blood. The body reacts rapidly to the abnormal proteins/antigens by producing the related antibodies. If pre-set levels are exceeded, the test will be positive.

Testing is only recommended for individuals in the target population that includes current and ex-smokers above the age of 40 who have smoked one pack or more of cigarettes per day. Also for anyone with two or more of the following: COPD, emphysema, environmental exposures, or a family history of lung cancer in a first degree relative. Anyone with a history of cancer, including skin cancer, is not eligible for this test. Lingering antibodies from a previous diagnosis could cause a false positive result.

Interpretation

Test results are reported as LOW, MODERATE, or HIGH level.

A LOW result indicates a lower likelihood of lung cancer than a moderate level. A MODERATE result indicates a lower indication of cancer than a HIGH result. A MODERATE or HIGH level test implies an eight times increase in the risk of cancer.

A LOW result does not mean that cancer is not present or will not develop. Continued monitoring is recommended along with a patient history and clinical findings.

 How to Obtain the Test

The test must be ordered by a physician. If your physician is not registered, ask him to contact Client Services at 888-583-9030 to become a test provider. Oncimmune will send a test kit upon request and include the materials for prepaid return overnight FedEx shipping to the lab.

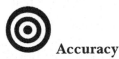 **Accuracy**

Oncimmune reports 98 percent accuracy for HIGH results within patients in the targeted population. They also report that the test has a 5 times better positive predictive value (PPV) than a CT scan and 7 times fewer false positives than a CT scan.

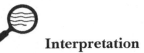 **Cost**

*   Oncimmune will bill Medicare Part B or your primary insurance carrier for the cost of the test. The appropriate

forms must be completed and photo copies of the front and back of your insurance card must be returned with the blood sample.

- If you do not have insurance, payment is required to be sent with the test.
- They accept credit cards, checks, or money orders.
- Financial assistance is available for the underinsured or Medicaid recipients.
- Out of pocket expenses may be reimbursable through Flexible Spending Accounts or Healthcare Spending Accounts.
- Cash or self-pay cost is approximately $150.

Process Time

Results take about one week and will be sent directly to the ordering healthcare provider.

Benefits

- The absence of detectible antibodies from patients in the target population can rule out the presence of lung cancer.
- Early detection.

Limitations

- The test is not effective on individuals with previous cancer. The body will have produced antibodies to previous cancers and those lingering antibodies can produce a positive result on this lung cancer test. If you receive a positive result and further investigation indicates that you do not have lung cancer, it is necessary to look

elsewhere in the body for cancer. A possible unknown cancer may be causing the positive result.
- Only available for individuals who qualify as part of the target population.

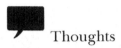 **Confidentiality**

Results are reported to ordering physician and become part of your medical record.

Thoughts

With approximately 85 percent of lung cancers being found late in the disease process, I am pleased to present this test as an addition to an early lung cancer detection plan for those in the high risk population. Cancers caught early translate to quicker intervention and higher survival rates.

This chapter is dedicated to my uncles, Don Behrend and Clarence Herzog. Both died after being diagnosed with very advanced lung cancer. This early detection test could have saved their lives.

Reference

References are available at www.oncimmune.com.

Chapter 12

Human Chorionic Gonadotropin (hCG) Test

Navarro Medical Clinic
Efren Navarro, MD
3553 Sining Street
Morningside Terrace
Santa Mesa, Manila 1016
Philippines
www.navarromedicalclinic.com
Evening phone calls after 6PM CST at 847.359.3634
Email: customer.service@navarromedicalclinic.com

*The following information was obtained from
www.navarromedicalclinic.com. Please refer to their
website for more information and updates.*

TEST

Summary and Explanation

Developed in the late 1950s by the renowned oncologist the late Dr. Manuel D. Navarro, the test detects the presence of cancer cells even before signs or symptoms develop. Dr. Navarro found hCG to be present in all types of cancers.

The test is based on a theory proposed by Howard Beard and other researchers who contend that cancer is related to a misplaced trophoblastic cell that becomes malignant. This school of thought looks at how cancer is similar to pregnancy in that from one cell comes many others.

A fetus starts as one cell which divides into many different kinds of cells – some cells become bones, others become organs, blood vessels, etc. But after pregnancy, that kind of frenzied division comes to an end and strict order begins. Once a bone cell, always a bone cell. In much the same way that cell division does not "play by the rules" during pregnancy, cancer cells do not play by the rules. Both cancerous cells and pregnant women secrete hCG. As a consequence, a measurement of the amount of hCG found in the blood or urine is also a measure of the degree of malignancy. The higher the number, the greater the severity of cancer.

Urine is the preferred specimen for the test because it is much harder to detect in the bloodstream. A 1980 study validated the use of the urine specimens for the hCG immunoassay. In 32 proven cancer cases, the immunoassay test gave 31 positive results using urine, while only 12 positive results were reported using blood.

The test detects the presence of brain cancer as early as early as 29 months before symptoms appear, 27 months for fibro sarcoma of the abdomen, 24 months for skin cancer, 12 months for cancer of the bones, and 24 months for metastasis from the breast cancer.

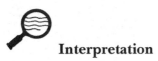 **Interpretation**

Interpretation of Readings

Index	International Units	Readings	Interpretation
0	zero	(-)	Negative
1-3	1-49	(+/-)	Doubtful
4	50-400	(+)	Faintly Positive
5	401-999	(++)	Definitely Positive
6	1000-3000	(+++)	Moderately Positive
7	3001-5000	(++++)	Markedly Positive
8	5001-10000	(+++++)	Very Markedly Positive
9	over 10000	(++++++)	Excessively Positive

Levels can reach up to 10,000 international units (IU) or more in some cancers. However, most cancers have results anywhere from 50 to 80 or 90 IU. Repeated testing can be used to monitor progress and response to treatment.

When a reading of index + 4 is made, it means that the result is above 50 IU and is positive, meaning cancer may be present. But if a reading of index +/-3 is made, it means that the result is below 50 IU and potential for cancer is essentially low.

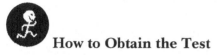

How to Obtain the Test

This test does not involve a kit. You will need the following locally available household items to prepare a dry extract from your urine sample. Instructions are simple and easy to follow.

- 7 oz. of acetone (nail polish remover is NOT A SUBSTITUTE).
- 1 teaspoon of alcohol – either ethyl or rubbing.
- One coffee filter – white or brown.
- One sandwich plastic bag.
- A glass container or glass jar.
- A glass measuring cup.
- Measuring spoon.

Follow the preparation and mailing instructions on the clinic's website: www.navarromedicalclinic.com/preparation.php

Before collecting the urine sample, make sure that there is NO sexual contact for 12 days for female patients, 48 hours for male. DO NOT SEND URINE IF THE PATIENT IS PREGNANT.

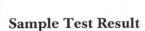

Sample Test Result

Dear Jenny,

Your HCG Test Result on 07/30/2013 is:

Index + 4,(51.8 Int. Units)

This is within the POSITIVE range (0 I.U. - negative, 1 to 49 I.U. - doubtful [essentially negative], 50 I.U. and above - positive). A POSITIVE result indicates the presence of Human Chorionic Gonadotropin, a hormone found in the urine of pregnant women. Numerous medical reports show this to be present in the urine of cancer patients. However, the result must be correlated with the medical information (X-rays, CT scans, utrasounds, MRIs, etc.,). A biopsy procedure confirms the diagnosis of cancer. The elevated HCG is possibly coming from remnants (microscopic or otherwise) of the breast cancer. This serves as the baseline result.

Results can go up to 10,000 int. units or more especially in testicular cancer, some uterine cancers (H mole and choriocarcinoma) and germ cell tumor. However, most other cancers have results anywhere from 50 to 80 or 90 IU. The result must be correlated with the medical history together with other pertinent medical information (X-rays, CT scans, ultrasounds, MRIs, etc.). The test cannot determine the stage of the cancer but when it is done on a serial basis, say once a month, one can follow and monitor the progress of the disease.

Wishing you the best of health, I remain.

Sincerely Yours,

Efren F. Navarro, MD

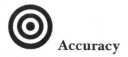

Accuracy

Research shows that in 32 patients with documented cancer, the immunoassay test gave 31 positive results using urine.

In serum hCG testing, blood is used. The Navarro Medical Clinic reports that results from a blood or serum sample are not as accurate because when hCG molecules pass through the liver, enzymes fragment them at which point the reagent may not be able to identify them. With the Navarro test, whole hCG molecules are in the urine sample.

Cost

$55 plus the cost of USPS 1st Class international mail. Payment instructions are online.

The household items needed cost around $10.

Process Time

Allow 3-4 weeks for test results to be available when mailing from USA, Canada, or Europe. Results are sent to the email address provided with the mailed test sample.

Benefits

- Affordable.
- Non-invasive screening test.
- Simple and can be done in the privacy of your home.
- Indicates the amount of cancer that may be present.

Limitations

- See "Precautions" on the test website for activities and medications that should be temporally stopped before urine sample is collected. Substances such as thyroid hormones, steroidal compounds (i.e. prednisone), female hormone supplements (estrogen, testosterone, progesterone), and vitamin D may interfere with results. If you are using these compounds you must stop taking them for 3 days prior to testing and resume after the urine is collected. AS ALWAYS, CONSULT YOUR PHYSICIAN PRIOR TO STOPPING ANY MEDICATIONS OR SUPPLEMENTS.
- The test is not organ or site specific.
- The test cannot determine the stage of the cancer.

NOTE: A positive hCG test result can be caused by pregnancy, malignancy, and some pituitary gland issues due to an hCG-like substance (HCGLS) that may occur rarely in peri-menopausal, post-menopausal women, and some older men.

Confidentiality

Results are sent directly to the patient's email address.

Thoughts

This test is affordable and can be done in the privacy of your home. It may seem silly to test for cancer with a coffee filter and a few household items, but I did it and thousands of others have done it before me. This test is another useful tool in evaluating your cancer status. I like that the test provides a numerical score that ranks the amount of hCG present as opposed to a simple positive or negative outcome. Increasing or decreasing levels can indicate the advancement or regression of disease. HCG is extremely sensitive; a tiny elevation in its level in women is highly indicative of cancer. In men, hCG is very good at diagnosing testicular cancer.

FYI – The hCG hormone is what many pregnancy tests are based upon. After conception, the body dispatches hCG to maintain the lining of the womb and enable the production of progesterone hormone, which is essential in the first trimester of pregnancy. If a home pregnancy test kit reads positive, it is reacting to an increased level of hCG.

This same hormone is attractive as a weight loss supplement because it can trigger the body's use of fat for fuel. Oncologists are not all of like minds on the issue of whether hCG used for weight loss has the potential to cause cancer. Some say that because hCG is secreted by tumors, it is a marker and should not be confused as the cause of the tumor. Others say we do not yet know all there is to know about hCG and cancer, hormones are very powerful, and we should not put additional hCG in the body. In an unrelated move, the U.S. prohibited the sale of over-the-counter and homeopathic hCG in 2011. The use of it now requires a prescription.

References

Williams RR, McIntire KR, Waldmann TA, et al. Tumor-associated antigen levels (CEA, HCG, alpha-feto protein) antedating the diagnosis of cancer in the Framingham Study. *J Natl Cancer Inst.* 1977 Jun; 58(6):1547-1551.

Chapter 13

Nagalase Test

Health Diagnostics and Research Institute (HDRI)
540 Bordentown Ave - Ste 2300
South Amboy, NJ 08879
Phone: 732-721-1234
Fax: 732-525-3288
E-mail: info@hdri-usa.com or lab@vitdiag.com
www.hdri-usa.com

> *Information on this test was provided by HDRI and by research*
> *done by the author. Please check the HDRI website for updates.*

TEST

Summary and Explanation

The test measures the activity of the enzyme α-N-acetylgalactosaminidase (nagalase) in blood. Nagalase accumulates in the serum of cancer patients and its activity correlates with tumor burden, aggressiveness, and clinical disease progression.

Nagalase is a crafty tool that cancer cells and viruses (HIV, hepatitis B, hepatitis C, influenza, herpes, Epstein-Barr virus, and others) make to ensure their survival.

Nagalase is an enzyme. Cancer and viruses secrete it to incapacitate the immune system.

The more cancers grow, they more nagalase they generate and we can measure the levels in the bloodstream. On the other hand, nagalase levels go down when the cancer or infection is being effectively destroyed. Any treatment that lowers the number of cancer cells or viral particles will lower nagalase levels. For example, nagalase levels will drop after surgery to remove all or a portion of a tumor.

Chemotherapy and radiation also reduce nagalase levels. In research studies, nagalase activity decreased to near tumor-free control levels one day after surgical removal of primary tumors from cancer patients, suggesting that the half-life of nagalase is less than 24 hours. The short half-life of nagalase is valuable for prognosis of the disease during various therapies.

Increased nagalase activity has been detected in the blood of patients with a wide variety of cancers including cancer of the prostate, breast, colon, lung, esophagus, stomach, liver, pancreas, kidney, bladder, testis, uterus, and ovary, mesothelioma, melanoma, fibrosarcoma, glioblastoma, neuroblastoma, and various leukemias. For various types of tumors, various levels of nagalase activity were found. It appears that the secretory capacity of individual tumor tissue varies among tumor types depending upon tumor size, staging, and the degree of malignancy or invasiveness.

Studies correlating nagalase levels with tumor burden suggest that the measurement of this enzyme can diagnose the presence of cancerous lesions below levels detectable by other diagnostic means.

Cancer patients with high levels of nagalase have been treated with the administration of GcMAF – that is a vitamin D cofactor called "group specific component macrophage activating factor." GcMAF is the protein the body makes to activate anti-cancer immune activity. But cancer, always clever in its effort to survive, ramps up the nagalase enzyme to disable GcMAF. So giving the body more GcMAF helps the immune system address the cancer.

Life Extension Foundation for Longer Life is exploring further clinical investigation into GcMAF's additive or synergistic effects when used with dichloracetate (DCA). GcMAF has demonstrated some complete remissions on its own in patients who participated in three separate trials on breast, prostate, and colorectal cancer. The mechanism of action involves resupplying the Gc protein (also known as vitamin D binding protein), which cancer cells destroy by secreting an abundance of the enzyme nagalase. GcMAF restores the deficiency (loss), which is a critical component in activating the macrophages, the immune system's cancer scavengers. It is interesting that vitamin D has such a potent anti-tumor effect that cancer cells produce the enzyme nagalase to prevent vitamin D from binding to cancer cells. GcMAF disables the ability of cancer cells to shield against vitamin D.

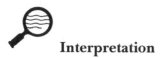

Interpretation

- Normal levels are considered to < 0.9.
- Levels higher than 4 are regularly found in cancer patients as well as in patients with chronic fatigue syndrome or Lyme disease.
- Levels > 0.9 and < 3 are commonly found in autistic children as well as in patients infected with various viruses.
- A nagalase test every 6-8 weeks gives an indication of whether your body is fighting the cancer.

How to Obtain the Test

- Must be ordered by a licensed clinician.
- For test kits please call, fax your request to 732-721-1234 or 732-525-3288, or email lab@vitdiag.com.
- If your clinician is not registered, have him contact the Health Diagnostics and Research Institute to register. HDRI must have a copy of their license on file.

Sample Test Result

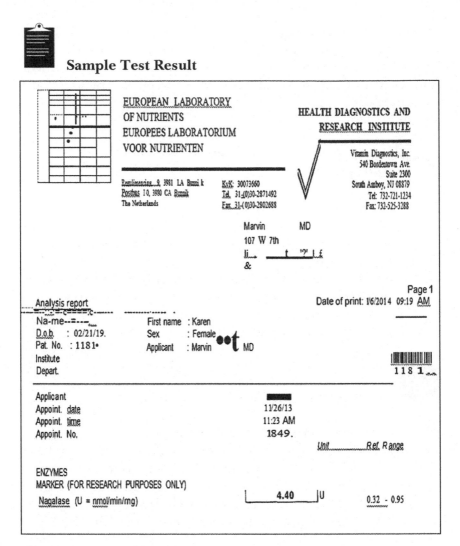

EUROPEAN LABORATORY
OF NUTRIENTS
EUROPEES LABORATORIUM
VOOR NUTRIENTEN

HEALTH DIAGNOSTICS AND
RESEARCH INSTITUTE

Vitamin Diagnostics, Inc.
540 Bordentown Ave.
Suite 2300
South Amboy, NJ 08879
Tel: 732-721-1234
Fax: 732-525-3288

Resmlicencing ..9, 3981 LA Bunni k
Postbus 10, 3980 CA Bunnik
The Netherlands

KvK: 30073660
Tel. 31-(0)30-2871492
Fax 31-(0)30-2802688

Marvin   MD
107 W 7th
li...   t   '?' l f
&

Page 1
Date of print: 1/6/2014 09:19 AM

Analysis report

Na-me--=---.	First name : Karen
D.o.b. : 02/21/19.	Sex : Female
Pat. No. : 1181•	Applicant : Marvin ●●t MD
Institute	
Depart.	

1 1 8 1

Applicant
Appoint. date   11/26/13
Appoint. time   11:23 AM
Appoint. No.   1849.

Unit   Ref. Range

ENZYMES
MARKER (FOR RESEARCH PURPOSES ONLY)

Nagalase (U = nmol/min/mg)   4.40   U   0.32 - 0.95

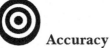

Accuracy

- Specificity: >95%.
- Limit of detection: 0.2 nmol/min/mg.
- Interassay precision: 92%.
- Intraassay precision: 96.6%.

Cost

$85 and includes overnight shipping within the United States only.

Process Time

Approximately 4 weeks.

Benefits

- Nagalase activity is directly proportional to viable tumor burden.
- The test can identify the presence of cancer.
- Nagalase in blood is a sensitive test for monitoring the efficacy of therapy in cancer. Your physician or oncologist can use results to obtain a better understanding of the therapy and to fine-tune your treatment.
- Because of the short half-life of nagalase, the method is suitable for monitoring various types of therapy.

Limitations

- The values may be affected by certain drugs used in the five days preceding blood draw. Drug use must be indicated on the questionnaire submitted with the requisition form.
- Does not identify specific organ or site of cancer.

Confidentiality

Results are reported to ordering physician and become part of your medical record.

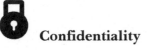

Thoughts

This test is a valuable tool in detecting the possible presence, progression, or regression of cancer. The presence of this enzyme seems to be proportional to tumor burden, thus allowing for early detection. It is reported to be sensitive enough to be able to pick up the presence of cancerous lesions before they are large enough to be detected by standard diagnostic tools. It is one of the more affordable early detection tests available.

Reference

References are available at www.hdri-usa.com under the Nagalase tab.

Chapter 14

ONCOblot® Labs
ENOX2 Protein Test

ONCOblot Labs
1201 Cumberland Ave., Suite B
West Lafayette, IN 47906
Customer Service:
972-510-7773
info@oncoblotlabs.com
www.oncoblotlabs.com

The information on this test was provided by
ONCOblot Labs. Check their website for updates.

TEST

Summary and Explanation

The ONCOblot® test is a highly sensitive blood test for cancer and can be used for early detection. The ONCOblot test can detect cancer before clinical symptoms appear. The test measures the ENOX2 protein that is found only on the surface of a malignant cancer cell. This protein is not a normal protein in blood serum. ENOX2 only exists in serum when cancer is present because these proteins have been shed by a tumor.

The ONCOblot test claims it can detect cancer consisting of 2 million cells compared to 4.5 trillion cells for a positive mammogram. A tumor the size of only 2 million cells is tiny and would be missed by most standard tests available today.

ENOX2 proteins are absent in noncancerous cells, and are not produced by benign or inflammatory conditions. So false positives, in principle, are eliminated. This test can tell us whether cancer is present, as well as tell us where in the body it is. ENOX2 proteins have molecular signatures such as the weight and isoelectric point (the pH at which a particular molecule or surface carries no net electrical charge) that are used to identify the source of the cancer. Approximately 96% of the time, the test will reveal the tissue of origin. If there is more than one tissue of origin, then more than one type of ENOX2 would be revealed and the results would indicate the origin of each tissue.

ONCOblot reveals the origin of malignant cells in more than 26 different kinds of cancer including: large cell lung, small cell lung, breast, prostate, colon, malignant melanoma, lymphoma/ leukemia, pancreatic, ovarian, and cervical.

ONCOblot became available in 2013 and meets the FDA requirements for a Laboratory Developed Test.

Interpretation

Test results indicate if the ENOX2 protein is present as a YES or NO. If present, the molecular weight and the isometric point (pH) are identified as well as the organ site.

The ONCOblot database, as of January 2014, includes the 26 most common forms of cancer. In the case of multiple cancers from different sites of origin, all are included. It is important to know that a cancer which has spread to other sites retains its original molecular weight and isometric point. For example, this would mean that cancer that was found in the liver that had spread from the breast, would have the same molecular weight and isometric point as the breast cancer (tissue of origin). The ONCOblot test only reveals tissue of origin, not metastasized cancers. The identification of the original data would confirm a metastasis and rule out a new cancer. NIDB (not in database) indicates either a molecular weight or an isoelectric point that is not yet associated with a specific malignancy in the company's database.

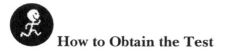

How to Obtain the Test

The test must be prescribed by a physician or clinician. There are three ways patients can get tested:

1. Have their personal physician order the test kit from www.oncoblotlabs.com.
2. Locate a physician who uses the test at www.oncoblotlabs. com under "How to Get Tested."
3. Make a phone appointment with the online physician at www.oncoblotlabs.com under "How to Get Tested."

Wait at least one month after completing chemotherapy or surgery before sending blood sample for testing to avoid a false negative report.

Cost

The cost for the ONCOblot test is $850.00 (Continental U.S. only and subject to change). This does not include the cost of the blood draw or physician fees. Note: Patients may use a lab of their choosing for the blood draw. Price varies, but estimates range from $25 - $50. Overnight domestic shipping of the patient's blood sample to the ONCOblot lab is included in the price of the kit.

Sample Test Result

LABORATORY REPORT   ONCOblot

PATIENT IDENTIFIER: XXX-DAL   ONCOblot: 406
DOB: 8/16/32   GENDER: F   DATE RECEIVED: April 3, 2013

ONCOblot° TEST RESULTS

ENOX2 proteins evident: Yes ☑ No ☐   ENOX2 proteins indicate cancer presence.

ENOX2	Molecular Weight (kDa)	Isoelectric Point (pH)	Organ Site
Protein 1	66	4.5	Breast

Molecular weights and isoelectric points given are within two times the standard deviations for the specific ENOX2 proteins listed, as being specific for a particular organ site.

Control Validation

Alpha Fetuin and Transferrin are reference proteins (controls) that validate that the ONCOblot[SM] test performed to standards.

Reference Protein 1 (Transferrin) present/in range: Yes ☑ No ☐

Reference Protein 2 (Alpha Fetuin) present/in range: Yes ☑ No ☐

Comments

Results and report have been reviewed and are approved for communication to the requesting clinician.

D. James Morré, Ph.D.   Date   Dorothy Morré, Ph.D.   Date
Director of Laboratory   Quality Assurance Officer

Test was performed at: ONCOblot Laboratories •1291C Cumberland Ave •West Lafayette, IN 47906

Additional sample test results and explanation of results are available at www.oncoblotlabs.com under the FAQ tab.

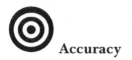

Accuracy

ONCOblot Labs reports the following, based on analyses of over 800 ONCOblots covering 26 different kinds of cancers with clinically confirmed diagnoses:

- 99.3% were positive for cancer based on ENOX2 presence.
- Of these, the organ site of the cancer was determined correctly in 96% of the samples.
- There were no false positives.
- There were less than 1% false negatives.

Process Time

10-15 business days from receipt of blood sample in the ONCOblot Labs.

Benefits

- Identifies the presence of cancer.
- Identifies site of origin 96% of the time.
- Can be used to monitor disease progression or recurrence.
- Processed with a small blood sample.
- Non-invasive.

Limitations

- Does not indicate size of tumor or stage of development.
- Not covered by most insurance companies at this time.
- Will not detect brain tumors or surface skin cancers.
- Cannot identify the location of metastasis of the original cancer.

Confidentiality

Results of your ONCOblot test will be sent back to the ordering physician/clinician and will become part of your medical record.

Thoughts

This test became available in January of 2013. It is based upon more than 20 years of research. The ONCOblot test was developed and created by Dr. D. James Morré and Dr. Dorothy M. Morré of Mor-NuCo, Purdue Research Park, West Lafayette, Indiana.

This test is said by some to be the biggest breakthrough in cancer identification today. I like that it has the power to catch many cancers at their absolute earliest stage of detection by locating and identifying the ENOX 2 proteins in the blood, which are unique to malignant cancer cells. Also, it is attractive because it is a simple blood test and it is radiation-free.

This chapter is dedicated to my friend Sam Raia, who was diagnosed with pancreatic cancer in August 2014. In each of the three prior years, he had received a PET scan. Each scan was positive – meaning it lit up for cancer. But biopsies also were taken each year and they came back negative so he was given cancer-free reports. Yet cancer was growing inside of him. When the final biopsy was done in 2014, the cancer had grown large enough that when the needle extracted cells, it actually got cancerous cells and Sam got the devastating news. An ONCOblot test could have verified his cancer status years earlier because it is an early detection test, and he would have had the diagnosis in time for intervention.

References

References are available at www.oncoblotlabs.com under the "How it Works" tab.

Chapter 15

Papanicolaou (PAP) and Human Papillomavirus (HPV) Tests for Cervical Cancer

The National Cancer Institute estimates that in the year 2013 there were 12,340 new cases of cervical/uterine cancer and 4,030 deaths from the disease. Many of these cases occur among women rarely or never screened for cancer. When cervical cancer is found early, it is highly treatable and survivable.

TEST

Summary and Explanation

The Papanicolaou (Pap) test is used to detect cell changes on the cervix that might become cancerous if not treated and to screen for existing cervical cancer. The Pap test can also find noncancerous conditions, such as infections and inflammation. Pap test screening is the most effective way to detect early abnormal cervical cell changes.

Human Papillomavirus (HPV) is a virus that causes almost all cases of cervical cancer. There are about 12 identified types of high risk HPV. HPV testing is used to look for the presence of viral DNA or RNA from high-risk HPV types in cervical cells. An infection from HPV is sexually transmitted and can also cause anal, vaginal, vulvar, penile, and oropharyngeal cancers.

The Pap test and HPV test can be done at the same time. During a pelvic examination, the doctor or nurse uses a small brush to collect a few cells from the cervix for testing. This takes only a few seconds. The collected cells are sent to a laboratory for analysis.

HPV infections are very common and are usually suppressed by the immune system within 1 to 2 years without causing cancer. The National Cancer Institute (NCI) reports that it can take 10 to 20 years or more for a persistent infection with a high-risk HPV type to develop cancer.

Current guidelines are as follows:

- Women should have a Pap test every 3 years beginning at age 21.
- Women ages 30-65 should have Pap and HPV testing every 5 years or a Pap test alone every 3 years.
- Women with risk factors may need to have more frequent screening or continue screening beyond age 65.
- Women who have had the HPV vaccine still need regular screening.
- Women who have had a hysterectomy may still need to be screened.

If cellular changes are detected on the Pap test, often treatment can be done to prevent cervical cancer.

Information on the National Breast and Cervical Cancer Early Detection Program is available at www.cdc.gov/cancer/nbccedp.

Interpretation

If your doctor says that your Pap test was "normal" or "negative," that means that there were no signs of cervical cancer, pre-cancer, or significant abnormalities found in your cervical cell sample. If your Pap test result is reported as anything other than this, it means that some type of abnormality was found. The possibilities include abnormal areas of tissue, possibly related to a HPV infection or even cervical cancer. An abnormality will not always indicate cervical cancer. However, the presence of "abnormal cells" can increase your risk of developing cervical cancer in the future.

Many abnormalities found by a Pap test go away by themselves. Because of this, some women will be asked to return for a repeat Pap test in three to six months. However, you need to talk with your doctor about what your results could mean for you and what you should do next. Your doctor may recommend further testing and treatment to reduce the likelihood that you will develop cervical cancer.

The NCI uses a system called the Bethesda system of classifying Pap tests. Lab specialists use this system to report the lab results to your doctor. The report lets your doctor know if the cells were normal, abnormal, or if there was an infection present. If the cells were abnormal, they are put in categories, or typed, based on how severe the problem is:

- Cells that show minor changes but the cause is unknown may be typed as ASC-US (atypical squamous cells of undetermined significance), ASC-H (atypical squamous cells that cannot exclude high-grade squamous intraepithelial lesion), or AGC (atypical glandular cells).
- Cells that show definite minor changes but aren't likely to become cancer may be typed as LSIL (low-grade squamous intraepithelial lesions).
- Cell changes that are more severe and are more likely to become cancer may be typed as HSIL (high-grade squamous intraepithelial lesions).

Follow-up screening options may include:

- Repeat Pap tests.
- Colposcopy: Allows your doctor to examine your cervix with a magnifying instrument.
- Biopsy or endocervical curettage: A procedure where a curette (a spoon-shaped instrument) is used to scrape the mucous membrane of the endocervical canal (the passageway between the cervix and uterus). This procedure obtains a small tissue sample, which is then sent to a pathology lab to be examined for abnormal cells.

If treatment is necessary a surgical excision procedure, cryotherapy (freezing of the cells), or laser therapy may be done, to remove or destroy the abnormal tissue and reduce the risk of cancer.

Most women with cervical cell changes or pre-invasive cancer have no symptoms. Screening tests, therefore, are very important.

The HPV test is reported as "negative" or "positive."

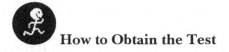 **How to Obtain the Test**

Pap and HPV tests are available at doctor's offices, medical clinics, and local health departments.

Do not do the following for 24 hours before the test: douche, have intercourse, take a bath, or use tampons. Showers are fine. Avoid scheduling your Pap test during your period (menstruation). Blood may make the Pap smear results less accurate. Tell your doctor if you might be pregnant.

A Pap test can be part of a routine gynecologic exam. During the exam a sample of cells from the cervix are collected. To perform a Pap or HVP test, your doctor will use a swab or small brush to collect samples of cervical cells from different areas of your cervix. These cells are sent to a laboratory where a technician examines them under a microscope for abnormalities. This procedure is sometimes referred to as a "Pap smear" because the cells obtained are "smeared" onto a glass slide to be examined under a microscope.

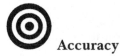 **Accuracy**

No test is 100% accurate, and it is possible for the Pap test to miss the presence of cancer. However, if abnormal cells are missed on one test, they are likely to be spotted during the next test. Generally, about 10 percent of Pap tests have abnormal results and only about 0.1 percent of the women who have these results actually have cancer. In most cases, abnormal cells are low grade and not likely to progress to cancer or are due to benign conditions, including natural cell changes after menopause.

 Cost

There are two costs involved in having a Pap and/or HPV test: the consultation with the doctor or nurse, and the Pap/HPV lab fee. Pap and HPV costs can vary based on the doctor.

The average rate can range from $50 – $250 without insurance for the tests and exam. Independently, the HPV test costs approximately $80 to $100 compared to $20 to $40 for Pap test. Many insurance plans cover a Pap and HPV test with an annual exam. Check with your provider for coverage and deductibles.

Medicare Part B covers Pap tests and pelvic exams once every 24 months for all women. As part of the exam, women at high risk for cervical or vaginal cancer, or who are of childbearing age with an abnormal Pap test in the past 36 months, are eligible for screening tests once every 12 months. Most states also provide coverage for testing through their Medicaid programs for low-income women.

The National Breast and Cervical Cancer Early Detection Program (NBCCEDP) provide free or low-cost mammograms and Pap tests to low-income women with little or no health insurance. Contact them through www.cdc.gov/cancer/nbccedp.

Process Time

Test results are usually reported in two to three weeks.

Benefits

- Pap tests done at regular intervals are very effective at detecting cervical cell changes before the changes become cancerous.
- Combining Pap and HPV testing improves detection rates.

Limitations

- False positives can lead to overtreatment of cervical cell changes that would never become cancerous.
- Routine screening is necessary due to the possibility of false negatives.

Confidentiality

Test results become part of your medical record.

Thoughts

The Pap smear has been in use since the 1940s to detect uterine and cervical cancer. Unlike mammograms and PSA screening tests, the Pap test has not been called into question as being plagued with a high rate of false results, or leading to too much unnecessary intervention. It is also free of radiation, dyes, or invasive procedures – it is simple. It is still considered a woman's gold standard for cancer screening.

Regular Pap and HPV tests are essential since they can spot abnormalities before they turn into cancer. Pap screening programs are attributed to the decline in the incidence of cervical cancer over the past 50 years. To protect your health, follow your doctor's recommendations regarding how often you should get tested. Cervical changes caught early can be easily treated and prevent the pain and expense of a late stage diagnosis. A Pap and or IIPV test can save your life.

References

National Cancer Institute. Cervical Cancer. Retrieved January 18, 2015 at: www.cancer.gov/cancertopics/pdq/genetics/colorectal/ healthprofessional. www.cancer.gov/cancertopics/types/cervical.

National Cancer Institute. Pap and HPV Testing. Retrieved January 15, 2015 at: www.cancer.gov/cancertopics/factsheet/detection/Pap-HPV-testing.

University of Maryland Medical Center. Retrieved January 2, 2015 at: www.umm.edu/health/medical/reports/articles/cervical-cancer#ixzz2qVoTNIJq.

CDC Website. National Breast and Cervical Cancer Early Detection Program (NBCCEDP). Retrieved January 29, 2015 at: www.cdc. gov/cancer/nbccedp/.

Chapter 16

Red Drop TK:
Thymidine Kinase Test

Red Drop TK Test
En Garde Labs
97 Mountain Way Drive
Orem, Utah 84058
Phone: 801-607-5096
www.en-garde.com/

The following information was provided by En Garde Labs.
Refer to their website for updates.

TEST

Summary and Explanation

The Red Drop TK test is a blood test for early cancer detection, and monitoring of treatment. It is patented and now available as a discrete, affordable blood test. Red Drop TK is a Swedish test which conforms to ISO certified technology. It is a valuable test for detecting cancer at its earliest stages, thereby increasing the chance of a better prognosis and effective treatment.

TK or thymidine kinase is an enzyme/functional protein that is common to all cells in your body which go through cell division. Most cancers have an increased rate of cellular division. TK levels increase when there is a rapid amount of cell division, thus providing a measurable indication of tumor growth. TK is responsible for DNA duplication during cell division and DNA repair. As cells become damaged or cancerous and multiply rapidly, the levels of TK in your blood increase.

Regularly monitoring TK levels in your blood can indicate when cancer is forming and provide an early detection tool. Changing TK levels can indicate whether your treatment is working, or give peace of mind when things are normal.

For the past 30 years, researchers from more than 30 countries have documented the direct correlation of TK levels to more than 18 different major categories of cancer. The evidence is clear and overwhelming – rising TK levels show a clear link to development and spread of cancer. The Red Drop Test website, www.reddrop.com/research, provides studies which show TK levels rising with cancer progression, decreasing with effective treatment, and low levels for those who are normal or in remission, including the majority of the common epithelial cancers. An epithelial cancer is one that begins in the cells that line an organ. These include:

- Breast cancer
- Lymphoma
- Myeloma
- Kidney cancer
- Thyroid cancer
- Cervical cancer
- Prostate cancer
- Non-Hodgkin's Lymphoma
- Colorectal cancer
- Ovarian cancer
- Head & neck cancers
- Esophageal cancer
- Lung cancer
- Leukemia
- Bladder cancer
- Melanoma
- Ovarian cancer
- Gastric cancer

The TK test cannot detect brain cancer due to presence of the blood brain barrier, or identify the specific type of cancer.

The Red Drop TK Test is licensed from Biovica, a bio-diagnostic company whose founder, Dr. Simon Gronowitz, has been at the forefront of TK research over the past 30 years. This highly sensitive and accurate test has been approved by regulatory authorities in Sweden and for use in the European Union. Further regulatory approvals are in process in other countries. The test has received CE and ISO certification, is patented in 40 countries, and is patent-pending in the USA.

Interpretation

Results are given as a score between 5 and 100,000. The higher the score, the more likely a cancer is present. The TK score is a measurement of thymidine kinase activity in the blood serum, which translates to a measure of the rate of cell division in the body, particularly in cells with some level of DNA damage.

Each type of cancer is quite different in terms of size, growth rates, aggressiveness, location, metastasis, etc. Some "wet" cancers such as lymphoma and leukemia have extremely high TK levels. Some solid tumors are small and grow at almost normal rates, so even a relatively low TK score could still be dangerous. Based on research of hundreds of people who are asymptomatic for cancer, Red Drop has established the following risk zones for "Normals" broken down by male and female.

Males
- 120 or higher would indicate a Severe Risk with the higher the score the higher the risk. TK scores that come back extremely high initially would be suspect for lymphoma or leukemia.
- 76 – 120 is High Risk.
- 41 – 75 is Elevated Risk.
- 21 – 40 is Moderate Risk.
- 20 or lower is Low Risk.

Females
- 120 or higher would indicate a Severe Risk with the higher the score the higher the risk. TK scores that come back extremely high initially would be suspect for lymphoma or leukemia.
- 66 – 120 is High Risk.
- 31 – 65 is Elevated Risk.
- 16 – 30 is Moderate Risk.
- 15 or lower is Low Risk.

Consistently rising TK scores indicate a need for further investigation and testing. Rising TK scores that your personal physician cannot explain, could mean that you are in a pre-cancerous phase where cells are being damaged or you could have early cancer cell development. In either case, this would be the time to be extra cautious with diet, exercise, and supplementation to see if you can proactively control the situation before it gets worse.

 How to Obtain the Test

Order at www.reddrop.com. The test can be ordered without a prescription or physician's order. You will be prompted to create your personal Red Drop account when you log in. The test kit will arrive in 3-5 days. Follow the instructions by going to a lab to have your blood drawn. The lab will have to spin the blood for 10 minutes to separate the serum from the blood cells. They will return your serum in the provided vial to you. The serum must remain cold. Use the provided ice packs and cooler. Return the serum sample via overnight FedEx to En Garde Labs in Utah. There is a kit instruction video available at www.youtube.com/myreddrop (www.youtube.com/watch?v=qUdgbbG5i5w). For questions call 801-607-5096.

Sample Test Result

Customer Name	Gender	Date of Birth	Risk Profile
Jenny Hrbacek, RN	F		

Last Collection Date	TK Score	Risk Level	Reference Intervals
Jul 31, 2013	16	Low risk	Female Reference Intervals
			Green - Low Risk 15 or under
			Yellow - Moderate Risk 16 - 30
			Orange - Elevated Risk 66 - 65
			Red - High Risk 66 - 120
			Purple - Severe Risk >120

 Accuracy

- Test is ultra-sensitive. A healthy person may have no TK detectable in their system. TK levels have been seen to rise in those with pre-cancer and through the various stages of cancer.
- At low levels of TK, accuracy is plus or minus 20 percent.
- At higher levels of TK, accuracy is plus or minus 2-3 percent.
- Factors other than a cancerous condition that may produce a high TK score: major wound healing, viral infections, and pernicious anemia (B12 deficiency).

Cost

The Red Drop TK Test is $299.95 plus shipping and handling. In addition, you will need to pay separately to have your blood drawn and prepared at a lab near you. That cost is typically $25-$50. At this time, insurance does not cover the cost of the Red Drop TK Test.

Process Time

After receiving the test kit it in the mail and returning it to Red Drop, you can expect an email in approximately 10 days, notifying you that your results have been posted to your account at www.reddrop.com. Log back in to retrieve your score. You will need to remember the user name and password you created when the test was ordered.

Benefits

- Useful as a wellness profile.
- A good early detection tool.
- Used to indicate progression or regression of disease.
- Indicates amount of cancer growth activity in relation to the TK score.
- Active form of TK that is measured has a short half-life so the test can be repeated weekly to monitor cancer or rapid cell growth activity.
- Red Drop reports that the test can indicate the aggressiveness of cancer; i.e., breast cancer score over 135 and up is aggressive.
- Remission can be confirmed and monitored.

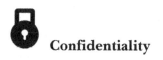

Limitations

- Does not diagnose cancer. High TK scores indicate that cancer is a possibility and should be further investigated.
- Requires additional testing to confirm and locate a possible cancer that is indicated by the score.
- Rare false positives can occur and be reported as higher scores. Reasons for this are injury healing, viral infection, or pernicious anemia.
- The TK score in and of itself can't help with the identification of origin site of any possible malignancy, except possibly for lymphoma of leukemia which report extremely high scores.
- Not covered as a diagnostic test under insurance, however, it may be covered under your wellness benefit.

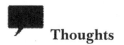

Confidentiality

Results are sent directly to the patients' personal Red Drop account that was created when the test was ordered. Accounts are password protected.

Additional Information

Red Drop recommends periodic re-testing to develop a baseline and monitor health status. See www.redddrop.com for recommendations.

Thoughts

The Red Drop TK1 test is a simple blood test that is private, convenient, and easily accessible without a physician's order. Even though it does not provide a definitive cancer diagnosis, it is a valuable monitoring tool that gives you an indication of the presence of rapid cell growth that is common with most cancers.

It is one of the more affordable tests presented in this book. Monitoring your TK1 levels can prove valuable to uncovering a potential problem early.

References

References are available at www.reddrop.com under the TK Research tab.

Chapter 17

Research Genetic Cancer Center Lab Tests

Circulating Tumor Count (CTC) Testing
Chemo Sensitivity and Resistance Testing
Natural Substance Sensitivity Testing
Immunity Test Panels
Metastasis Marker Tests

Research Genetic Cancer Center, R.G.C.C., U.S.A., LLC
Branch office for the USA, North America, Canada
3105 Main Street
Rowlett, Texas 75088
214-299-9449
Email: info@rgccusa.com

This information was provided by Research Genetic Cancer Center, R.G.C.C., U.S.A., LLC. Check their website for updates.

TEST

Summary and Explanation

Research Genetic Cancer Center (R.G.C.C.) is a world class laboratory that specializes in cancer genetics and circulating tumor cell counts. The lab is composed of the most advanced and innovative technologies focusing on molecular oncology. R.G.C.C. offers several different tests that are used for:

- The early detection and diagnosis of new cancers (years before most cancers would be detected).
- Monitoring of existing cancers.
- Prognosis – providing information about the risk of recurrence of a current or previous cancer.
- Development of a personalized cancer treatment plan geared to achieve the best treatment outcome.
- Blending the very best of alternative and traditional therapies.

Unlike other tests discussed that identify factors in the blood when cancer is present, the R.G.C.C. lab has a very sensitive test that allows it to isolate and count circulating tumor cells (CTCs) in a blood sample – these are cancer cells that have broken away from the primary tumor and have entered the blood stream.

R.G.C.C. prefers blood sample for testing, however, the testing can be done with tumor tissue samples as well. Once cancerous tumor cells are circulating freely in the body, they have the potential to generate metastatic disease. R.G.C.C. has a proprietary technology that allows it to remove CTCs from a blood sample and grow them in the laboratory for further testing. This brings the tested substances into direct contact with each individual's own isolated cancer cells, not just a few cells from biopsied material. The lab also evaluates genetic markers (72 tumor related genes) on the tumor cells to predict outcomes of treatments and prognosis. R.G.C.C. can provide the following information:

- A count of circulating tumor cells present in the blood, which may indicate tumor burden.
- Identification of several specific types of cancer. Approximately 95 percent of the time when markers are positive, they can identify melanoma and sarcoma cancers and the site of origin for kidney and prostate cancers.
- Chemosensitivity testing – Identification of chemotherapy drugs that demonstrate the most effective kill rate to a person's individual cancer cells.
- Identification of chemo-resistance – Identification of chemotherapy drugs that will not be as effective for treatment.
- Assessment of natural substances and plant extracts for potency against the cancer patient's isolated CTCs. Mechanisms of action and percentages of effectiveness are included.
- Identification of immunity factors and metastatic risk.
- Tests for all cancers with circulating CTCs and cancer stem cells (CSCs). Not effective for the brain and central nervous system cancers.
- Data on how an individual will react to specific chemotherapy agents. An individual's genetic makeup

determines whether they are "accumulators" or "rapid metabolizers" of certain drugs. This can play a critical role in determining how effective a specific drug treatment is likely to be, and how significant the side effects will be.

- Tests 72 tumor related genes and four resistant factors that can be used by the physician to determine the nature and aggressiveness of the cancer.
- Identification of specific markers on the tumor cells to assist the physician in forming a targeted approach.

R.G.C.C. International was established in 2004 by Ioannis Papasotiriou, M.D., Ph.D. Dr. Papasotiriou worked in the department of Experimental Physiology and Biochemistry in the Medical School of Thessaloniki in Greece. R.G.C.C. is a growing, innovative, and pioneering company in the area of chemosensitivity/chemo-resistance testing with branches and representatives all over the world. The company's headquarters are in Switzerland with laboratories located in Northern Greece. Branch offices are in the U.S.A., United Kingdom, Germany, Cyprus, Hungary, and Australia.

 Interpretation

Results are presented in a written report that your doctor can use to help guide your treatment options and choices. This test requires an experienced clinician to fully interpret the results. For ease of understanding, sensitivity results are presented in graph form.

If the submitted blood sample is negative for CTCs, no further testing can be done. The patient has a good prognosis as no cancers cells were detected.

How to Obtain the Test

- Call R.G.C.C.-U.S.A. Branch Office at 214-299-9449 to schedule an appointment for a consultation and testing.

Callers can also be directed to a registered network practitioner in their area.
- More information and sample tests can be located at www. rgccusa.com. Email info@rgccusa.com with questions.
- Payments can be made online. They accept credit cards and payments are made in Euros. Euro to dollar conversion rate is calculated at time of payment.
- R.G.C.C. recommends that patients with active CTCs re-test with an ONCOCOUNT (CTC count) every 3 - 6 months to monitor disease and effectiveness of treatment. Check with your ordering physician for specific recommendations.

Accuracy

R.G.C.C., Ltd. of Greece in April 2012 received international validation from the Hellenic Accreditation System S. A. (Accreditation Certificate No. 860). The lab is accredited for the following methods:

- CTC/CSC isolation and immunophenotyping.
- Cancer cell culture viability/cytotoxicity assays after exposure to substances.
- Gene expression assays.

Cost

The fees below are for laboratory work only. They do not include physician consultation and test interpretation.

- ONCOCOUNT: CTC count only; 550 euros (about $670 - $742 USD).*
  This test only provides the number of CTCs in the provided blood sample and does not provide any other information.
  See Sample Test Result #1

* See www.usforex.com/currency-converter for current conversion estimations.

- ONCOTRACE: CTC count and immunophenotype; 650 euros.
  This test provides the number of CTCs in the provided blood sample and an index of cell markers for all types of cancers.
  See Sample Test Result #2

- ONCOTRAIL: CTC count in the provided blood sample and an index of markers for a specific cancers; 625 euros. Available for breast, prostate, colon, melanoma, lung, sarcoma, gastrointestinal cancers.
  This is a tailor made test for the specific type of malignancies. This test includes relevant markers and is used as a tool for follow up control.
  See Sample Test Result #3

- ONCOSTAT: CTC count and chemosensitivity for cytotoxic drugs; 1600 euros.
  This test includes a CTC count in the provided blood sample and a chemosensitivity/chemo-resistance assessment for cytotoxic drugs. New drugs are added periodically. As of 2014 the list is:

Alkylating Agents
ACNU – Nimustine
BCNU – Carmustine
Bendamustine – Treanda
Bleomycin – Blenoxane
Carboplatin – Paraplatin
CCNU – Lomustine
Chlorambucil – Leukeran
Cisplatin – Platinol
Cyclophosphamide – Cytoxan
DTIC
Estramustine – Emcyt
Hydroxyurea – Droxia/Hydrea
Ifosfamide – Ifex
Melphalan – Alkeran
Mitomycin – Mitomycin C
Nedaplatin – Aqupla

Oxaliplatin – Eloxatin
Procarbazine – Matulane
Temozolomide – Temodar
Treosulfan
Trofosfamide – Ixoten

Epothilones
Ixabepilone – Ixempra

Inhibitors of Topoisomerase I
CPT11 – Irinotecan
Gimatecan
Topotecan – Hycamtin

Inhibitors of Topoisomerase II
Amrubicin-Hydrochloride – Calsed
Dactinomycin – Cosmegen
Daunorubicin – Cerubidine
Doxorubicin – Adriamycin
Epirubicin – Pharmorubicin
Etoposide – Vepesid
Idarubicin – Idamycin
Liposomal Doxorubicin – Doxil
Mitoxantrone – Novantrone

Nucleus Spindle Stabilizer I
Abraxane – Paclitaxel
Cabazitaxel – Jevtana
Docetaxel – Taxotere
Eribulin – Halaven
Paclitaxel – Taxol

Nucleus Spindle Stabilizer II
Vinblastine – Velban
Vincristine – Oncovin
Vinorelbine – Navelbine

Nucleoside Analogues
5FU – 5-Fluorouracil
Capecitabine – Xeloda
Cytarabine – cytosine arabinoside
Fludarabine – Fludara
FUDR – Floxuridine
Gemcitabine – Gemzar
MTX – Methotrexate
Pemetrexed – Alimta
Raltitrexed – Tomudex
UFT – Uracil – Tegafur

- ONCOSTAT EXTRACTS: CTC count, and sensitivity for natural substances; 1400 euros.
  This test includes the assessment of natural substances and plant extracts for potency against cancer patients isolated CTCs. New substances can and are added periodically.
  As of 2014 the list of 46 natural substances tested on every patient is:

AHCC (Active Hexose Correlated Compound)
Amygdalin (B-17, Laetrile)
Anvirzel™ Oleander Extract
Arabinoglactan
Aromat8-PN™
Artecin®
Artemisinin
Ascorbic Acid (Intravenous)
Bio Ae Mulsion Forte®
Bio-D-Mulsion®
Cellular Vitality
Cruciferous Complete
C-Statin
Curcuma Sorb (formally MERIVA®)
CV247
DCA (dichloroacetate)
Dextrol
Epimune Complex
Fermented Soy Extract
Fucoidan
Genistein
Indo 3 Carbinol
Intenzyme Forte™
Lycopene
Mammary PMG®
Melatonin
Metformin
Mistletoe
Naltrexone
Nrf2 Activator™
NuMedica Minellized D3®
OPC Synergy™
Paw-Paw
PME (poly mannose extract from aloe vera)
POLY-MVA®
Proteo-Xyme™
Quercetin

Retenzyme Forte®
Resveratrol
Salicinium™
Salvestrol
Superoxide Dismutase
Thymex®
Ukrain
Virxcan™
Vitanox®

Results give the percentage of effectiveness for each substance. Substances are added yearly, and those that no longer show efficacy are deleted. See the website www.rgccusa.com for the most recently tested agents.

- ONCOSTAT PLUS: 1900 euros.
  This is R.G.C.C.'s most comprehensive test. It includes everything in the ONCOSTAT and ONCOSTAT EXTRACTS, plus the following:

  Resistance Factors
  MDR1
  MRP
  LRP
  GST

  Biological Modifiers Tested
  5-Azacytidine – Vidaza
  Abiraterone – Zytiga
  Alemtuzumab – Campath
  Anastrozole – Arimidex
  Bevacizumab – Avastin
  Bortezomib – Velcade
  Brentuximab Vedotin – Adcetris
  Catumaxomab – Removab
  Cetuximab (225) – Erbitux
  Crizotinib – Xalkori
  Dasatinib – Spryce
  Erlotinib – Tarceva
  Everolimus – Afinitor, Zortess
  Fulvestrant – Faslodex
  Gefitinib – Iressa
  Gemtuzumab Ozogaminic – Mylotarg
  Goserelin – Zoladex

Ibritumomab – Zevalin
Imatinib-Mesylate – Gleevec
Lapatinib – Tykerb
Leuprolide – Eligard, Lupron Depot
Nilotinib – Tasigna
Octreotide – Sandostatin
Ofatumumab – Arzerra
Olaparib – AZD-2281
Panitumumab – Vectibix
Pazopanib – Votrient
Pertuzumab – Perjeta
Rituximab – Rituxan
Semaxanib – SU5416
Sorafenib – Nexavar
Sunitinib – Sutent
Tamoxifen
Tositumomab – Bexxar
Trabectedin – Yomdelis
Trastuzumab – Herceptin
Vandetanib – Caprelsa
Vemurafenib – Zelboraf
Vorinostat – Zolinza

Tumor Related Genes – Growth Factors & Proliferation Stimuli
SS-r
Progesterone Receptor
Estrogen Receptor
p180
COX2
5-LOX
NFkB
IkB(a,b,c)
EGF
Ras/Raf/MEK/Erk
mTOR
c-erb-B1
c-erb-B2
Bcr-abl
ALK
EML-4-ALK
NPM-ALK
CD 117(c-kit)
RET
IGF-r 1
IGF-r-2
NR3C4-A Testosterone receptors
NR3C4-B DHT receptors

Self-repair Resistance
HSP 27
HSP 72
HSP 90
Gamma GC (gene for drug resistance)
DNA Methyltransterase-1
DNA Demethylase
06-METHYL-DNA-TRAN
TGF-b (transforming growth factor-beta)
Histone deacylase dipeptide
HDAC
HAT

Angiogenesis
VEGF (vascular endothelial growth factor
FGF (fibroblast growth factor)
PDGF (platelet derived growth factor)
ANG 1
ANG 2

Cell Cycle Regulation & Immortalization/Apoptosis
E2F1
P27 (gene of the cycle-dependent kinase inhibit
P53 (gene; DNA gene guardian)
P16 (tumor suppressor gene; stops tumor cell death)
BCL-2
H-TERT Human Telomerase M2

Angiogenesis-Metastasis
KISS-1-r
Nm23 nonmetastatic gene 23
MMP (matrix metalloproteinase)
c-MET

Drug Metabolisms & Targets
CES1&2 carboxyesterase
DPD dihydropyrimidine dehydrogenase
UP Uridine phosphorylase
NP Nucleoside phosphorylase
TP (thymidine phosphorylase)
TS
DHFR (dihydrofolate reductase)
SHMT serine Hydroxymethyl- transferase)
GARFT
RIBO-Nucleoside Reductase
CypB1
ERCC1
RRMI

Markers
CD33 Myeloid Cell Origin
CD52 Leukemia Marker
CD20 Lymphoma Related Antigen
EPCAM Epithelial Marker

Sample Test # 1 ONCOCOUNT

R.G.C.C.-RESEARCH GENETIC CANCER CENTRE LTD

Florina, __ / __ / 2013

Dear Colleague,

We send you the results from the analysis on a patient Ms/Mr_____ suffering from _____ carcinoma stage _____. The sample of 20ml of whole blood that contained EDTA-Ca as anti-coagulant, and packed with an ice pack .

In our laboratory we made the following:

• We isolated the malignant cells using Oncoquick with a membrane that isolates malignant cells from normal cells after centrifugation and positive and negative selection using multiple cell markers .

The results during the isolation procedure are presented below :

Table of markers:

CD45 positive cells (Hematologic origin cells)		CD45 negative cells (non Hematologic origin)	
CD34	NEGATIVE	CD133	POSITIVE
		CD44	NEGATIVE

Index of marker: CD45: Hematologic origin cell marker, CD133, CD44: tumor stem cell marker, CD34: hematological stem cell and blast cell marker, epithelioid sarcoma marker.

Conclusion: We notice that after isolation procedure there are remaining malignant cells. The concentration of these cells was _____ cells/ml, SD +/- 0.3cells.

Sincerely,

Ioannis Papasotiriou M.D., PhD
Head of molecular medicine dpt of
R.G.C.C.-RESEARCH GENETIC CANCER CENTRE LTD

Index of circulating cells number: (upper limit : progress of disease, lower than limit: beginning of disease or stable of disease when the patient is on treatment plan)
Breast cancer: 5cell/7.5ml , Prostate cancer 20cells/ml , Sarcoma: 15cells/6.5ml,Colon cancer: 5cells/ml, Lung cancer (Lc=0, r=0.99): 10cell/ml

*This test will NOT DETECT cancers of the brain or other cancers that have been "encapsulated" by the body, not releasing circulating tumor or stem cells (CTC, CSC) into the blood stream or if any of these cells are dormant. We still recommend the use of known blood markers and/or various scans with this test when cancer is suspected or known to exist. No test is 100% accurate

Ms/Mr _____
ADDRESS : Florina-GR P.O. 53070
TEL : +30-24630-42264 , FAX: +30-24630-42265
Web site : www.rgcc-genlab.com E-mail :Papasotiriou.ioannis@rgcc-genlab.com

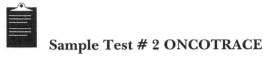

Sample Test # 2 ONCOTRACE

R.G.C.C.-RESEARCH GENETIC CANCER CENTRE LTD

Florina, __/ __ /2013

Dear Colleague,

We send you the results from the analysis on a patient Ms/Mr _____ suffering from _____ carcinoma stage _____. The sample of 25ml of whole blood that contained EDTA-Ca as anti-coagulant, and packed with an ice pack .

In our laboratory we made the following:

* We isolated the malignant cells using Oncoquick with a membrane that isolates malignant cells from normal cells after centrifugation and positive and negative selection using multiple cell markers .

The results during the isolation procedure are presented below :

Table of markers:

CD45 positive cells (Hematologic origin cells)		CD45 negative cells (non Hematologic origin)	
CD15	NEGATIVE	CD34	NEGATIVE
CD30	NEGATIVE	CD99	NEGATIVE
BCR-ABL	NEGATIVE	EpCam	POSITIVE
CD34	NEGATIVE	VHL mut	NEGATIVE
CD19	NEGATIVE	CD133	POSITIVE
		CD44	POSITIVE
		Nanog	POSITIVE
		OKT-4	NEGATIVE
		Sox-2	POSITIVE
		PSMA	NEGATIVE
		c-MET	NEGATIVE
		CD31	NEGATIVE
		CD19	NEGATIVE
		MUC-1	NEGATIVE
		CD63	NEGATIVE
		panCK	POSITIVE

Index of marker: CD45:Hematologic origin cell marker, BCR-ABL, CD30, CD15: hematologic malignancy marker , CD133, Sox-2, OKT-4, Nanog, CD44: tumor stem cell marker, CD19: lung cancer cell marker (NSCLC), CD31: endothelial cell membrane antigen, CD34: hematological stem cell and blast cell marker, epithelioid sarcoma marker, CD63: melanoma cell marker, CD99: sarcoma marker, EpCam: epithelial origin marker, MUC-1: lung cancer cell marker (SCLC), PSMA: prostate specific cancer stem cell membrane antigen, VHL mut: renal carcinoma marker, c-MET: membrane antigen that regulates the mesenchymal to epithelial transition, panCK: epithelial origin cell marker .

Conclusion: We notice that after isolation procedure there are remaining malignant cells. The concentration of these cells was ___cells/ml, SD +/- 0.3cells.

Sincerely,

Ioannis Papasotiriou M.D., PhD
Head of molecular medicine dpt of
R.G.C.C.-RESEARCH GENETIC CANCER CENTRE LTD

Index of circulating cells number: (upper limit: progress of disease, lower than limit: beginning of disease or stable of disease when the patient is on treatment plan)

Breast cancer: 5cell/7.5ml , Prostate cancer 20cells/ml, Sarcoma: 15cells/6.5ml, Colon cancer: 5cells/ml, Lung cancer (Lc=0, r=0.99): 10cell/ml.

*This test will NOT DETECT cancers of the brain or other cancers that have been "encapsulated" by the body, not releasing circulating tumor or stem cells (CTC, CSC) into the blood stream or if any of these cells are dormant. We still recommend the use of biopsy, blood markers and/or various scans with this test when cancer is suspected or known to exist. No test is 100% accurate .

Ms/Mr _____
ADDRESS : Florina-GR P.O. 53070
TEL : +30-24630-42264 , FAX: +30-24630-42265
Web site : www.rgcc-genlab.com E-mail :Papasotiriou.ioannis@rgcc-genlab.com

Sample Test # 3 ONCOTRAIL - Breast Cancer

R.G.C.C.-RESEARCH GENETIC CANCER CENTRE LTD

Florina , __ / __ /2013

Dear Colleague,

We send you the results from the analysis on a patient Ms _____ suffering from breast stage ___.
The sample of __ml of whole blood that contained EDTA-Ca as anti-coagulant, and packed with an ice pack .

In our laboratory we made the following:
- We isolated the malignant cells using Oncoquick with a membrane that isolates malignant cells from normal cells after centrifugation and positive and negative selection using multiple cell markers .

The results during the isolation procedure are presented below:

Table of markers:

CD45 positive cells (Hematologic origin cells)		CD45 negative cells (non Hematologic origin)	
NANOG	NEGATIVE	NANOG	POSITIVE
OKT-4	NEGATIVE	OKT-4	POSITIVE
SOX-2	NEGATIVE	SOX-2	NEGATIVE
		MUC-1	POSITIVE
		EPCAM	POSITIVE
		CD133	POSITIVE
		C-MET	NEGATIVE
		CD31	NEGATIVE
		CD44	POSITIVE
		PANCK	POSITIVE

Index of marker: CD45: Hematologic origin cell marker, Nanog: tumor stem cell marker, OKT-4: tumor stem cell marker, Sox-2: tumor stem cell marker, MUC-1: Breast cancer cell membrane antigen, EpCam: Epithelial origin marker, CD133: tumor stem cell marker, c-MET: membrane antigen that regulates the mesenchymal to epithelial transistion, CD31: endothelial cell membrane antigen, CD44: Hematologic origin cell marker, PanCK: epithelial origin marker.

Conclusion: We notice that after isolation procedure there are remaining malignant cells. The concentration of these cells was __cells/7.5ml, SD +/- 0.3cells.

Sincerely,

Ioannis Papasotiriou M.D., PhD
Head of molecular medicine dpt of
R.G.C.C.-RESEARCH GENETIC CANCER CENTRE LTD

Index of circulating cells number: (upper limit : progress of disease, lower than limit: beginning of disease or stable of disease when the patient is on treatment plan)
Breast cancer: 5cell/7.5ml , Prostate cancer 20cells/ml , Sarcoma: 15cells/6.5ml, Colon cancer: 5cells/ml, Lung cancer (Lc=0, r=0.99): 10cell/ml.

*This test will NOT DETECT cancers of the brain or other cancers that have been "encapsulated" by the body, not releasing circulating tumor or stem cells (CTC, CSC) into the blood stream or if any of these cells are dormant. We still recommend the use of biopsy, blood markers and/or various scans with this test when cancer is suspected or known to exist. No test is 100% accurate

Ms _____
ADDRESS : Florina-GR P.O. 53070
TEL. : +30-24630-42264 , FAX: +30-24630-42266 Web site: www.rgcc-genlab.com E-mail :papasotiriou.ioannis@rgcc-genlab.com

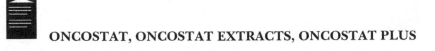

ONCOSTAT, ONCOSTAT EXTRACTS, ONCOSTAT PLUS

These three test results involve far too many pages to attempt to reproduce here. Please see www.rgccusa.com for the sample test results. They are presented in easy-to-read charts.

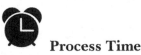

Process Time

Results take approximately two weeks and are emailed directly to the ordering practitioner.

Benefits

- CTCs can be detected long before cancer will be seen on a scan – this is early detection. Cancer cells often invade the blood stream when the tumor size is only 1-2mm or about 1/4 to 1/2 the size of a BB pellet.
- Number of CTCs has shown to be directly related to disease progression/regression in most cases.
- If CTCs are present, a personalized cancer treatment plan can be developed using the ONCOSTAT PLUS Test.
- R.G.C.C. has a proprietary process that allows them to grow trillions of isolated cancer cells in a calf serum culture for sensitivity testing. This process keeps the identical genetic, epigenetic, and phenotype of the patient's cancer stem cells.
- Drugs and natural substances are tested by direct contact with the patient's tumors cells, unlike predictive genomic tests where there is no contact between the cancer cells and tested substance. Remember all testing is done in triplicate, never single or double, as this assures unquestionable accuracy.

- Gives percentages of effectiveness or resistance for each tested drug and nutrient.
- Money and energy can be focused on substances that are the most effective.
- R.G.C.C. can provide the patient with a list of the most effective chemo agents and natural substances for their particular cancer. In the traditional setting, the patient would not be able to find out if a different chemotherapy would be more potent or effective at killing their cancer cells. (For example, a patient with breast cancer may be more effectively treated with a drug for prostate or even colon cancer).

LIMITATIONS

Limitations

- Cannot identify brain or central nervous system cancers because of the blood/brain barrier. Actual tissue samples of a brain tumor must be provided to the lab for testing.
- Cannot identify tumors that are encapsulated.
- The sensitivity tests for drugs and nutrients should be repeated every 1-3 years. This must be done to allow for changes due to genetic mutations that cancer cells make during replication and growth. For example, substances or drugs that were effective on the individual's original test may no longer be effective.
- Not every practitioner is trained to interpret the results, but the number is growing. As of late 2014, there are approximately 350 doctors using this test in the United States, Canada, and North Central America. Others are using this worldwide now.
- Most conventional U.S. oncologists are not familiar with this test and can dismiss the test results/recommendations unlike Europe where this test is more widely used and accepted.
- Cost can be a limiting factor; this test is not currently covered by insurance.

Confidentiality

The results are presented in a written report and become part of your medical record.

A Note from
Ray Hammon, D.C., N.M.D., D.C.B.C.N

My Personal Experience with RGCC Cancer Testing

Over the past 11 years I have been using the R.G.C.C. Ltd. cancer test for all of our cancer patients and screening those who want to know if they have cancer. At this time I have 36 years of experience in private clinical practice. We have performed well over 1,000 R.G.C.C. tests during these years. During the past 3 years our branch, R.G.C.C. USA (serving the U.S., Canada, and North Central America), has overseen many hundreds more tests administered by more than 425 health care providers serving this region. We have worked with more than 30 different types of cancers as of January 2015.

It never ceases to amaze me how different each test result is. Results from the same types of cancers, even amongst family members, will yield different results. I can accurately say that the results of every test are at least 30-60% different from every other. This is what really makes the R.G.C.C. cancer test in a league of its own. I have yet to see any test that gives this much diverse and useful information about every individual as this one, and I have looked at many over these years.

This is the very reason our results for most of the patients we have worked with have approximately a ≥ 35% survival/stabilization rate. This is not just by looking at the tumor shrinkage only, but the CTCs/CSCs that are responsible for 95%+ of all metastases, which are responsible for 90%+ of all cancer related deaths. I feel it is crucial to target more than just the tumor. Circulating tumor and stem cells must be addressed. The testing provided by R.G.C.C. allows the health care provider to offer the cancer patient a true, unmatched Personalized Cancer Care. It has also allowed me to give my patients many options and design a program just for them. My outlook on treating cancer has changed. I now feel that cancer can be managed much like other chronic diseases utilizing this vast amount of accurate, scientific, and patient specific information.

I am privileged to have been associated with R.G.C.C. Ltd. and Dr. Papasotiriou for 11 years and to have been the first clinic on this continent to use this test. For the past 4 years we have owned and operated R.G.C.C. USA. Our responsibilities are many to the health care providers of the USA, Canada, and North Central America. It is my pleasure to be a part in assisting patients and their physicians to learn about the many benefits that R.G.C.C. Ltd. of Greece has to offer. I truly believe that R.G.C.C. has met the challenge and passed the test by providing the testing necessary to develop a **Personalized Cancer Care Program**.

I can assure everyone we have learned a great deal from Dr. Papasotiriou regarding his testing procedures, the accuracy, the technology, and the clinical application of this test. It is a continued pleasure to share these years of experience with those who want to learn a better way to care and support cancer patients. I share in the opinion of many patients and colleagues around the world that R.G.C.C. is the very best world class laboratory in the field of oncology testing and development.

Dr. Papasotiriou is one of the very few true scientists I have known in my lifetime and the only one whom I have had the pleasure of working with. I can speak highly of his integrity, knowledge, humility, desire for accurate scientific methods, and complete dedication to his work.

"Discovery consists of seeing what everyone has seen and thinking what nobody else has thought."

– Albert Szent-Gyorgyi

Sincerely,

Ray Hammon, D.C., N.M.D., D.C.B.C.N.
Integrative & Functional Health Center
Rowlett, Texas, USA

■◤ Thoughts

Unlike other tests that identify factors in the blood that may indicate the presence of cancer, the basic ONCOCOUNT test isolates and counts circulating tumor cells that are present in the blood sample submitted. These cells are important because they often lead to a metastatic recurrence. Unlike other labs that require a tumor sample to do chemo and nutrient sensitivity testing, this is a blood test. This test is sensitive enough to pick up circulating tumor cells before they can form a tumor large enough to be seen on a scan.

NOTE: A positive test result can be alarming because it may be the first time you have been told you have cancer. Standard oncology methods of testing are not as sensitive. This is why this kind of early detection test is so valuable – it allows you to intervene years before you might have otherwise.

If the ONCOCOUNT/CTC is "0," there is a low probability that the patient has cancer. A "0" also can confirm that any prior cancer treatment has been effective. However, I recommend that this test be used on an annual basis to monitor for a possible increase in CTCs and for early detection. Utilizing the testing for natural substances is financially beneficial because you can focus on taking only the substances that have the highest percentage of effectiveness and the chemosensitivity testing will identify the most effective chemotherapy drugs for the tested sample.

Please understand that chemotherapy is a treatment, not a cure, and is toxic to both healthy and cancerous cells. I included in Treatment Options and Complementary Therapies chapter information about insulin potentiated therapy (IPT), a low dose, less toxic, method of giving a 10-20 percent dose of standard chemotherapy. Many practitioners using IPT are using the R.G.C.C. chemo sensitivity panel to identify the most effective chemo drugs for IPT.

It is important to note that R.G.C.C. may find CTCs years before the primary tumor can be seen on a PET scan. This is true early detection. An integrative physician can then be consulted to help you implement therapies to reverse, halt, or slow the cancer growth. This test is money well spent. It is my hope that the CTC test offered by R.G.C.C. will become the standard for early detection.

Part 2

Tests to Detect Cancer:

Non-Early Detection

The focus of this book is to inform the reader
of early detection testing options for cancer.
In this chapter, we present two tests we feel are
worthy of discussion, even though they are not
generally utilized for early detection of cancer.

(Prices for tests subject to change.)

208

Chapter 18

Biofocus Tests

Detection of Circulating Tumor Cells
Chemotherapeutic Drugs and
Alternative/Natural Agents Sensitivity Tests
Immune CELLULAR NK Test

Biofocus®
www.Biofocus.de
Biofocus Gesellschaft für biologische Analytik mbH
Berghäuser Str. 295
45659 Recklinghausen
Germany
Phone: +49 2361 3000-130
Please call from 7:00 am – 5:00 pm GMT
Fax: +49 2361 3000-162
EMAIL for Dr. L. Prix: prix@biofocus.de

The following information was obtained from
www.Biofocus.de and by the staff at Biofocus.
(The Biofocus website has an icon that can be utilized to view the content in English).

TEST

Summary and Explanation

Biofocus® is a laboratory located in Recklinghausen, Germany that specializes in molecular detection of circulating tumor cells in the blood stream. It uses a proprietary technique to isolate these cells. Results are based on measurements of gene expression in the enriched circulating tumor cells.

Biofocus's Institute for Laboratory Medicine is under the direction of Dr. Doris Bachg and Dr. Uwe Haselhorst. The results are presented by email in English to the ordering practitioner and can be used as a guide for treatment option and choices.

The test requires that a blood sample be sent to Biofocus.

- The Biofocus test is a CTC detection test and does not provide a numerical value of the cancer cells or CTCs present in the blood. It gives a "yes" or "no" answer as to whether CTCs are present, but if "yes" there is no measurement of how much.
- This test is preferably used for monitoring of patients with known cancer. Not necessarily an early diagnostic test.
- Useful in monitoring response to therapy.
- Provides information about the risk of recurrence.
- Used for development of a targeted, patient-specific therapy utilizing the identification of chemotherapy drug targets that demonstrate the best response to an individual's cancer cell based on the predicted genetic expression of the cell, also known as chemo-sensitivity testing.
- Identifies drug resistances to aid in the selection of appropriate therapies.
- Utilized to assess the effectiveness of natural/alternative substances thru the genetic expression of the cancer patient's isolated CTCs.
- Identifies immune activating agents.
- On average, Biofocus detection rates for CTCs in advanced stage carcinoma are 80%.
- The test is used for different types of cancer. Not recommended for central nervous system/brain tumors due to the blood brain barrier and because these tumors rarely shed cells into the blood stream.
- Limited detection rates (40% – 50%) in soft tissue sarcomas (except synovial sarcoma).
- Test is not suitable for T-cell lymphomas. Acceptable for B-cell lymphomas.
- Results take approximately 2 weeks.

Biofocus offers the following four different tests examining the identified gene expression on the isolated CTCs. An additional 60 Euros is charged to cover shipping costs. Biofocus accepts Visa, MasterCard, and American Express.

- Test option #1: Molecular detection of circulating tumor cells (CTCs) in blood. (490 Euros)
- Test option #2: Molecular detection of circulating tumor cells (CTCs) in blood plus testing for use of chemotherapeutic drugs and alternative/natural agents. (1890 Euros)
- Test option #3: Molecular detection of circulating tumor cells (CTCs) in blood plus testing for use of alternative/natural agents in conjunction with standard chemotherapy. Identifies the most effective alternative/natural substances. (1330 Euros)
- Test option #4: Immune Function Testing by the CELLULAR NK (natural killer) test. This test identifies immune system stimulators that aid the immune system in the breakdown of the tumor cell. (190 Euros)

Thoughts

The Biofocus CTC test is very useful for detecting the presence of circulating tumor cells in the blood. Unlike other tests, you do not have to send a tumor sample for the test to be done. This makes the test very attractive for those not wanting to have a biopsy or surgery.

I originally thought this test included a numerical value for the number of CTCs in the tested blood sample. However, I found this not to be the case. Dr. Lothar prix at Biofocus told me:

It is possible for us to correlate these figures with an absolute count of tumor cells. There may be fewer cells expressing the gene strongly, or more cells expressing weaker. So, comparing between different individuals is not possible, but follow up testing in the same individual may find indications for rise or fall of tumor cell burden.

With that said, my research does indicate that obtaining a CTC count is valuable because increasing or decreasing counts can provide a tool for evaluating treatment and disease progression or regression. I feel that this test falls a bit short because no CTC count is given and the results are based on predicted genetic expression and not the actual reaction of physically bringing the isolated CTCs in direct contact with the test drug or natural substance.

I like this test because it does examine both chemo and natural substances sensitivities; Biofocus is one of a handful of labs in the world that realize the efficacy of using natural substances to treat cancer and I applaud them for their work in this area.

Chapter 19

CELLSEARCH

Circulating Tumor Cell Test

CELLSEARCH®
Janssen Diagnostics, LLC (Formerly Veridex Corporation)
700 US Highway Route 202 South
Raritan, NJ 08869 USA
www.cellsearchctc.com
877-837-4339 or 585-453-3240
Email: JDxMedicalAffairs@its.jnj.com

The following information was obtained from representatives of CELLSEARCH and from www.cellsearchctc.com. Janssen Diagnostics is a part of the Johnson & Johnson Corporation.

TEST

Summary and Explanation

The CELLSEARCH® CTC test is the first and only clinically validated, FDA-cleared blood test for enumerating or counting circulating tumor cells (CTCs) in patients with metastatic breast, colorectal, and prostate cancer. The CELLSEARCH CTC test acts as a real-time liquid biopsy that predicts prognosis at any time during a patient's course of treatment.

The test requires a blood sample that is sent to a registered CELLSEARCH lab for analysis.

- The CELLSEARCH test has not been identified as an early detection test.
- The test is used in the conventional oncology setting as a supplemental test.
- It is used in the assessment of disease status in conjunction with laboratory analysis, imaging, biopsies, or other standard methods of monitoring known cancer.

- Is used to identify changes in disease status based on predictive prognosis at any time during cancer treatment.
- It increases the predictive accuracy of prognosis when other clinical parameters are conflicting.
- The test is available at several labs around the U.S. including Quest Diagnostics and LabCorp.
- The cost of the test may be covered by insurance. If insurance is not used, the cash price from Quest Diagnostics (as of January 2015) is $746.30 for one test – either breast, colon, or prostate.

Clinical studies have demonstrated that the number of circulating tumor cells (CTCs) correlates to disease prognosis and can provide an important marker for assessing patients' status throughout the continuum of treatment.

Thoughts

The information on CELLSEARCH is included because this is presently the only FDA approved circulating tumor cell (CTC) count test available from a lab located within the U.S. This is the test that you will likely receive if a recurrence of cancer is suspected in the conventional treatment setting.

CELLSEARCH does not promote this test as early detection because the test will only detect metastatic cancer of the breast, colon and prostrate.

The confusion begins when a patient is told that their CTC from CELLSEARCH is "Zero." This can lead to a misunderstanding of their condition. They may still have cancer, just not enough cancer for this particular test's ability to pick it up. I recommend that you look into a more sensitive test such as the "ONCOCOUNT" test provided by R.G.C.C. labs, because it can detect cancer at its earliest stages and long before it has metastasized to other organs.

References
Provided By the Company

Cristofanilli M, Hayes DF, Budd GT, et al. Circulating tumor cells: a novel prognostic factor for newly diagnosed metastatic breast cancer. *J Clin Oncol.* 2005; 23(7):1420-1430.

de Bono JS, Scher HI, Montgomery RB, et al. Circulating tumor cells predict survival benefit from treatment in metastatic castration-resistant prostate cancer. *Clin Cancer Re*s. 2008 Oct 1; 14(19):6302-6309. doi: 10.1158/1078-0432.CCR-08-0872.

Cohen SJ, Punt CJA, Iannotti N, et al. Relationship of circulating tumor cells to tumor response, progression-free survival, and overall survival in patients with metastatic colorectal cancer. *J Clin Oncol.* 2008; 26(19):3213-3221.

Henry NL, Hayes DF. Uses and abuses of tumor markers in the diagnosis, monitoring, and treatment of primary and metastatic breast cancer. *Oncologist.* 2006; 11(6):541-552.

Monteil J, Mahmoudi N, Leobon S, et al. Chemotherapy response evaluation in metastatic colorectal cancer with FDG PET/CT and CT scans. *Anticancer Res.* 2009 Jul; 29(7):2563-2568.

Metser U, You J, McSweeney J, Freeman M, Hendler A. Assessment of tumor recurrence in patients with colorectal cancer and elevated carcinoembryonic antigen level: FDG PET/CT versus contrast-enhanced 64-MDCT of the chest and abdomen. *AJR Am J Roentgenol.* 2010 Mar; 194(3):766-771.

Lee DK, Park JH, Kim JH, et al. Progression of prostate cancer despite an extremely low serum level of prostate-specific antigen. *Korean J Urol.* 2010 May; 51(5):358-361.

Part 3

Functional Tests:

Providing Early Warning Signs

Chapter 20

Biological Dental Exam

Screening For Heavy Metals, Infection, Energy Blockages

TEST

Summary and Explanation

A biological dentist office is a fluoride-free, mercury-free, and mercury-safe environment. It should utilize individual testing for the biocompatibility of dental materials to be used with each patient.

Years of traditional dental work can leave a person with a mouth full of toxic metals, unsuspected sites of infection deep in the bone, and interrupted flow of the body's natural energy pathways. The complex relationships of oral and systemic health within the whole person are inseparable.

Biological medicine considers the health of the whole body to determine the cause of disease, instead of just treating symptoms. This approach focuses on restoring the body to equilibrium, thereby ending symptoms and optimizing health. Foreign objects in the month will often set the body up for a chronic inflammatory response. Dental issues in the mouth are often reflected elsewhere in the body and vice versa. Poor oral health can compromise and distract the immune system from looking for cancer cells.

Conventional medicine has largely ignored the relationship of the mouth to the rest of the body; however, there are three important areas to assess:

Heavy Metal Toxicity

Amalgam or silver fillings contain about 50 percent mercury plus other toxic metals. A large filling may contain as much mercury as a thermometer. Mercury vaporizes easily at room temperature, and in this state it is odorless and tasteless. This vapor can be inhaled and easily absorbed into the bloodstream. Mercury is a powerful neurotoxin. Research demonstrates that mercury is more toxic than lead and arsenic, therefore no amount of mercury exposure should be considered harmless.

In 2001, the U.S. National Health and Nutrition Examination survey of 31,000 adults, NHANES III, found that the number of dental fillings correlated to the incidence of cancer, mental conditions, thyroid conditions, neurological issues (including multiple sclerosis), diseases of the respiratory system, and diseases of the eye.[1] A 2005 German risk assessment study of mercury from dental amalgams found it may lead to nephrotoxicity, neurobehavioural changes, autoimmunity, oxidative stress, autism, skin and mucosa alterations, Alzheimer's disease or multiple sclerosis, and that "removal of dental amalgam leads to permanent improvement of various chronic complaints in a relevant number of patients in various trials."[2] Amalgam risk assessments conducted in 1995, 2010, and 2012 by Dr. G. Mark Richardson, an expert to the European Union's Scientific Committee on Health and Environmental Risks, revealed that toxic levels of mercury were released from dental fillings.

The American Dental Association's position is that there is no scientific evidence validating the harmful health effects of dental mercury fillings. The International Academy of Oral Medicine and Toxicology (IAOMT), however, has catalogued hundreds of scientific studies dating back over a century demonstrating that mercury in dental fillings is hazardous to human health.[3] As long as the ADA tenaciously holds to its position, it will be at odds to the growing body of science, and the desire of growing numbers of people to relegate mercury fillings to history. Norway, Sweden, and Denmark have banned the use of amalgam fillings for environmental and health reasons.

Mercury fillings that have remained in a person's mouth for many years have an accumulative effect. Mercury is able to bind with cellular DNA and interfere with the cells' function. It is also absorbed by the roots of the teeth as well as the surrounding bone and adjacent gum tissue. Symptoms of chronic metal intoxication include numbness, fatigue, joint pain, and headaches. Mercury has also been associated with a number of emotional and psychological problems, such as memory loss, mood swings, anxiety, and depression, to name a few.

Blood testing for mercury is usually non-conclusive because the mercury quickly binds to the tissues and organs and will no longer be circulating freely in the blood. The better method is a urine test where a physician administers a chelating agent (an agent that binds metals) followed by a urine collection for several hours. A laboratory will analyze the sample for mercury and other heavy metal levels.

Nickel is another metal commonly used in crowns and bridges. It is known to cause cancer, birth defects, and suppress the immune system. Thomas Rau, M.D., of the Paracelsus Clinic in Switzerland, conducted research on 150 women with breast cancer. He found that 147 (98 percent) of them had a root canal on a tooth related to the breast meridian. Just as energy flows thru the meridians, Dr. Rau's research demonstrated that mercury also flows to organs on the related meridians. He did this by testing mercury levels in breast cancer tumor tissue and found that the tumors contained high levels of the toxin. For more information on his work, see www.drrausway.com.

Infection or Cavitation Assessment
A chronic infection of a tooth may cause a person no readily identifiable symptoms. Acute and chronic infections create disruptions on the entire energy meridian and can affect the related organs. Even placing a crown on a tooth can leave the tooth no way to breathe or detoxify. This many times leads to chronic degeneration.

Root canals are the only case in modern medicine where a dead body part is left in the body. The problem with root canals is the inability to achieve a complete, long-lasting seal around the dead root (periodontal ligament) left in the canal. Your teeth are living organisms that are connected to the rest of your body with over 3 miles of tubules, canals in each tooth from which toxic bacteria can chronically drip into the body. These tubules are not fed by the blood supply, so antibiotics cannot reach them. Sealing a dead tooth creates an incubator for chronic infection to fester inside these tubules.

Cavitations can also be a problem. A cavitation is the empty space that remains after a tooth has been pulled. It is a hidden pocket of infection deep in the jaw bone that harbors infection and leads to bone loss. Cavitations are not visible by X-ray until there is about 30 percent bone loss. A biological dentist can use special detection scans and X-rays to assess for cavitations, clean them out, and reseal them. Experience tells us it is particularly difficult even for biological dentists to successfully rid a cavitation site of infection.

Another area of infection is in the gums. This can develop into periodontal disease involving both the gums and the bone supporting the teeth. It is estimated that 50 percent of adults have some form of periodontal disease.

Electrical/Energy Blockages

The tooth-body connection is based on the science behind the 12 meridians (energy pathways) that are a vital component of the body's electrical structure. When looking at a meridian tooth chart, you can locate the organs that correspond with each of the 32 teeth.

The body is an environment composed of both chemical and electrical fields. Think of how the chemistry of alcohol, for example, affects the brain. Then think of how nerve endings use electrical charges to fire in the brain. Our cells conduct the electrical charges created by our central nervous system. A compromised electrical system results in faulty communications throughout the body.

Dawn Ewing, Ph.D. and Director of the International Academy of Biological Dentistry and Medicine, uses the example of an electrocardiograph (EKG) to explain how the body uses electricity: During the EKG procedure, sticky pads are put on the patient's, chest, arms and legs. Electricity is introduced and an image of where the infarcted (dead) tissue is located after a heart attack is produced because electricity will not pass thru dead tissue. Oral conditions such as dead teeth, infections, and jaw bone deterioration likewise can interfere with energy flow. A test called a Meridian Stress Assessment (MSA), or electrodermal oral screening, can be used to measure the body's current state of health by looking at energy flow and levels. A MSA is used to determine where and to what degree energy is excessive, lacking, or blocked. The test is done in a medical or dental office by a specially trained dentist or integrative physician. It uses no needles, just electrodes.

Some integrative physicians believe patients with cancer and other chronic illness will not make significant advances in their health until dental issues are resolved; they ask patients to make that a first priority. The metal toxicity and chronic infections interfere with the ability of most other healing efforts you might initiate.

How to Obtain the Test

Locate a Biological Dentist:

- Contact the International Academy of Biological Dentistry and Medicine at www.iabdm.org or 281-651-1745
- Contact the International Academy of Oral Medicine Toxicology at www.iaomt.org or 407-298-2450
- Price-Pottenger Nutrition Foundation at www.ppnf.org or 800-366-3748 (U.S.) or 619-462-7600

Heavy Metal Toxicity Test:

- To get tested, find a local integrative physician or naturopath

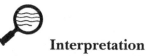

Interpretation

The information you receive as a result of the electrodermal testing and a thorough biological exam will be interpreted individually, as well as with all components of the body.

Digital X-rays should be utilized as they use approximately 80 percent less radiation than conventional films. They produce a computer generated image that provides greater contrast and enables the dentist to enlarge hard-to-see areas.

As with most test interpretation, the skill level of the interpreter is very important.

Test results for the heavy metal toxicity test are given in numerical values indicating the level of toxicity.

Cost

The cost for a new patient with a biological dentist will vary. The visit should include a comprehensive oral exam, digital X-rays, and materials compatibility testing. Most appointments last approximately 2 hours and include an in-depth discussion of your dental situation and care. We found prices ranging from no charge for an initial consult to $400 for a complete first visit and assessment.

Oral meridian stress assessment testing is approximately $150.

Heavy metal toxicity testing varies in price. Sometimes an office visit is required plus laboratory fees for the urine challenge test. Some doctors use hair analysis for toxicity testing.

The cost of a biological dental exam may be covered on your dental insurance and the charges for heavy metal removal may be approved by your health insurance, so check with your providers.

Process Time

- A dental exam by a biological dentist can usually be completed in one visit.
- Heavy metal toxicity testing takes several hours for urine collection and the specimen must be sent to a lab for processing. Results are usually received in 2 weeks.
- Meridian Stress Assessment lasts about an hour and checks burdens stemming from root canals, crowns, fillings, and cavitations (extraction sites). It requires a current panorex, an X-ray showing a full view of the oral cavity, less than 90 days old with no dental work having been done in the interim. Results are immediate.

BENEFITS

Benefits

- A complete dental evaluation including aspects of the whole person's health are considered and addressed.
- Improvement in overall health with the discovery and treatments of unrecognized dental toxins and hidden dental infection.
- Dental work can be completed with the use of biocompatibility dental materials thus reducing the potential for immune reactions to the materials utilized, which could create health problems.
- Energy blockages can be identified and addressed.

LIMITATIONS

Limitations

Thorough research must be conducted by the patient to insure that the biological dentist is trained to address important issues of toxicity, safe removal of amalgams, biocompatibility of dental materials, hidden infections, and energy blockages. Not all biological dentists offer all of these services.

Confidentiality

Tests ordered by a dentist will become part of their/your dental record.

Thoughts

It is time for the patient's total health to be considered. During your yearly physical, your general practitioner will listen to your lungs and heart, but very rarely does he look at your gums and teeth, or consider the impact of mercury fillings, or the occasional flare up of bleeding and sore gums. Biological dentists are trained to recognize the impact oral health and understand how it relates to your physiological health. It's time to stop isolating body parts and look at them as components that make up who we are as a whole.

A healthy body will try to reject dead or dying teeth and that presents a strain on the immune system. This process produces a stressed and weakened body. Addressing oral issues can be a big factor in halting the progression of disease, removing blocks to healing, and restoring health.

It is becoming an accepted suspicion that root canals and oral cavitations are associated with breast cancer. Look into it yourself.

Remember, insurance companies are in business to make money. So don't retreat if your insurance will not pay for biological dentistry work, the investment is worth it. Find a good biological dentist for you and your family. Better yet, only use a biological dentist and prevent the need for clean-up work later.

I will finish with the words of John Parks Trowbridge, M.D.:[*]

> The deep, dark secret in modern dentistry is that people get relief from their immediate pain but get sicker and sicker and sicker because of the toxic metals and chemicals their dentists have poured into their mouths. Dentists reassure patients that "there's nothing wrong" when, indeed, the answers are there to be found by professionals using the advanced techniques and treatments of the NEW dentistry.

> Lest you misunderstand that I'm talking about discomforts and problems in your mouth, let me assure you that I'm talking from the perspective of a "wholistic" physician, taking care of the "whole patient." Ours is an era of devastating diseases that relentlessly claim the comfort and independence of their victims – diseases such as diabetes, heart disease, hardening of the arteries, liver failure, MS (multiple sclerosis), myasthenia gravis and so on. A startling number of these problems can improve dramatically – beyond a patient's fondest dreams –

when enlightened medical and dental practitioners team up to remove toxic metals and chemicals, remove unsuspected sites of infection, restore nutritional balance and employ advanced techniques of "biological dentistry."

* Taken from the forward of Dr. Dawn Ewing's book, *Let the Tooth Be Known* (2012). Ewing is a Doctor of Integrative Medicine in Spring, Texas. The book is available as a download at www.drdawn.net. Dr. Trowbridge has served as president or director of professional organizations including the American College for Advancement in Medicine, the International College of Integrative Medicine, the American Board of Clinical Metal Toxicology, the International Academy of Biological Dentistry and Medicine, and the American Preventive Medical Association, among others. His practice is in Humble, Texas.

References

1 NHANES III Screening – 35,000 Americans. Raw data retrived January 30, 2015 at: www.flcv.com/NHanes3.html.

2 Mutter J; Naumann J, et al. Amalgam: Eine Risikobewertung unter Berücksichtigung der neuen Literatur bis 2005" [Amalgam risk assessment with coverage of references up to 2005]. *Gesundheitswesen* (Bundesverband der Arzte des Offentlichen Gesundheitsdienstes (Germany). 2005 Mar; 67(3):204-216. English abstract Retrieved January 30, 2015 at: www.ncbi.nlm. nih.gov/pubmed/15789284.

3 Press release April 2, 2013. International Academy of Oral Medicine and Toxicology Challenges ADA's Claim that Mercury Fillings Are Safe. Retrieved January 12, 2015 at: www.prnewswire. com/news-releases/international-academy-of-oral-medicine-and-toxicology-challenges-adas-claim-that-mercury-fillings-are-safe-201014311.html.

Chapter 21

Biological Impedance Analysis

TEST

Summary and Explanation

Biological impedance analysis, or bio-electrical impedance analysis (BIA), is a method of assessing your body composition, meaning the measurement of body fat in relation to lean body mass. This test measures fat, muscle, bone, and water and is extremely important because it paints a different picture than the number on your bathroom scale. It is an integral part of a health and nutrition assessment.

Research has shown that body composition is directly related to health. A normal balance of body fat is associated with good health. Excess fat in relation to lean body mass can greatly increase your risk for disease. A BIA allows for early detection of an improper balance in your body composition, which signals the need for intervention and prevention.

This is a non-invasive test that involves the placement of electrodes on the right hand and right foot. A low level, unnoticeable, electrical current is sent through the body. The flow of the current is affected by the amount of water in the body. The device measures how this signal is impeded through different types of tissue. Tissues that contain large amounts of fluid and electrolytes, such as blood and lean tissue, have high conductivity, but fat and bone are low in fluids and slow the signal down. The BIA determines the resistance to flow of the current as it passes through the body. This measurement is used to provide several estimates relating to the volume of body water.

For example one measurement that is calculated is the "phase angle." It is a measurement that relates to the body's overall health and can be a predictor of outcome and indicate the course of disease. Phase angle is based on total body resistance and reactance. Lower phase angles appear to be consistent with either cell death or a breakdown of the cell membrane. Higher phase angles appear to be consistent with large quantities of intact cell membranes and body cell mass.

All living substances have a phase angle. In fresh uncooked vegetables, the phase angle can exceed 45. In cooked vegetables, the phase angle is 0 because they are dead. As you get older, phase angles will decrease and will be approximately four or less at the time of death. Fit adolescents may have a phase angle greater than 10.

Low phase angles are consistent with:

- Malnutrition.
- Infection.
- Chronic disease.
- Cancer.
- Sedentary lifestyle.
- Chronic alcoholism.
- Old age (over 75).

 How to Obtain the Test

BIA testing is offered by many allopathic and nutritionally minded natural practitioners. Check with your local medical community to find a center offering this test.

The procedure is quite simple. You will be asked to remove your shoes and socks. Electrodes will be placed on your right hand and on your right foot. Once the lead wires are hooked up to the electrodes, the test only takes a few seconds and the BIA data will be input into a computer.

Prior to the test:

- All metal jewelry should be removed.
- Empty your pockets and remove any heavy clothing.
- Avoid exercise or other activity that would make you sweat at least 8 hours before your test.

- Avoid caffeine or alcohol in large quantities12 hours before the test.
- Go to the bathroom to get rid of any waste products.

NOTE: Measuring under consistent conditions (proper hydration and at the same time of day) gives the best results. The test should be done within a few minutes of lying down, as there is evidence that impedance values rise sharply after a few minutes of lying on your back.

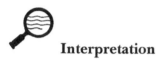 **Interpretation**

BIA measures the impedance or resistance to the electrical signal as it travels through the water that is found in muscle and fat. The more muscle a person has, the more water their body can hold. The greater the amount of water in a person's body, the easier it is for the current to pass through it. The greater the amount of body fat, the more resistance is recorded by the current. Resistance produces inferior results. Results are gender specific.

BIA provides the following key measurements:

- Fat Free Mass % – This is the percentage of the body that is not fat. This represents metabolically active tissue of muscles, bones, cartilage, organs, and blood.
- Fat % – This is the percentage of the body weight that is fat.
- Total Body Water – The complete volume of fluids in the body.
- Intracellular Water – This is the amount of water volume inside the cell. Healthy cells maintain their integrity and hold their fluid inside. Low levels can indicate poor health.
- Extracellular Water – Amount of water volume outside of the cell. Higher values may be related to fluid retention, toxicity, allergies, stress, poor absorption, or insulin resistance.

- Phase angle – Energy production from working cells indicating cellular health. This level is associated with aging. Higher values indicate good health and lower values indicate acute or chronic illness.
- Basic Metabolic Rate – This number represents the number of calories burned at a normal resting state over a 24 hour period. It represents the amount of energy that your body requires to perform its most basic functions.

Accuracy

Studies show that BIA is quite variable at providing estimated body composition measurements; however factors such as dehydration and previous exercise must be taken into consideration.

Cost

Average cost is $40 - $50.

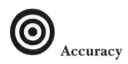

Process Time

The test takes only a few minutes. A report is generated immediately after the test.

Benefits

- A fast, accurate, and safe way to measure six key body composition elements.
- Measures long-term changes in body composition.
- An effective tool in measuring progress.

- Identifies if the body is functioning properly, aging well, or has an increased risk of illness.
- Measurements can be utilized to create an effective, personalized program to improve your health status, thereby assisting you to maintaining function, productivity, immunity, physical performance, and longevity.

Limitations

- If a person is dehydrated, the amount of fat will likely be overestimated. Hydration can be effected by the failure to drink enough water, hormonal changes, food, caffeine or alcohol consumption, strenuous exercise, stress or illness, or taking prescription drugs.
- It does not take into account the location of body fat.
- Cannot diagnose any specific disease.
- People with pacemakers are not candidates for this test.
- BIA is not recommended for competitive athletes, body builders, pregnant or lactating women.

Confidentiality

Results become part of your medical record.

Thoughts

BIA can be a good tool to assess your current state of health. Deficiencies found can be utilized as early detection and interventions can be made. Improving your BIA measurement, or maintaining a healthy BIA, can help aid your body and support proper body functions and reduced your risk to illness.

I recommend that the personalized nutrition and exercise plan that is offered as a result of a weak BIA test be taken very seriously and followed. Cancer patients almost always have a weak BIA.

If you get a poor or less than desirable result, implement good nutrition and consistent exercise and IMPROVE YOUR SCORE!

Reference

Dehghan M, Merchant AT. Is bioelectrical impedance accurate for use in large epidemiological studies? *Nutrition Journal.* 2008 July; 7:26.

Chapter 22

Biological Terrain Assessment

TEST

Summary and Explanation

A biological terrain assessment (BTA) analyzes small amounts of blood, urine, and saliva to provide data about the current state of the building blocks of the body. BTA was invented by Louis-Claude Vincent, professor of hydrology, and has been utilized since 1946. His method allows the practitioner to take a broad-spectrum view of the body chemistry beyond specific symptoms that a patient may have.

The BTA process itself is simple, quick and noninvasive. Blood, saliva, and urine samples are taken, tested, and analyzed by a computer. The results show which biological systems are in good shape and which are vulnerable, weakened or compromised. This information leads to the implementation of specific therapies to improve the terrain, and thereby support the body's innate ability to maintain health and fight disease.

The following components are included:

* Acid/Alkaline pH Challenge Test
* Adrenal Stress Urine Test
* Calcium Urine Test
* ChemStrip Urine Test
* Free Radical/Oxidata Urine Test
* Vitamin C Urine Test
* Zinc Taste Test

A skilled practitioner has the ability to pick up pre-pathological changes in the body that predispose one to infections, as well as many chronic diseases. BTA is a powerful health screening instrument that provides valuable biochemical information about cellular function and cellular metabolism in the tissues, organs, and systems of the body. This includes such data as oxygen transport, nutrient delivery, waste removal, mineral retention, cellular absorption, and multiple metabolic chemical interactions. More specifically, it measures the acid/base balance, the degree of oxidative stress, and the concentration of minerals in the body fluids.

The goal of a BTA is to gain a deeper understanding of the in-depth elements within the patient's chemistry and prescribe the exact forms of treatment to help the patients regain and maintain a healthy internal biochemical environment.

A BTA provides a wealth of information about the state of the body's cells, organs, and biochemical balance including:

- Level of acidity of the cells and fluids of the body.
- Blood alkalinity as a compensation for tissue acidity.
- Tendency of the blood to thicken and become sticky.
- Ability of the kidneys to excrete acids and other waste products.
- Ability of the cells to produce energy.
- Free radical activity in the body.
- Mineral deficiencies or excesses in the body.
- Digestive enzyme deficiency or efficiency.
- Sufficient anti-oxidants in the body.
- Liver toxicity.
- Lymphatic congestion.
- Heavy metal toxicity.
- Dehydration.
- Immune system breakdown.
- Tendency towards degenerative disease.

Also, results can be compared with known norms and an estimation of your biological age as opposed to your chronological age can be made.

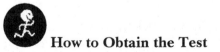 **How to Obtain the Test**

BTA testing is offered by many allopathic and nutritionally minded practitioners. Check with your local medical community to find a center offering this test.

The procedure is quite simple, you may be asked to follow a few simple instructions prior to testing:

- 3 Days prior to testing – stop taking all alkalinizing agents.
- 2 Days prior to testing – stop taking vitamins supplements. Continue life-supporting medicines (heart, blood pressure, or diabetes medications).
- Fast for 12-14 hours. Complete your dinner prior to your test no later than 7 PM the night before. After dinner, brush your teeth. Then refrain from eating or drinking anything until after your test. Refrain from using any toothpaste, mouthwash, or mouth rinses both at bedtime and on the morning of your test. Also avoid using any lipstick or makeup around your mouth and lips. Such substances can change the chemistry of the mouth and saliva.
- On the morning of your test, obtain a sample of your first morning urine. Try to obtain a mid-stream specimen.

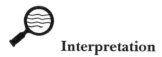 **Interpretation**

All values are then analyzed and plotted by computer software onto a report that contains graphs and charts. The data are then assessed by the practitioner and used as a teaching guide to share with the patient.

All three bodily fluids are analyzed. The saliva measurements reflect liver function very well, since most of the saliva is lymph, and most lymph is produced in the liver. Urine measurements reflect how well the kidneys are functioning, since the kidneys filter the blood. Whatever is in the first morning urine should represent overages in the body. The blood measurements are good indicators of cell function throughout the body.

The following are explanations of each sub-test:

- Acid/Alkaline PH Challenge Test – Acid-alkaline balance is extremely important. When pH is not in balance, enzymatic reactions slow down and oxygen delivery to the cells is impaired. Pathogens such as viruses, bacteria, and yeast can grow more readily. Also, cancer tends to prefer an acidic, oxygen-deprived environment. This test is used to monitor mineral reserves that the body uses to maintain pH. These minerals are needed by virtually every cell enzyme activity. Each enzyme reaction requires mineral co-factors for optimum efficiency. The degree of adaptability of the body's alkaline buffer system reflects the state of mineral reserves. Results can indicate potential adrenal stress, cell rigidity, and organ problems.

- Adrenal Stress Urine Test – The adrenal stress urine test measures chloride displacement in the urine. Minerals such as sodium, potassium, and magnesium – all bound to chloride – are displaced due to high tissue and serum acidity (> H+ ions). High acidity is the result of a hyper-stimulated sympathetic system, which directly stimulates the adrenals. Results can help determine the degree of adrenal weakness, energy output, kidney dysfunction, stress levels, and probable magnesium, potassium, and calcium deficiencies.

- Calcium Urine Test – The calcium test measures calcium in the urine. Calcium is the most abundant mineral in the body. It is important because it plays a role in heart and muscle contraction, nerve impulse conduction, neurotransmitters and their enzymes activation, blood pressure regulation, blood clotting, hormone production, energy metabolism, saliva production, and more.

- ChemStrip Urine Test – The chemstrip urine test is a simple dip-stick urine test that screens for gross pathology in 13 categories of screening: color, transparency, odor, specific gravity, pH, leukocytes, nitrites, protein, glucose, keytones, urobilinogen, bilirubin, and blood.

- Free Radical/Oxidata Urine Test – The free radical urine tests looks for molecules that have an uncoupled electron. This uncoupling occurs as a by-product of normal metabolic reactions and xeno-toxic reactions (foreign to the body). Many chronic diseases are implicated with free radical damage.

- Vitamin C Urine Test – Vitamin C in the urine is assessed in this test. The role of vitamin C is now well established. It is involved in literally hundreds of biological processes in the body. The following is a partial list of vitamin C's most important functions:

  o Essential to production of collagen and connective tissue.
  o Provides support and protection of blood vessels, bones, joints, organs and muscles, eyes, teeth, ligament, cartilage and skin.
  o Essential to antibody production.
  o Increases white blood cell activity.
  o Essential to the manufacture of neurotransmitters, particularly the conversion of tryptophan to serotonin, and of tyrosine to dopamine and adrenaline.
  o Protects against high blood pressure.
  o Appears to reduce the risk of cancer, particularly esophageal, larynx, stomach, colon, and lung.
  o High levels of vitamin C reduces the risk of cataracts and the oxidation stress of diabetes.
  o Vitamin C, when combined with bioflavonoids, reduces histamine reactions.
  o Important to the transport of iron across the cell membranes.

- Zinc Taste Test – Zinc is essential to the production of hydrochloric acid (necessary for digestion), antibodies, white blood cells, and thymus hormonal function. It provides nutritional support for teeth, bones, nails, hair and skin, and it produces carbonic anhydrase, the primary enzyme for the conjugation of CO_2. Zinc is essential to the conversion of linoleic acid (LA) to gamma linolenic acid (GLA) and is involved with metabolism of the testes, pituitary, thyroid, and adrenal glands. It is also an essential co-factor in the production of seminal fluid. Many people tested are zinc insufficient.

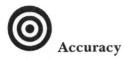

Accuracy

BTA produces estimated ranges and results. Practitioners use the full body of data collected to compile a diagnostic picture. Locate a practitioner who is skilled in BTA testing and interpretation, and implements it into their practice.

Cost

Prices can vary, usually around $150.

Process Time

A BTA can be performed in one office visit and results are generated at the time of the test.

BENEFITS

Benefits

- Estimates the overall health and strength or weakness of the body.
- Where abnormalities are found the system will suggest possible causes and suggest remedial action to be taken.
- Test data can impart objective analytical guideposts about the function of the lymphatic and liver systems, the kidneys, and the blood itself.
- Provides objective data to determine if a course of treatment is supporting or hindering progress.

Limitations

Does not diagnose any specific illness.

Confidentiality

Results become part of your medical record.

Thoughts

When you know how the chemistry of your body is functioning, you can make lifestyle adjustments that support improvements in your health. Information obtained from a BTA provides valuable guidelines for the treatment of illness and the maintenance of health. Each of the tested chemical levels translates to the vitality and health to every cell, tissue, organ and gland.

Implementing steps to improve bodily functions will make it much easier to heal from cancer or to prevent disease. In particular, the oxidation-reduction values indicate the state of oxygen in the body and we know that cancer cells are aerobic (do not use oxygen). So get proactive, increase your oxygen levels, and irritate those cancer cells!

Chapter 23

C-Reactive Protein (CRP) Test

Inflammation Test

TEST

Summary and Explanation

A C-reactive protein (CRP) test is a blood test that measures the amount of this particular protein in your blood. This protein is produced by the liver and measurements provide a gauge of the levels of inflammation in the body. Conditions such as cancer, arthritis, lupus, inflammatory bowel disease, or an infection can cause elevated CRP. Chronically elevated inflammation causes damage to the body. The test does not show where the inflammation is located or indicate the cause. Other tests are needed to find the cause and location of the inflammation. C-reactive protein levels are often higher in people who have recently had a heart attack.

The *Journal of Clinical Oncology* reported in 2009 the following study results:

Elevated levels of CRP in cancer-free individuals are associated with increased risk of cancer of any type, of lung cancer, and possibly of colorectal cancer. Moreover, elevated levels of baseline CRP associate with early death after a diagnosis of any cancer, particularly in patients without metastases.[1]

Once a high level is documented, repeated testing can be used to monitor the body's response to treatment to see if what you are doing is actually lowering CRP levels.

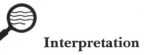

 Interpretation

Normal results should fall within the following range: 0 – 1.0 mg/dL or less than 10 mg/L, increasing slightly with age.

Normal value ranges may vary slightly among different laboratories.

 How to Obtain the Test

The C-reactive protein test is a simple blood test and it is available at most laboratories. You can eat and drink normally before the test. Tell your doctor all of the medicines you are taking, because some medicines can affect the results. For insurance reimbursement, a doctor's order is usually required.

Direct to consumer lab testing is available at www.requestatest.com. This lab offers a C-reactive protein (CRP) quantitative test. To order the test, log onto the site and create a user name and password. You will be given a secure profile in which to view your results when available.

Sample Test Result

TEST	RESULT	FLAG	UNITS	REFERENCE INTERVAL
C-Reactive Protein, Quant	1.1		mg/L	0.0 - 4.9

 Cost

Medicare and insurance usually cover the test when ordered by a physician. Check with your provider.

The best direct-to-consumer price found was at www. requestatest.com for $59.

Process Time

Results are usually available with 24 – 48 hours.

Benefits

- Elevated levels may indicate the need for further testing and investigation.
- Once an evaluated CRP is detected, exercise, diet, medications, and supplements may be used to decrease the level.

Limitations

- Any condition that results in sudden or severe inflammation may increase your CRP levels.
- Do not have the test if you have just exercised, have an infection, have an intrauterine device (IUD), had a recent heart attack, or if you are pregnant. These may alter the tests accuracy. Also, positive CRP results will occur during the last half of pregnancy or with the use of birth control pills (oral contraceptives).

Confidentiality

Tests ordered by a physician will become part of your medical record. Tests ordered from a direct to consumer lab will be reported to you.

Thoughts

Given that higher CRP levels are associated with decreased cancer survival, reducing CRP levels in cancer patients is very important to improving outcomes. I had an elevated CRP level and was able to reduce it with diet, anti-inflammatory supplements, and aerobic exercise. Checking your CRP may seem like a small detail, but I encourage you to use every tool necessary to be cancer free.

Reference

1   Allin KH, Bojesen SE, Nordestgaard BG. Baseline C-reactive Protein Is Associated With Incident Cancer and Survival in Patients With Cancer. *J Clin Oncol*. 2009 May 1; 27(13):2217-2224.

Chapter 24

Dark Field Microscopy

Live Blood Cell Analysis

TEST

Summary and Explanation

Hippocrates believed that bodily fluids were an important factor concerning health and that disease would manifest in these fluids. History has proven him to be correct, and we know that the blood plays a central role in the overall health of every person. Whole human blood consists of red blood cells, white blood cells, and platelets that float in plasma, a straw-colored liquid made up of about 90 percent water. The plasma also contains electrolytes, proteins, nutrients, hormones, and other substances.

When technicians and doctors send your blood work off to the lab, the technician will be looking at dead blood cells. Heat or chemical fixatives preserve the sample for examination. A small sample is smeared onto a slide, stained, and then observed under the light of a microscope. Images stand out against a bright, white background. A traditional blood analysis is often looking for chemical composition and cell counts.

Dark field microscopy is the only way to observe *live* blood cells. It is often referred to as a "live blood cell analysis." A freshly-drawn, live blood sample is put on a slide and put under a dark-field microscope where it is magnified, viewed through a sideways beam of light, and projected onto a computer screen. The dark field microscope allows nearly invisible microorganisms within the blood to be "lit up" and stand out against a contrasting dark field.

A live blood analysis sees the blood in motion and is typically used to view the interaction of live blood cells with other factors such as fibrin, spirochetes, viruses, and elements of the immune system.

The examination usually includes a CD of the live blood visualized on the computer screen.

How to Obtain the Test

You may find it challenging to locate doctors who use this technique. The FDA does not approve of dark field microscopic blood analysis; therefore, insurance does not cover it. Dark-field microscopy is an accepted tool, but it is considered an "unestablished" laboratory test.

Some doctors offering it believe that it falls within the scope of their license to practice medicine and it should not be regulated under the 1988 Clinical Laboratory Improvement Amendments (CLIA), since the "conventional" lab group feels threatened by dark field analysis.[1] It would be a bit like having chiropractors or acupuncturists regulated by medical doctors who typically do not have the training or disposition to appreciate the other techniques.

Dark field microscopic blood analyses are offered by many allopathic and nutritionally minded practitioners. Check with your local medical community to find a center offering this test.

Prior to the test:

- Fast for 4 hours prior to the analysis.
- Drink water during the fasting period as you need to be well hydrated for an accurate analysis.
- Continue prescription medications.
- Schedule your appointment for at least 3 hours after taking supplements.

It is recommended that you wait for a period of one month before your appointment if you have had any of the following: ultrasound, mammogram, MRI, CAT scan, bone scan, X-ray, flu shots, vaccinations, or anesthetic.

Sample Test Result

The test is usually recorded on a CD. The movement of the live blood is quite remarkable.

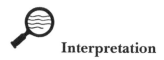

Interpretation

The condition, shape, behavior, vitality, and quantity of the components of the blood are analyzed.

For example: Red blood cells (RBCs) should be round and freely floating in plasma. If they are irregular, spiked, or hooked together in chains (looking like a roll of coins), they have a reduced capacity to carry oxygen and may be open to free radical damage and pathogens (causative agents of disease, such as bacterium or virus). If RBCs are clumped together, they are not able to flow through the capillaries and deliver oxygen and nutrients throughout the body.

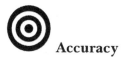

Accuracy

The accuracy of the interpretation relies solely on the level of competency of the examiner, so do your research and find a qualified practitioner. An increasing number of health professionals have found that the use of this technique allows for inspection of cellular dynamics, which normally escape analysis using standard non-living blood tests.

Cost

Price estimates range from $60 – $150 and may include a CD or photos of your analysis.

Often a follow-up analysis is recommended to assess for improvements or changes at the cellular level.

Process Time

A typical blood analysis will last 30 to 40 minutes. Results are immediate.

Benefits

The presence and causes of many health problems escape detection through conventional blood chemistry analysis alone. Live cell microscopy can show the following and more:[2]

- Free radical damage.
- Indications of heavy metal toxicity.
- Bacteria in various stages of development.
- White blood cell activity.
- Red blood cell activity.
- Fungi (yeast/Candida).
- Abnormalities associated with hormonal imbalances.
- Folic acid and vitamin B12 deficiency.
- Iron deficiency.
- Uric acid crystals (possible risk for gout).
- Poor circulation and abnormal blood clotting.
- Liver stress.
- Bowel toxicity.
- Plaque.
- Essential fatty acid deficiency.
- Predisposition to chronic and degenerative disease.

Limitations

- Using blood as a sole measurement of micronutrient status (fats, proteins, and carbohydrates) is not recommended.
- Nutrient quantity, shapes of cells, and cell metabolites in the blood do not always reflect their storage or biological function.
- It is possible to have normal results and still have gross deficiencies of nutrients in the cell, or have abnormal results when in fact the analysis is a function of misinterpretation or human error. Blood analysis has great medical diagnostic value and helps save many lives; however, it should not be used out of context or alone to determine health status.

Confidentiality

Results of the analysis are given directly to the patient.

Thoughts

Claims that blood microscopy can reveal a long list of issues and diagnose diseases like cancer are controversial.

Remember Masaru Emoto's book, *Hidden Messages in Water*, that created such a sensation? He took pictures of water crystals that actually change their structure and shape after being exposed to different words, different music, and even different thoughts. Emoto's microscope revealed, and the camera recorded, what appeared to defy science. How could a water crystal exposed to the classical music of Tchaikovsky change shape after exposure to a selection of heavy metal music? Dark field microscopy shares some of the same incredible reaction; some in the medical community reject it while others embrace it.

Dark field microscopy has a somewhat limited exposure to the medical community in North America, where patients typically are not allowed in the lab, and thus fresh blood is not available to those who work with microscopes. Dark-field microscopes are not radically different from microscopes already approved by the FDA for other diagnostic purposes. The controversy lies in the interpretation.

I feel that dark field microscopy can give skilled practitioners a way to evaluate overall terrain and to monitor progress. It seems hard to understand why live blood analysis is not used more frequently. Our blood is crucial to good health and is worthy of attention and examination.

The key message here is not to rely on just one type of diagnostic test or screening procedure, but to utilize several different testing methods to gather the information necessary to objectively evaluate your existing state of health or risk of disease. The outcome of each test forms a piece of a diagnostic puzzle required to complete the whole picture. The more pieces you can gather, the better picture you will have available to make informed choices. Disease imbalances occur over time, and the idea is to modify and improve suboptimal patterns before serious trouble such as disease arises.

. . . because the life of every creature is its blood.

Leviticus 17:14

Resources

1   Department of Health and Human Services. Office of the Inspector General. CLIA Regulation of Unestablished Laboratory Tests. July 2001. Retrieved January 9, 2015 at: http://oig.hhs.gov/oei/reports/oei-05-00-00250.pdf.
2   Denks S. Microscope Training Workshop: Live Blood and Dry Layer Perspectives.

Chapter 25

Electrodermal Screening

Meridian Energy Analysis

TEST

Summary and Explanation

Electrodermal screening is also called EAV, electroacupuncture, bioelectric functional diagnosis, and meridian energy analysis. It is energy medicine if you prefer, applied to diagnostics. This test combines modern technology with Chinese medicine. It is a form of computerized information gathering, based on physics, not chemistry.

Throughout the long history of the healing arts, it has been understood that the body is not only made up of tissue, blood, bone, and organs, but also a vast array of tiny electrical charges produced by every cell in the body.

The Chinese eloquently laid out for us the energy pathways of the body, the twelve primary meridians that serve as electrical resistance points. Each of these points can be measured and if an abnormal energy reading is found, it indicates inflammation or deficiency.

In 1951, Yoshio Nakatani, M.D., Ph.D., developed a method of examining the meridian system of the body through electronic measurements. This altered the way acupuncture would be practiced throughout Japan, Europe, Australia, and North America. Dr. Reinhold Voll of Germany continued this work in the 1950s. Dr. Voll explained that the body has at least 1000 points on the skin which follow the 12 lines of the classical Chinese meridians. He found, for example, that patients with lung cancer had abnormal readings on the acupuncture points referred to as lung points. He developed a non-invasive test he called electroacupuncture which has been since refined and is very much in use today.

During an electrodermal screening, the patient will hold a probe in one hand, while a second probe is touched to an acupuncture point. This completes a low-voltage electrical circuit, and a computer screen or a needle on a gauge reads out a number between 0 and 100. The input of voltage begins at the electrode in the hand and the reading is generated at the acupuncture point. The electrical discharges from these points are seen as information signals about the condition of the body's organs and systems. The electrical current used is too small to be felt by the patient.

The degree to which energy is excessive, lacking, or blocked can be assessed. This testing is similar to the electrical readings that are generated by the commonly used EKG to show heart function or an electroencephalogram to show brain activity. The recorded information is useful to physicians in evaluating conditions in the body and developing a treatment plan.

Electrodermal testing is also used to aid in the prescription of homoeopathic and herbal remedies. This is effective because all matter, even medications and herbs, vibrate at a specific frequency. When an electrical current passes through the tested substance, it carries the vibrational signal of the medicine with it into the body. This vibrational information then reacts with vibrational patterns already existing within the body, resulting in a constructive or destructive resonance. Electrical changes can be measured instantaneously.

In a test for food allergies, for example, the patient would be asked to hold a vial of, say wheat, and the machine would register the constructive or destructive resonance. Or the patient may be asked to hold a supplement to see how the body reacts. Different substances are tested until one is found that "balances" the energy disturbance. Electrodermal screening is used as an adjunctive diagnostic tool.

Many integrative practitioners are recognizing the importance of cellular energy and are including the area of energy medicine in their practice. Burton Goldberg, known as the "voice of alternative medicine," is particularly adamant about the positive contribution of this kind of testing. He had this to say:

You must find disease before it manifests and then get to the root cause. Any physician who does not utilize electrodermal screening is guilty of malpractice.

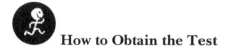

How to Obtain the Test

Electrodermal screening is offered by many chiropractors as well as allopathic and nutritionally minded practitioners. Check with your local medical community to find a center offering this test.

Note: Electrodermal testing devices measure galvanic skin responses. They have not been approved by the Food and Drug Administration for assessment of nutritional deficiencies, food allergies, the presence of toxins, Candida, Epstein Barr virus, or the weakness of organs and glands. Use of a device for these purposes is legal but "inconsistent" with FDA approval. Electrodermal testing devices are a Class II device approved for biofeedback and lie detection.

Western medicine has not embraced electrodermal screening because it is based both on new principles of quantum physics and old traditions of energy medicine, neither of which is taught in Western medical schools.

Interpretation

The electrodermal reading is a measurement of how much energy makes it through the circuit – the lower the resistance, the higher the reading. Readings taken usually are described using two values: the initial reading (generally the highest value), and the indicator drop (ID). An initial reading of approximately 50 followed by little or no indicator drop is considered "good." Initial readings below 45 or above 60 and substantial IDs are all considered negative signs.

Testing methods do vary; however, a typical examination begins with the four quadrant measurements (hand to hand, foot to foot, right hand to foot, and left hand to foot) which are measurements of whole-body energy levels. These are followed by a check of the several minor energy pathways to be used as control measurement points (CMPs). These measurements give an indication of the overall condition of every body part and function. The other points along a meridian are called branch points and are checked if the CMP reading is poor to gain more specific information.

During the testing, the body becomes an integral part of a closed circuit. The conductance circuit touches two areas on the body being tested. In the first point of contact, the ground electrode is held in the palm of the opposite hand to be tested. In the second place the test probe touches the specific acupuncture or conductance points on skin. After completing this closed circuit, a known amount of electric current is emitted from the instrument through the probe. The instrument then measures the conductance from baseline to peak and return to baseline through the conductance point that is being tested by the probe. This represents a dynamic conductance value.

It is considered that inflammation of an organ may cause increase ion concentration and the increase of ions enhances the flow of electrons causing resistance to decrease while the conductance may increase. On the other hand, a degeneration of an organ may cause decease in ion concentration that hinders the flow of electrons, so as the resistance increases conductance decreases.

Information obtained should be used in conjunction with other testing to develop a full clinical picture.

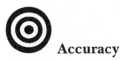 **Accuracy**

Results can be affected by the experience, skill, and medical intuitiveness of the person performing the test. Many integrative practitioners consider this testing a valuable part of a health assessment. Conventional physicians question the efficacy and accuracy.

 Cost

An electrodermal screening analysis price will vary depending on the practitioner and their experience. Prices generally range from $99 - $200.

Process Time

The exam should take no more than an hour. Some points can take up to 60 seconds to acquire a reading.

Benefits

Electrodermal screening has the ability to address the body holistically for a number of reasons:

- It enables the detection of disease before it becomes apparent.
- A standard examination enables the practitioner to quickly, painlessly, and safely collect information on the body's individual systems.
- The electrical signal reading is a very direct and true description of the condition of the body because it is created by the body.
- The meridian network regulates or at least participates in every type of bodily function, so naturally it is a very good means by which to monitor the function of the whole body.
- By identifying energy imbalances, steps to rebalance energy for optimal functioning can be taken.
- Useful for substance testing by allowing the practitioner to test medications, vitamins, herbs, metals, etc., for each individual patient, thus preventing possible side effects with no risk to the patient.

Limitations

- Should only be used only as an adjunctive tool along with conventional diagnostic methods. Valuable as a subset of the entire clinical picture.
- Not available for individuals with pacemakers.

Confidentiality

Results are given to the patient and become part of your medical record.

Thoughts

We don't think twice or question the validity of an EKG, but most people are resistant to considering the idea that other areas of the body are affected by electrical charges, not just the heart or brain. The Chinese have known of the power of the meridians for centuries. But in America, if we cannot see it or touch it, we seem to ignore it.

Why does simply holding a substance – in other words, putting the substance in our circuit – result in measurable electrical resistance? Because all matter vibrates at a specific and unique frequency as a result of the electric charges of the particles at the atomic level. These vibrating, electrically charged particles emit electromagnetic waves which have their own unique electromagnetic signature. That's modern physics. Cellular biology tells us that all cells have two types of antenna-like receptors on their surface, one to detect biochemical substances such as hormones and nutrients, the second to receive electromagnetic signals from the surrounding environment. Leading cell biology researcher Bruce Lipton, Ph.D., tells us cells are actually a hundred times more sensitive to electromagnetic signals than chemical signals. This is why many people are so worried about the effects of wireless technology that surrounds us and impacts us in ways we may not yet appreciate.

Every function in the body depends on the correct energy. Dr. Jerry Tennant of the Tennant Institute in Texas teaches doctors around the world how to incorporate into their practice a better understanding of the body's energy system. He encourages doctors to "think like an electrician, and to identify the power supply to the organ in question." He also teaches patients how to add energy, how to re-charge the 70-100 trillion cells in the body. Check out his web site at www.tennantinstitute.com and his Biomodulator that infuses the body with energy for healing.

From Dr. Tennant I learned:

* Every cell in the body is designed to run at -20 to -25 millivolts. To heal, we must make new cells. To make a new cell requires -50 millivolts. Chronic disease occurs when voltage drops below -20 and or you cannot achieve -50 millivolts to make new cells. Thus chronic disease is always defined by having low voltage.
* +30 millivolts is where cancer occurs.

Energy also can be used to diagnose. Electrodermal screening is a useful adjunctive tool in the hands of a skilled practitioner. It can determine functional imbalances or disturbances in the health of any patient and often finds the cause of an illness when conventional testing methods are unable to do so.

Knowing that the chemical/surgical approach is not always successful, why not try treating with energy? It does not have the negative side effects of drugs which can essentially poison a pathway to relieve a symptom. I feel it is very worthy of consideration.

An example of how the body is intricately affected by electrical patterns was demonstrated when my husband came home from work and asked me to sit down, then lift my right leg and move it in a circular, clockwise motion. At the same time, I was to draw a number 6 in the air with my right hand. I could not do it! A few days later, I was having an electrodermal analysis done by Carla McEwan, C.P.T. of Flexible Anatomy in McKinney, Texas and she explained it this way:

When you try to draw the number 6, you find your leg begins to take the pattern of your arm. This has to do with the way your brain codes for movement using the kinetic chains of movement and the myofascial lines. Basically, the body's electrical flow works in a crisscross or figure 8 pattern. You were trying to redirect the natural flow of energy, because you could have easily drawn the number 6 if you used the opposite arm.

Carla went on to explain about the motor cortex of the brain and how it uses a "turning curve." Her continuing explanation reflected years of study and work in quantum physics and the workings of the body. She did say that with practice, I could do it, but it's incredibly difficult. I tell this story because it is important that we understand the complexity of the body – not just the part we can see, but the unseen electrical activity.

Let me add something here because several times in this book, I say that results will likely vary upon the skill of the practitioner. Medicine is part art, part science. In Western medicine, the art often gets pushed aside in an attempt to reach a "science-based" understanding of things. That has upsides and downsides. A big downside is that it fosters a one-size-fit-all chemical approach to a metabolic disease like cancer, and this has not served us well. Patients are diagnosed literally by the book, prescribed by the book, dosed by the book . . . and yet we are unique beings with individual needs. The *art* of medicine is where personalization, medical intuition, innovation, and challenges to the status quo can more readily take place. The use of energy machines in medicine is very much a situation where results may vary based on the skill of the person working with you – the practitioner is not merely writing the umpteenth prescription of the month for statins because your cholesterol number fits within a certain metric.

References

International Health Technologies Website. Retrieved January 12, 2015 at: wwww.biomeridian.com/electrodermal-analysis.htm
BioRenew Website. A History of Electrodermal Testing. Retrieved January 8, 2015 at: http://biorenew.com/history_of_electrodermal_testing.

Chapter 26

Estrogen Profile

Estrogen Metabolite Test

Estrogen Profile
Meridian Valley Lab
6839 Fort Dent Way, Ste. 206
Tukwila, WA 98188
Email: info@meridianvalleylab.com
www.meridianvalleylab.com

*The following information was provided by Meridian Valley Lab.
Refer to their website for more information and updates.*

TEST

Summary and Explanation

Our hormones work together like a symphony – each hormone is like an instrument in that symphony. What happens when a hormone becomes off-key? Just as the music would be disrupted, many critical functions in the body are disrupted.

Estrogen is a powerful hormone that can exhibit both protective and detrimental effects on estrogen sensitive tissues. When our levels are low, symptoms such as hot flashes, fatigue, headaches, night sweats, and weight gain develop. Prolonged hormonal imbalance opens the door to disease.

The Estrogen Profile measures many estrogen metabolites, through a 24-hour urine collection sample, including the ratio of 2-OH estrone and 16a-OH estrone. Considerable evidence indicates that this ratio can be used to evaluate relative risk for estrogen-sensitive diseases including breast and cervical cancers, osteoporosis, and recurrent respiratory papillomatosis.

Dr. Jonathan V. Wright, founder and medical director of Tahoma Clinic in Renton, Washington commented, "The human papilloma virus (HPV), which causes (among other things) cervical cancer, has been proven sensitive to changes in the '2/16' ratio, growing faster when it's lower, growing more slowly when it's higher. It's higher when we eat broccoli, cauliflower, cabbage, bok choy and any of the other cruciferous vegetables. Every woman may have an interest in discovering if her own '2/16' estrogen ratio is low, especially as she can change it and lower her cancer risk herself! And just in case diet isn't sufficient, there are natural diet supplements that will do this job.

"The estrogen profile also accurately measures levels of two proven anti-carcinogenic metabolites, estriol and 2-methoxyestradiol. These metabolites can also be increased by diet changes, lifestyle changes, and supplements, with no drugs required."

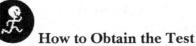 **Interpretation**

Upon completion of the test, the ordering physician will receive a complementary consultation to review the results with a Meridian Valley Lab physician. During the consult, the lab's expert physicians will assist with interpretation and recommend treatment options for the patient.

How to Obtain the Test

The Estrogen Profile requires a physician prescription. Your physician must set up an account with Meridian Valley Lab and order the test for you. Once ordered, you will receive very specific urine collection instructions as well as a hormone symptoms questionnaire and a return shipping label.

Sample Test Result

	Amount Excreted in 24hrs			Adult Reference Range
CREATININE	0.2 gm/24hr LOW			0.5-2.0 gm/24hr
TOTAL VOLUME	1500 mL			
STEROID	If Creatinine Value is out of normal range, results may be affected.			Female
	Amount Excreted in µg/24hr	Phase	Day	µg/24hr
ESTRONE	11.9	Luteal	17-26	3.3 - 44.6 *
		Follicular	27-11	2.0 - 39
		Mid-Cycle	12-16	11.0 - 46
		Post Menopausal		1.0 - 7.0
ESTRADIOL	5.5	Luteal	17-26	1.4 - 12.2 *
		Follicular	27-11	1.0 - 23
		Mid-Cycle	12-16	4.0 - 45
		Post Menopausal		0 - 4
ESTRIOL	6.5	Luteal	17-26	6.1 - 32.4 *
		Follicular	27-11	3.0 - 48
		Mid-Cycle	12-16	20 - 130
		Post Menopausal		0 - 30
Total Estrogens	23.9	Luteal	17-26	10.8 - 89.2 *
		Follicular	27-11	7.0 - 110
		Mid-Cycle	12-16	38 - 221
		Post Menopausal		0 - 41
Estrogen Quotient	0.4	Estriol / (estrone + estradiol)		>1.0
2-OH ESTRONE	9.8	Luteal	17-26	3.8 - 38.1 *
		Post Menopausal		0.2 - 5.4 *
16α-OH ESTRONE	2.8	Luteal	17-26	2.1 - 7.9 *
		Post Menopausal		0.15 - 3.5 *
2 / 16α Ratio	3.5	Luteal	17-26	1.8 - 5.5 *
		Post Menopausal		0.6 - 5.0 *
4-OH ESTRONE	1.8	Luteal	17-26	0.8 - 5.9
		Post Menopausal		0.05 - 1.1
2-METHOXYESTRONE	7.9	Luteal	17-26	2.2 - 14.4 *
		Post Menopausal		0.3 - 4.1
2-METHOXYESTRADIOL	0.9	Luteal	17-26	0.1 - 2.2 *
		Post Menopausal		0.03 - 0.54

* Reference range revised based on the reference range study in September, 2006

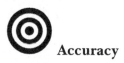 **Accuracy**

Hormones are secreted in small "bursts" throughout the day. By collecting urine for a full 24-hour period, this test captures the hormonal peaks and valleys and provides an accurate assessment of your hormone levels. Other methods, such as serum or saliva, only capture the hormone levels that circulate in the body at the moment of collection.

Cost

Meridian Valley Lab offers an abundance of affordable 24-hour urine hormone profiles. The Estrogen Profile can be ordered individually or can come as part of a larger profile. Please talk with your physician to identify which profile is right for you. Your physician can obtain pricing directly from the lab. MVL does not accept insurance, however, you may check with your insurance carrier for reimbursement. Meridian Valley Lab offers a variety of hormone panels ranging in price from approximately $250 to $700.

Process Time

Results will be sent to the ordering physician within 10-14 business days after receipt of the test at the lab.

Benefits

- Noninvasive.
- Results can be used to develop interventions allowing you to take an active role in preventing estrogen driven cancers or their recurrence.

Limitations

Meridian Valley Lab reports no limitations to this test.

Confidentiality

The Estrogen Profile will become a part of your medical record with your personal physician.

Thoughts

Breast and prostate cancers are two of the most prevalent cancers in the 21st century. Both are scientifically linked to hormones and are often fueled by estrogen, therefore, it only seems prudent to look into this issue. I encourage you to leave no stone unturned, especially if you are concerned with estrogen-related cancers. Remember, with the test results, you are given a recommended protocol to implement to improve your estrogen metabolism function.

Although the science of testing for estrogen metabolites is still in flux, my research indicates that increasing lean body mass, increasing intake of cruciferous vegetables, Di-indolylmethane (DIM), and fiber can help to balance estrogen.

Let us not forget that our world today is infiltrated with many chemicals that act as estrogen mimickers in the body – these include pesticides, products associated with plastics like BPA, ordinary household products like detergents, food additives like propyl gallate, phthalates in cosmetics, non-stick cookware, and triclosan in antibacterial soap. We are also affected by the wide spread use of hormones in the beef, diary, and lamb industries. This much excess estrogen in our daily world makes it hard to ignore the need for proper estrogen levels.

I like that Meridian Valley Lab uses a 24-hour urine test because it accounts for the full day and night of hormonal secretion. This eliminates the possibility of falsely elevated or depressed levels that may be obtained when a single point collection occurs at a peak or valley of an individual's secretory cycle. Also, not all technical methods of urine assay are equally accurate. This lab uses highly sophisticated gas chromatography in tandem with mass spectrometry which I feel is emerging as the method against which all other methods will be measured.

Because our hormones interact like a musical symphony, I want to point out another test offered by Meridian Valley Lab that may be helpful: the 24 Hour Urinary Melatonin Testing. Melatonin is the hormone that works while we sleep to, among other things, help the body clear out cancer cells. Studies show that melatonin may inhibit the growth of breast cancer cells by interacting with estrogen-signaling pathways.

NOTE: Estrogen receptor positive breast cancer patients are treated with prescription drugs such as Tamoxifen and aromatase inhibitors. These drugs are estrogen inhibitors and work by blocking the estrogen receptors on the cancer cells. They do not address any impairment in estrogen metabolism or unhealthy estrogen levels.

References

Stanczyk FZ, et al. Standardization of steroid hormone assays: Why, how and when? *Cancer Epidemiol Biomarkers Prev.* 2007 Sep; 16(9):1713-1719.

Bradlow HL, et al. 2-hydroxyestrogen: the 'good' estrogen. *J Endocrinol.* 1996 Sep; 150(Suppl):S259-265.

Saeed M, et al. Formation of depurinating N3Adenine and N7Guanine adducts by MCF-10F cells cultured in the presence of 4-hydroxyestradiol. *Int J Cancer.* 2007 Apr 15; 120(8):1821-1824.

Fuhrman BJ, et al. Estrogen metabolism and the risk of breast cancer in postmenopausal women. *J Natl Cancer Inst.* 2012 Feb 22; 104(4):326-339.

Falk RT, et al. Relationship of serum estrogens and estrogen metabolites to postmenopausal breast cancer: a nested case-control study. *Breast Cancer Res.* 2013 Apr 22; 15(2):R34.

Siominski A, Baker J, et al. Metabolism of serotonin to N-actylserotonin, melatonin, and S-methoxytryptamine in hamster skin culture. *J Biol Chem.* 1996, 271:12281-12286.

Bhatti P, Mirick DK, Davis S. Racial differences in the association between night shift and melatonin levels among women. *Am J Epidemiol.* 2013 Mar 1; 177(5):388-393.

Chapter 27

Galectin-3 Test

Inflammation Test

TEST

T Summary and Explanation

The galectin-3 test is a blood test that measures the amount of a specific lectin (carbohydrate-binding protein) molecule. Normally, galectin-3 is found in small amounts in our blood; however, scientific research indicates that higher than average levels of this molecule in our blood stream can reflect the presence of a wide array of serious health concerns. Increased galectin-3 levels are linked to increased inflammation, risk for cardiovascular disease, and cancer progression.

This test has traditionally been used for the detection of heart disease, but today we are learning that high levels of galectin-3 in the body, and the inflammation it indicates, are also associated with the progression of metastatic cancer, ulcerative colitis, rheumatoid arthritis, diabetes type II, and other debilitating diseases.

Dr. Isaac Eliaz of the Amitabha Medical Clinic & Healing Center in Santa Rosa, California has done most of the current research on galectin-3 and the use of modified citrus pectin (MCP) to act as an antagonist to control unhealthy levels of this lectin. A number of published studies demonstrate that the over-expression of galectin-3 is directly involved in cancer proliferation and metastasis. Therefore it is important to reduce its harmful effects.

Cancer patients typically have high levels of both inflammation and galectin-3. Galectin-3 is found to be over-expressed on the surface of cancer cells, acting as sticky protein on the surface of the cell, which allows the cancer cells to aggregate (tumorigenesis), then disperse throughout the circulatory system and attach elsewhere (metastasis). This is a primary mechanism by which cancers grow, proliferate, metastasize, and advance angiogenesis (blood vessel formation) to feed active tumors. Dr. Eliaz uses MCP because published research demonstrates it blocks the activity of galectin-3 and inhibits the damage caused by excess galectin-3 throughout the body. More information on MCP is provided in chapter Nutrients – Critical Components.

Like the C-reactive protein test, the galectin-3 test gives a measurement of inflammation present in the body, but also can reveal the process of fibrosis (scaring and thickening of the tissues) and potential for cancer progression.

 Interpretation

- Levels above 17.8 are considered to be an extreme risk factor.
- Levels between 14.0 and 17.8 are considered to be a high risk factor.
- Levels below 14 are considered ideal for the general population.
- Levels below 12 are considered ideal for cancer and cardiac patients.
- Dr. Isaac Eliaz reports that when a level changes by 20 percent within 3 months, these changes correlate with an increase or decrease in disease progression or mortality risk.

 How to Obtain the Test

- May be ordered by a licensed clinician.
- May also be ordered without the assistance of a licensed clinician at www.lifeextension.com. Log on and search for the "Galectin-3 test."

Accuracy

* Specificity: >99%.
* Sensitivity: >99%.

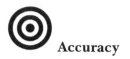

Cost

* Tests ordered through a licensed clinician may be eligible for insurance coverage; check with your provider.
* Tests ordered directly through LifeExtension are $120. An additional discounted price is available for LifeExtension members. Upon receipt of your test results, a LifeExtension physician will review your results by telephone at no additional charge.·

Process Time

Results are available within 10-14 days.

Benefits

* Can identify the presence of inflammation that fuels cancer cell growth.
* Can be used to identify disease progression and can play a significant role in tracking treatment success.
* A simple blood test that requires no special preparation.

Limitations

Does not identify the presence of cancer, only the presence of inflammation that accompanies cancer and the potential for the spread of cancerous cells.

Confidentiality

Results ordered through a licensed clinician are reported to ordering clinician and become part your medical record. Tests ordered through LifeExtension will be reported to you directly from LifeExtension.

Thoughts

It is critical to expose the underlying causes and fuels for cancer. Since cancer does not show up with visible symptoms until the disease is fairly well along, this test is a valuable tool in detecting the inflammation necessary for the potential presence, progression, or regression of cancer. Even better yet, if higher than normal levels are detected, modified citrus pectin can be utilized to bring levels down. I can only recommend PectaSol-C by ecoNugenics, as this is the form used in the vast majority of the studies that confirmed the effectiveness of MCP.

References

Gazella, K. New Twist on Health – Modified Citrus Pectin for Cancer, Heart Disease, and More. Published by CHAT, Inc., 2014.

www.dreliaz.org

Chapter 28

Hemoglobin A1c Test

Estimated Average Glucose Level

TEST

Summary and Explanation

Hemoglobin A1c is a blood test that checks the amount of sugar/glucose bound to the hemoglobin in red blood cells. Hemoglobin is the protein in red blood cells that carries oxygen. Sugar is sticky and a coating of sugar forms on the hemoglobin when it binds with glucose. That coat gets thicker when there is more sugar in the blood. The test measures how thick the coat has been over the past 3 months, which is how long a red blood cell lives, thus indicating the *average* blood sugar levels during this period. The relationship between sugar and it ability to fuel cancer makes this test a valuable tool in the effort to slow cancer cell growth.

A hemoglobin A1c test is routinely used to diagnose pre-diabetes or diabetes and to monitor the long-term control of blood glucose levels. This test in not like the home blood glucose tests that measure the level of blood glucose at a given moment.

Increasingly, the studies tell us that excess insulin increases the risk and progression of certain cancers. In 2012, researchers at the University of Texas Health Science Center in San Antonio reported:

> Diabetes is believed to be a contributing factor to several types of cancer, and new research in San Antonio patients reveals an association with kidney cancer. The study of data records of 473 patients who underwent surgery for renal cell carcinomas found that 25 percent had a history of diabetes. The strong message is that if you're diabetic, have your

hemoglobin A1c tested every three months by a physician and keep your blood glucose level as normal as you can on a daily basis.[1]

A 2013 study found a high prevalence of liver cancer in type 2 diabetics. Researchers noticed that liver cancer developed in these patients within the first 5 years after diagnosis of type 2 diabetes, which is when insulin levels are extremely high.[2]

Another 2013 study showed over a 10 year period that type 2 diabetics treated with any kind of insulin-augmenting drug had up to an 80 percent increased risk of experiencing cancer, an adverse cardiac event, or death from any cause compared to patients who only received the drug metformin, which lowers insulin levels.[3]

The hemoglobin A1C test goes by many other names, including glycated hemoglobin, glycosylated hemoglobin, A1C and HbA1c.

 How to Obtain the Test

The hemoglobin A1c test is a simple blood test and it is available at most laboratories. The test requires no special preparation and you can eat and drink normally before the test. For insurance reimbursement, a doctor's order is usually required.

Direct to consumer lab testing is available at www.requestatest. com. This laboratory has locations around the county and offers a "hemoglobin A1C with eAG test." This test includes a calculation for estimated average glucose (eAG). The eAG measurement indicates your average daily blood sugar level, which is reported in the same units a person with diabetes would see from a glucose meter they use to measure their own blood sugar. To order the test, log onto the site and create a user name and password. You will be given a secure profile in which to view your results.

Sample Test Result

Test	Result	Flag	Units	Reference Interval
Hgb A1c with eAG Estimation				
Hemoglobin A1c	5.4		%	4.8 – 5.6
Increase risk for diabetes: 5.7 – 6.4				
Diabetes: >6.4				
Glycemic control for adults with diabetes: <7.0				
Estim. Avg Glu (eAG)	108		mg/dL	

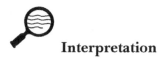

Interpretation

The goal is to keep the blood glucose levels near the normal range of 70 to 120 mg/dL before meals and under 140 mg/dL 2 hours after eating. Hemoglobin A1c levels are reported in percentages. A non-diabetic person will have a hemoglobin A1c between 4% and 6%.

The following is the correlation between hemoglobin A1c levels and average blood sugar levels as reported by the Mayo Clinic:[4]

Hgb A1c	Average Blood Glucose Level
5 percent	97 mg/dL (5.4 mmol/L)
6 percent	126 mg/dL (7 mmol/L)
7 percent	154 mg/dL (8.5 mmol/L)
8 percent	183 mg/dL (10.2 mmol/L)
9 percent	212 mg/dL (11.8 mmol/L)
10 percent	240 mg/dL (13.3 mmol/L)
11 percent	269 mg/dL (14.9 mmol/L)
12 percent	298 mg/dL (16.5 mmol/L)
13 percent	326 mg/dL (18.1 mmol/L)
14 percent	355 mg/dL (19.7 mmol/L)

The higher your hemoglobin A1c level, the poorer your blood sugar control is. A high result may indicate a need to discuss blood glucose management with your doctor. The normal range for A1c results may vary somewhat among labs.

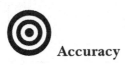 **Accuracy**

It must be noted that the results reflect the *average* blood sugar level for the past three months. It will not match up to any one time home glucose test result.

 Cost

Medicare and insurance usually cover the test when ordered by a physician. Check with your provider.

The best direct to consumer price found was at www.requestatest.com for $29.

Process Time

Results are ready in approximately 24 – 48 hours.

Benefits

The benefit of measuring hemoglobin A1c is that is gives a picture of what is happening over the course of approximately 3 months with blood sugar levels. The value does not fluctuate as much as finger stick blood sugar measurements.

- The test can also help you and your doctor identify high blood glucose levels.

- The need for steps to be taken to manage blood glucose levels can be identified.
- Blood sugar levels can be monitored and kept low to reduce the fuel source for cancer cells.

Limitations

The effectiveness of A1C tests may be limited in certain cases. For example:

- Heavy or chronic bleeding, or a recent transfusion, may deplete your hemoglobin stores making the test results falsely low.
- Iron-deficiency anemia may falsely increase the result.
- If you have an uncommon form of hemoglobin (known as a hemoglobin variant), your A1c test result may be falsely high or falsely low. This type of hemoglobin variant is most often found in Blacks and people of Mediterranean or Southeast Asian heritage.
- Chronic kidney disease, liver disease, and vitamin B12 deficiency can also affect the test.

Confidentiality

Tests ordered by a physician will become part of your medical record. Tests ordered from a direct to consumer lab will be reported to you.

Thoughts

Any attempt to prevent or treat cancer that does not include a low sugar diet is missing a vital component. Blood glucose levels must not be chronically high because cancer cells use a process of sugar fermentation for their fuel. The standard American diet is high in sugar and contributes to the prevalence of cancer and diabetes. The connection between diabetes and an increased risk of developing cancer has been well established. For cancer patients and for those at risk of developing cancer, maintaining normal blood glucose levels is critical. Many alternative and integrative physicians are paying special attention to the hemoglobin A1c levels in their patients with cancer. So eat your veggies and pass on the dessert.

Footnotes

1   The University of Texas Health Science Center at San Antonio press release January 25, 2012: One-fourth of South Texas kidney cancer patients have diabetes. Retrieved January 15, 2015 at: http://uthscsa.edu/hscnews/singleformat2.asp?newID=4063.
2   Yang WS, Shu XO, Gao A, et al. Prospective evaluation of type 2 diabetes mellitus on the risk of primary liver cancer in Chinese men and women. *Ann Oncol.* 2013 Jun; 24(6):1679-1685.
3   Currie CJ, Poole CD, et al. Mortality and other important diabetes-related outcomes with insulin vs other antihyperglycemic therapies in type 2 diabetes. *J Clin Endocrinol Metab.* 2013 Feb; 98(2):668-677.
4   Mayo Clinic website. Tests and Procedures: A1C Test-results. Retrieved January 14, 2015 at: www.mayoclinic.org/tests-procedures/a1c-test/basics/results/PRC-20012585.

Chapter 29

Lymphocytic Response Assay

Environmental and Food Inflammatory Testing

Lymphocyte Response Assay (LRA)
ELISA/ACT® Biotechnologies, LLC (EAB)
109 Carpenter Drive, Suite 100
Sterling, VA, 20164
800-553-5472
www.ELISAACT.com

The following information was obtained from
ELISA/ACT Biotechnologies LLC.

TEST

Summary and Explanation

Lymphocytes are small white blood cells that play a large role in defending the body against disease. These are your immune system's "soldiers."

A lymphocytic response analysis (LRA) is a test to identify immune responses to 491 common substances. This testing is important because if unknown reactive substances are allowed to come into contact with the body and produce chronic inflammation, the immune system will become overburdened and exhausted. This leaves the body unprotected and susceptible for diseases such as cancer because the immune system is tied up with other distractions.

One of the recent major advancements in medicine is our expanded understanding of the immune system and its important role in general health and wellness. Medical science has come to recognize that the immune system has defense as well as repair components. If either the defense or repair function becomes overburdened or overstressed, immune dysfunction and chronic disease may result.

Recent studies have shown that when the defense elements (lymphocytes) are constantly mobilized to fight off foreign antigens that cause disease, the vital repair process is deferred. Think of it as a case of the repairmen sitting on the sidelines, waiting for the soldiers to finish battle. Without repairmen on the job, however, organs and tissue weaken over time, and the disease state progresses.

Digestive remnants and environmental antigens are the most common assaults that pose the greatest burden to our immune system on a daily basis. When digestive remnants – food particles not completely digested – pass through the gut and enter the blood, they and excite the immune system. We call them circulating immune complexes (CICs) and they are often associated with autoimmune diseases. Other digestive remnants make it to the digestive tract where they putrefy and form toxins that are absorbed into the blood. Environmental antigens are the non-pathogenic antigens; common ones are mold, animal dander and secretions, and dust mites.

By identifying these harmful antigens and eliminating exposure, the immune burden can be reduced or eliminated, allowing the defense and repair systems to return to optimal function. The result is improved, sustainable health.

Lymphocyte response assay (LRA) by ELISA/ACT® is a comprehensive and reliable test that can identify the causes of delayed allergy/hypersensitivity reactions. You might know you have an allergy to shrimp, for example, because your respiratory system reacts immediately when you eat that food. But less dramatic reactions can occur hours or weeks after exposure. You may develop achiness or joint pain long after a food or chemical exposure and not make the connection. These reactions can be instrumental in provoking chronic conditions and autoimmune dysfunction.

The effect of immune system dysfunction can be chronic inflammatory and autoimmune diseases that often defy treatment. Many affected people go from doctor to doctor trying to find out what is wrong with them and how to fix it. Unlike treating disease symptoms, this test will identify the root cause of inflammation. The test is a valuable tool that physicians can use to examine the state of an individual's immune health by monitoring delayed hypersensitivity responses to common substances. A personalized treatment plan is also provided along with the test results to help with the overall program.

The LRA by ELISA/ACT methodology can evaluate all three delayed hypersensitivity pathways: reactive antibody, immune complex, and cell mediated reactions. The LRA method, looking directly at lymphocytes, is able to screen out protective antibodies and identify only those reactive and symptom-provoking responses to items tested. Accurate testing is possible because of a specialized blood drawing system that keeps the lymphocytes in the blood sample from being activated before analysis.

The following general testing categories are available:

- Foods.
- Dander, hairs, and feathers.
- Additives/preservatives.
- Medications.
- Environmental chemicals and toxic minerals.
- Therapeutic herbs.
- Molds.
- Food colorings.

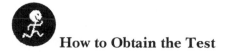 **How to Obtain the Test**

The LRA test is available through healthcare professionals. To locate a healthcare professional in your area who is currently utilizing the LRA by ELISA/ACT tests and treatment plans, contact client services department at 800-553-5472 or clientservices@ELISAACT.com.

LRA tests are also available directly through:
www.BetterLabTestsNow.com

Note: A 12-hour fast is required prior to the test as well as other specific and simple instructions that must be followed.

Sample Test Result

ELISA/ACT® LRA RESULTS   **Patient, Sample 65056**
                                        September 1, 2011

Strong Reactions   *Avoid for at least 6 months.*
· **Blueberry**   · **Cotton Oil**   · **Pepper, Black**

Cottonseed Oil

History/Discussion: Cottonseed oil is extracted form the seeds of cultivated cotton. It is used in the manufacture of soaps, creams and lubricants and at times is used in food processing. Cottonseed oil is known to cause many allergic reactions, and is considered to be an inferior grade oil for human use.

Sources of Exposure: Cottonseed oil is found in many foods, especially salad oils, margarines, mayonnaise, and chips and other fried foods. Lesser grades of olive oil, many hard candies, chocolate candy, furniture polishes, and paint may well contain cottonseed oil. Sardines may be packed in cottonseed oil, and lard compounds and lard substitutes may contain it as well. It may also be used to polish fruit at stands. In addition, cottonseed oil is used in cosmetics, baby creams, nail polish remover and body creams.
Cottonseed flour is used for human food, notably fig newtons. It is also used in the manufacture of Xylose, a sugar substitute which may be used in gum and soft drinks.
Cotton linters are short fibers that cling to the cotton sees after the long fibers have been removed. These linters contain fragments of cottonseeds and thus have some cottonseed oil. Linters, as well as cotton itself, is used in cotton wadding or batting found in cotton pillows, comforters and mattresses. Cottonseed linters are also used in some varnishes, artificial leather and weather proofing.
Cottonseed cake and meal are used as fertilizer. It is also used as feed for cattle, poultry, horses, swine and sheep. Barns and other places where animal feed is kept may bring exposure. Careful avoidance of all cottonseed oil containing foods and materials is important for people sensitive to cottonseed oil.

Substitutions: Any of the many other high quality, non-reactive oils.

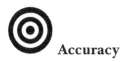

Interpretation

Lymphocytic response is measured via an *ex vivo* (outside of the body) system, however, it tests lymphocytic reactions as though they are still in the bloodstream being exposed to specific foreign invaders. Reactions are reported as strong, moderate, or non-reactive.

Accuracy

EAB reports 97+ percent accuracy (no more than 3 percent day-to-day variance), less than 0.1 percent false positives, and less than 1 percent false negatives.

The lab is a CLIA accredited clinical testing laboratory.

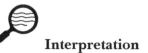

Cost

EAB offers several different combinations of test panels. Fees range from $100 - $2,000 depending on the number of requested substances and the fees of the practitioner who is ordering the test. Some insurance companies are starting to cover this type of testing, so check with your carrier.

Test results include:

- A detailed report identifying up to 491 substances as nonreactive, moderately reactive, and/or strongly reactive.
- An easy-to-use guide explaining each reactive item, along with suggestions for avoidance and substitutions.
- Individualized nutritional supplement and behavioral recommendations based on the patient's health assessment questionnaire completed prior to the test.

- "Alkaline Way" guide available via download explaining the LRA by ELISA/ACT program and how to easily and effectively incorporate the program into the patient's lifestyle.
- A 30 minute consult with an EAB nutritionist is included with a test panels valued at more than $250.

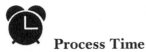 **Process Time**

Because the LRA tests require live cell, the blood samples must be shipped to the lab overnight. The samples are processed the same day they arrive at the lab. A full report is delivered to the ordering practitioner within 7-10 business days.

BENEFITS **Benefits**

- Identification of inflammatory substances.
- Provides a plan to address immune system dysfunction.

LIMITATIONS **Limitations**

Additional reactive substances may be present that are not included in the test.

Confidentiality

Results are returned to the ordering physician and become part of your medical record.

Thoughts

The immune system is your body's "defense system." Its main responsibility is to protect your body from various foreign invaders, such as environmental toxins, chemical residues from processed foods, viruses, germs, and cancer cells. I have often wondered why my immune system didn't attack and kill my cancer early on. Could it be that it was busy dealing with repeated doses of substances that we think are harmless, but it viewed as a threat? Sinus pressure, joint pain, or fatigue could be manifestations of a simmering immune system weakness.

It is much easier to strengthen your immune system before it falters and misses that first cancer cell that can grow into a life changing problem.

Take care of your immune system and it will take care of you.

Reference

Case studies and references are available at www.ELISAACT.com.

Chapter 30

Parasite Urine and Stool Test

Dr. Raphael d'Angelo
Center for Holistic & Integrative Medicine
ParaWellness Research Program
18121 E. Hampden Ave - Unit C #123
Aurora, CO 80013
303-680-2288
Email: info@parawellnessresearch.com
www.parawellnessresearch.com

Information for this test was provided by the Center for Holistic & Integrative Medicine. Check their website for updates.

The Importance of a Parasite Test

A study published in *The Lancet Oncology Journal* in June 2012 reported that approximately one in six of all cancer cases started out as preventable or treatable infections caused by bacteria, viruses, or parasites. Each year, these infections cause about two million cancer cases worldwide resulting to 1.5 million deaths.[1]

"Infections with certain viruses, bacteria, and parasites are one of the biggest and preventable causes of cancer worldwide," said study co-authors Catherine de Martel and Martyn Plummer of the International Agency for Research on Cancer in France.

The late Dr. Hulda Clark and others put great significance on toxins such as parasites, fungus, and bacteria for the treatment of cancer. Dr. Clark was one of the early voices to say it is a misconception that only people living in Africa or South America have parasites. Rather, she said, about 85 percent of the entire world's population is infected by different types of parasites and worms – it is the nature of life.

With our global economy and the importation of foods from around the world, we are not only sharing in other culture's cuisines but we are also sharing their organisms. You don't have to be a world traveler to be infected with parasites. Therefore, we can no longer feel safe from third world infectious diseases.

Even though the following quote from the American Cancer Society states that they do not believe organisms such as parasitic worms are a problem in the United States, they do admit that they are a concern in the development of cancer.

Certain parasitic worms that can live inside the human body can also raise the risk of developing some kinds of cancer. These organisms are not found in the United States, but they can be a concern for people who live in or travel to other parts of the world.[2]

The CDC reports on its website:

Parasites are also a cause of waterborne disease in the United States. Both recreational water (water used for swimming and other activities) and drinking water can become contaminated with parasites and cause illness. Recreational water illnesses (RWIs) are diseases that are spread by swallowing, breathing, or having contact with contaminated water from swimming pools, hot tubs, lakes, rivers, or the ocean.

The most commonly reported RWI is diarrhea caused by parasites, such as *Cryptosporidium* and *Giardia intestinalis*. *Giardia intestinalis* is also a common parasite found in drinking water. Both *Cryptosporidium* and *Giardia intestinalis* are found in the fecal matter of an infected person or animal. These parasites can be spread when someone swallows water that has been contaminated with fecal matter from an infected person or animal. Individuals with compromised immune systems who come into contact with these parasites can also be at greater risk for serious illness.[3]

TEST

Summary and Explanation

This test requires the submission of stool and urine specimens. Meticulous processing is coupled with extensive microscopic examinations which result in a detailed test report.

The types of parasites often recovered fall into various categories including roundworms, tapeworms, flukes, protozoa, and yeast. It is important that all such infestations be addressed so the body can restore and maintain good health. The presence of these microscopic organisms will compromise any immune system trying to fight off cancer.

The definition of a parasite is any organism that uses another organism for some aspect of its life cycle. Humans can become infected with parasites in various ways: the bite of certain insects, the food or liquids we consume, penetration of the skin or other body orifices such as when going barefoot or swimming, and pets and domesticated animals can transmit infection.

Parasites should be eliminated as they accumulate in and on tissues creating inflammation, toxin production, and in some cases, blockages of ducts or destruction of tissue. Parasite activity in the gut has been known to produce symptoms such as reflux, nausea, gas, bloating, cramping, loose stools, foul-smelling stools, constipation, and diarrhea. Some people harbor parasites without any symptoms.

The ParaWellness Research Program is a private membership research program run by Raphael d'Angelo, M.D. For testing, you are required to sign a request to be a Research Associate. This protects your right to investigate and manage your health as you see fit. As a Research Associate, you are entitled to submit specimens for parasite analysis and to receive full disclosure of the result of this research along with recommendations to improve your health in light of the findings.

Raphael d'Angelo, M.D., is a holistic medical doctor who provides consultative services in various areas of natural health. He received his medical degree from the University of Oklahoma in 1976. He has more than 45 years of experience and proficiency in medical microbiology and parasitology and has conducted research in various aspects of infectious diseases. Dr. d'Angelo is certified in family medicine, integrative holistic medicine, medical microcurrent, clinical aromatherapy, and medical technology.

Interpretation

The comprehensive evaluation of stool and urine samples generates a report that includes the specific names and amounts of parasites found, and an explanation of what these results are really saying. Also included in your report are specific details of each parasite in regard to how they are commonly acquired and what can be done to eliminate them. The cost of the test also includes a phone consultation with Dr. d'Angelo, so he can answer questions and provide more information about the findings and possible treatments.

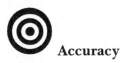 **How to Obtain the Test**

Order a parasite test kit online at www.parawellnessresearch. com or call 303-680-2288. The kit will be sent to you by UPS or Priority Mail.

Fill out the requested information, collect the urine and stool samples, and return them to PWR. Once placed in the container with the preservative, specimens are stable for approximately 2 months without refrigeration, so they will be well preserved when sent by mail.

When testing is complete, the report will be sent to you by U.S. mail, and if you choose, an email report may also be sent to you.

Accuracy

An accurate result requires many different aspects of collection and testing to come together properly and precisely. Over the years, microbiology testing has taken many turns as technology has improved. With parasite testing, microscope diagnosis is still the gold standard. Inexperience, inattention to detail, and insufficient time spent looking through the microscope are the usual reasons why negative test results are often reported when parasites are actually present.

ParaWellness Research gives every effort to ensure that no possible parasite is overlooked. In fact, if the testing comes out completely negative, PWR will request additional collection samples from the individual for further testing before a true negative result is reported. PWR brings more than 45 years of experience to this process.

 Sample Test Report

Report of Parasite Testing for Patient: John Doe, December 2012

Dear John,

The analysis of your urine and stool revealed the following results:

I did not detect any parasites in the microscopic examination of urine.
I did detect parasites in the microscopic examination of stool:
  • Iodamoeba butschii cysts (protozoa) – moderate amount observed
  • Ascaris lumbricoides ova (roundworm) – 2 ova (eggs) observed
  • Yeast organisms (fungi) – elevated levels present
These organisms are considered pathogenic in that they can cause or contribute to tissue inflammation and destruction. It is best practice to work on eliminating them.

I have enclosed information on each of the parasites and specific remedies to address the problem.
This information is provided to you as a research associate member.
I am often asked about the role of nutrition in the treatment or resolution of chronic health challenges.
I would invite you to the books and literature at www.RAVEdiet.com.

Thank you for the opportunity to be of help. In my prayers, I have added your name that you may have full restoration of your health.

Best wishes for optimal health,
                    Raphael d'Angelo, MD, MT(AAB)
                    ParaWellness Research Program

Memberships: American Association of Bioanalysts, American Society for Parasitology, American Society for Tropical Medicine & Hygiene, & the American Society for Microbiology.

Methodology: Gross examination, direct smear plus Wheatley's Gomori Trichrome Blue Stain, Modified Kinyoun's Acid Fast Stain, Trichrome Blue Microsporidium Stain, selective immune antigen testing.

Cost

- $297 for the initial comprehensive parasite testing kit with. This includes a phone consultation with Dr. d'Angelo on the findings and suggested treatment specific to the findings.
- $200 for the repeat test kit after treatment. Although optional, it is recommended to confirm that the parasites were completely eliminated after the completion of treatment.
- Testing is not usually covered by health insurance programs. A few health savings accounts and flex spending programs have covered the testing and/or treatment. ParaWellness Research is a private health research program and open only to those who agree to be research members.

Process Time

The turnaround time from receipt of specimens until the report is generated is approximately 10 to 14 days.

Benefits

- Reduction of the burden on the immune system by implementing a personalized treatment plan that is recommended based on the test results.
- Resolution of symptoms associated with the parasite and/or yeast infection.
- When protozoa are eliminated, the absorption of food, nutrients, medications, and supplements is improved.
- Elimination of worms and flukes will allow for repair of damaged and inflamed tissues.

Limitations

Anti-parasitic or anti-yeast treatments can affect the results and should be stopped for seven days prior to collection of specimens.

Confidentiality

The results of all research and testing on your specimens are provided directly to you. If you so indicate, a copy will be sent to your doctor or health practitioner.

A note from Dr. Raphael d'Angelo
Cancer and the Parasite Connection
©2011, 2013 Raphael d'Angelo, M.D., all rights reserved.
Reprinted with permission.

As an integrative medical doctor I want to share with you the connection between cancers and parasites. Few doctors give much attention to the possibility of parasitic infection when it comes to initiation or continuation of cancers. A partial reason for this is that doctors and patients are under a false belief that our public health and sanitation is effective enough to prevent parasite problems.

Any veterinarian will tell you that our soil and surface water are just as parasite infested as any other part of the world. Some benefit is achieved by water purification. But our food, insect and airborne exposures put us on par with our neighbors in less developed countries of the world.

In practical terms, doctors believe that most people do not really have a parasite problem. This is fostered by the large number of stool parasite tests that are reported negative by conventional labs. As a medical lab technician in my earlier years, I can tell you that the responsibility to examine specimens for parasites under the microscope is relegated to a low time and effort priority given all the other testing that labs must accomplish in the course of a day. This is really unfortunate because parasites are present in most people when the specimens are prepared properly and adequate time is spent examining multiple microscope slides thoroughly.

Diagnostic medical parasitology is the branch of medical science that examines body fluids and tissues for the presence of parasites. I have been involved in this since 1966 when I served as an Air Force microbiology technician in Viet Nam. After medical school and a residency in family medicine I continued my career as a parasitologist by setting up and running labs in practices where I worked. Now that I am partially retired, I specialize in parasite exams for people who want to know what is really happening to them.

This brings us to the connection between parasites and cancer. A true statement is that chronic inflammation is a seedbed for chronic degenerative diseases including cancers. In my work with cancer patients, I found that at a certain point in recovery the healing process will plateau and may not advance until we uncover and correct any existing parasite problems.

Parasites come in many forms. Some are actual worms such as tapeworms and roundworms. Others are flukes. Many are single celled protozoans. The fungi such as yeast and molds along with pathogenic bacteria and viruses are parasites. These organisms fulfill the criteria that part or all of their life cycle require the human host for protection, nutrition or reproduction.

Most parasites produce toxic waste. Some of them destroy our cells. Some invade our tissues. Some steal our food. Some do all of these things. As tissues become inflamed from such things happening, cancers can arise. One way to think of cancer is an attempted healing response gone awry.

Gastrointestinal symptoms commonly found with parasites are flatulence, diarrhea, abdominal bloating, abdominal cramping, constipation, malabsorption, maldigestion, bloody or odorous stool, mucus and leaky gut. Systemic symptoms can be one or more of the following: fatigue, nervous/sensory disorders, pain, skin disorders, allergies, nausea, muscle weakness/pain, immune deficiencies, headache, fever, insomnia, night sweats and weight changes.

Who needs a good parasite exam? The truthful answer is – we all do. Let's take some examples of how we can become parasitized.

The oral route is the most common route into the body. Parasites can be found in the soil that clings to our vegetables. Protozoan single cell parasites like Cryptosporidium and Giardia can be recovered in drinking water as some resist the chemical treatment and filtration processes. Tapeworms or their eggs can be present in uncooked meats and fish and adhere to our skin during preparation. The pets we love can get us infected when they lick us. Barefoot activities outside can be a source of opportunity for roundworms such as Ascaris to directly penetrate skin. Insects are known to carry a whole host of parasitic organisms. Even treatments such as taking antibiotics can promote difficulties with yeast like Candida.

In a recent month I tested 54 stool specimens. Roundworm eggs were present in 25 people; half were infested with yeast and most had one or more protozoans. What is remarkable is that all the cancer patients had parasites and of those without cancer only one was parasite free! What we think is happening is that the parasites create tissue inflammation and destruction which bogs down the immune system and provides fuel for cancer growth and invasion by yeast. The yeast feed on the dying tissue and they secrete more toxins that further destroy tissue keeping the cycle of inflammation (which promotes cancer) going. By eliminating the parasites and the yeast the immune system is freed up to do its job of attacking and resolving the cancer.

My mission continues to be raising awareness of the actual level of our parasite problem and the natural ways of parasite elimination.

Sincerely,

Dr. Raphael d'Angelo

Thoughts

This test is included in the book because microbes and fungus can be a very real drain on the body and thus the immune system, deterring the healing process. The body must be detoxified and the immune system must be supported to fight cancer. In conducting the research for this book, I came across many studies linking parasites to cancer. Most cancer patients test positive for parasites.

We are no longer isolated from organisms and infectious diseases from other parts of the world due to the importation of foods and global travel. I encourage you to not overlook this important step in your quest for health.

Additional Source for Parasite Testing:

Parasitology Center, Inc.
Parasitology Center specializes in the diagnosis and management
of parasites and is under the direction of Parasitologist Dr. Omar
M. Amin.
11445 E. Via Linda, # 2-419
Scottsdale, AZ 85259-2638
Phone: 480-767-2522
Fax: 480-767-5855
www.parasitetesting.com

Footnotes

1   De Martel C, Ferlay J, et al. Global burden of cancers attributable
    to infections in 2008: a review and synthetic analysis. *The Lancet
    Oncology*. 2012 June; 13(6):607-615.
2   American Cancer Society website. Infectious Agents and
    Cancer. Retrieved January 5, 2015 at: www.cancer.org/
    cancer/cancercauses/othercarcinogens/infectiousagents/
    infectiousagentsandcancer/infectious-agents-and-cancer-parasites.
3   CDC website. Parasites: Water. Retrieved January 15, 2015 at:
    www.cdc.gov/parasites/water.html.

Chapter 31

PH Alkaline/Acid Test

TEST

Summary and Explanation

PH testing is a simple method of measuring how acidic or alkaline your body is. The pH scale goes from 0 – 14. A pH less than 7 is acidic and more than 7 is alkaline. When healthy, the pH of blood, spinal fluid, saliva, and urine should be around 7.365. A pH reading indicating high acid or alkaline levels can indicate a health problem.

PH is short for potential hydrogen. Hydrogen ions create acidity. When the pH is low or acidic, there is reduced binding potential of hydrogen ions, therefore hydrogen levels remain high in the body which translates to an acidic environment. Measuring saliva or urine provides a snap shot of the body's extracellular pH.

The test is done by exposing the test strip or test paper to a few drops of saliva or urine. A color change will indicate the pH level. The pH scale logarithmic, which means that each step is ten times the previous. In other words, a pH of 5 is 10 times more acid than 6, 100 times more acid than 7. In this light, you can understand how a slight change in your pH value can have an impact on your internal environment, and, ultimately, your health.

Cancer patients commonly have an acidic pH. Once a tumor develops, it creates its own acidic environment through the process of glycolysis (sugar fermentation for energy), which produces lactic acid. This means that cancer is generating acidity in the body. Acidic pH measurements may indicate the presence of lactic acid production by cancer cells. Cancer patients often experience water weight gain, edema, or swelling. This is a result of the body sending fluid to the cancerous area in an attempt to dilute the lactic acid build up. Therefore, it can be useful for a cancer patient to monitor their pH and work towards being pH neutral or slightly alkaline.

An important part of healing is the body's ability to release stored toxins from the cells. Cancer causes a significant release of acidic products in the body. The fluid around the cells begins to resemble a toxic waste site and it is an acidic area. So the body will actually hold onto some toxins as a self-protective mechanism – the body doesn't want to release even more acidic waste into already acidic soup.

It is believed that acid wastes thicken the blood, and the coagulated blood cannot carry the quantity of nutrients and oxygen the organs need to function efficiently. Also, when the body is acidic, you have a decreased ability to absorb minerals and other nutrients, decreased energy production in the cells, decreased ability to repair damaged cells, decreased ability to detoxify heavy metals, and increased ability for yeast overgrowth, especially Candida Albicans.

Many proponents of alkaline diets profess that they fight cancer. Personal experience made me see those arguments in a new light. At one point, I embarked on a program designed exclusively to make my body alkaline. And I did indeed become alkaline. That daily litmus paper was blue, meaning it measured 8-10 on the pH scale and that is about as alkaline as you can get. After 3 months, I had the R.G.C.C. lab run the test to measure my circulating tumor cells once again. The news was bad. Before I had started the alkalinizing protocol, my CTC count was a low 3.1 (per 7.5 ml of blood). After the 3 months of the protocol, my numbers were up to a worrisome 4.7. I say this because I want you to know that there is more to it than what we know, because cancer obviously thrived as I strove to be more alkaline.

One mistaken idea is that eating alkaline foods makes your blood alkaline. It doesn't. Some metrics in the body are wide ranging, such as cholesterol levels. But blood pH is a very strict metric. The body has a built in homeostatic mechanism that works to maintain a constant pH of about 7.36 to 7.44. The body keeps the blood pH within that narrow range by withdrawing and depositing acid and alkaline minerals from the bones, soft tissue, and body fluids.

Eating "acid-forming" foods is not going to necessarily make you acid either. We think of lemons, for example, as being acidic. However, in the body, they become alkaline. People love to create lists of alkaline and acidic foods, but according to the nutrition experts of the Weston A. Price Foundation, a lot of that preaching may be just plain wrong:

> After a meal rich in proteins, the blood will become more alkaline for a short period, which is in effect a balancing reaction to the secretion of large amounts of hydrochloric acid in the stomach. Following this, the blood then undergoes a short-lived increase in acidity, which is again a balancing reaction to the heavy secretion of alkaline enzyme-rich solutions from the pancreas. These reactions are completely normal and should in no way be interpreted as justification for avoiding high-protein, "acid forming" foods.

> Under the vast majority of conditions, high-protein foods, such as meat and eggs do not cause the blood to be pathologically acidic. On the contrary, good quality protein is needed for the body to maintain the proper pH values of the blood and extra cellular fluids and to maintain the health and integrity of the lungs and kidneys, those organs which have the most to do with regulating the pH values of the blood.[1]

I feel whether the food is on a list as being alkaline or acid is not as important as the **quality** and **quantity** of that food. If you are eating the standard American diet with its heavy dose of sugars, bad fats, depleted grains, and meat from animals fed drugs and unnatural diets, you are not giving your body what it needs to detox and repair. Cancer patients need to eat a high quality, non-processed, nutrient rich, balanced diet to nourish their bodies. That is going to include abundant organic vegetables; low glycemic fruits such as green apples, berries, and cherries; small portions of clean fish, organic chicken, and grass fed meats; organic butter and cream; coconut, olive, sesame, and avocado oils; nuts; herbs and spices; sea salt with all its minerals;

and ample amounts of clean water. Adding a good mineral supplement and a green vegetable product can also be helpful. And it should go without saying at this point: **Don't eat sugar!**

Cancer patients must avoid the high glycemic sugary processed foods that create stress and an increased burden for the body's built in homeostasis mechanism.

PH testing is one of the least expensive and easiest methods to gauge how your body's homeostasis mechanisms are coping.

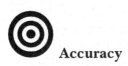 **Interpretation**

Most significant urine and saliva readings are taken first thing in the morning, upon rising, before you eat, drink, or brush your teeth. You will find that your body is more acidic during the first morning readings, because it is detoxifying and repairing during the night. Going to bed with a full stomach will add to morning acidity, so try to have diner 3-4 hours before bedtime. Several readings can be taken throughout the day, at least two hours after eating or drinking to obtain an overall average. Instructions and indicator color changes vary by brand.

How to Obtain the Test

Litmus paper for pH testing is available from many sources. Check your local health food store or order online.

Accuracy

The pH testing provides an overall indication of extracellular pH. Do not use old test strips or test strips that have been stored in high temperatures as they may not produce an accurate reading. I found this out through trial and error by using older ones stored in a box in the garage and compared them to fresh new ones. The older ones can degrade and become inaccurate.

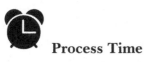

Cost

Approximately $10 - $15 for up the 100 test strips (about 10-15 cents per test strip) or $10 - $12 for a roll of litmus test paper. You will need about 1 ½ inches of test paper for each test.

Process Time

It takes only a few seconds to perform the test. Please refer to your specific tests instructions.

Benefits

- Results of pH tests are expressed as an approximate numerical value.
- Low cost.
- Easy to use.
- Easily accessible.
- May indicate a need to support the body's pH management.

Limitations

- Does not give an exact number. Most brands indicate a specific range varying by 0.2.
- Readings fluctuate based on food and beverage intake.
- Does not diagnose disease, only the need for attention or corrective measures.

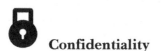

Confidentiality

Testing can be performed in the privacy of your home, making the results confidential.

Thoughts

The notion of being pH balanced has become quite popular and is showing up in magazines, diets, and health related books. However, underneath this trend is an important concern that lifestyle factors play a huge role in maintaining homeostasis. Most Americans are overloaded with highly processed, sugary, acid-forming foods. These foods tip the body's pH toward acidity. Our bodies have the ability to balance out a certain amount of acidity; however, the effects of standard American diet overwhelms that ability to buffer the acids in our diets – particularly when other acid-promoting factors such as stress enter the picture.

The monitoring and management of pH is useful for someone fighting cancer or trying to prevent it. If pH readings are consistently acidic, diet *must* be addressed. Tracking your urine or salivary pH on a daily basis over the course of a week or so will provide a window into what is going on in your internal environment.

When pH is off, pathogenic microorganisms thrive, enzyme efficacy decreases, and cellular oxygen is decreased. Chronic acidity, left unchecked, interrupts cellular activities and increases overall inflammation. We also know that the overgrowth of organisms such as yeast adds to the body's acidic burden.

Detoxification is important as acids start to build up if you don't eliminate them. One of the simplest ways to cleanse toxins from body is by drinking plenty of clean water, or other non-acidic beverages, and eating a balanced diet. The Institute of Medicine has determined that an adequate intake for men is roughly 3 liters (about 13 cups) of total beverages a day and the adequate intake for women is 2.2 liters (about 9 cups) of total beverages a day. Your body is 60 percent water; even cartilage and bone have water content. So make what you drink clean and full of minerals.

PH testing is simple, affordable, and can empower you to take steps with diet and lifestyle to adjust and lessen the body burden.

Footnote

1   Fallon S, Enig M. *Nourishing Traditions*. New Trends Publishing, Inc. Revised second edition. 2001, pages 59-60.

Chapter 32

Self-Assessment of the Heart

TEST

Summary and Explanation

Most physicians are fearful to tread into issues of the heart and emotions. In an attempt to be politically correct, they tend to overlook the issue. Whether you are Protestant, Catholic, Jewish, or a member of another religion, it is commonly accepted that we are body, mind, and spirit. Overlooking emotional wounds can impede healing.

According to famed holistic physician Dr. C. Norman Shealy, the most prevalent ongoing emotion leading up to cancer is depression, while chronic anger is the most likely emotion to cause heart disease and high blood pressure. These findings parallel those of former Stanford University scientist Dr. Bruce Lipton, whose research shows that chronic stress is a primary cause of more than 95 percent of all types of disease conditions.[1] Our emotions affect our bodies. Many believe that resolving emotional conflict is the first step to healing disease. Dealing with and healing this type of stress requires a focused effort.

Hans Selye, an endocrinologist born in 1907 and known for his pioneering work, coined the term "stress." He identified the three stages of stress as the alarm stage, resistance stage, and the exhaustion stage.

During the alarm stage, the body produces at burst of adrenaline hormones. It is not the occasional short burst, but the prolonged chronic release of these hormones into the body that create destruction and take a toll on your health.

During the resistance stage, the body is under prolonged stress. The adrenal glands produce cortisol and levels remain high, often producing problems such as fatigue, insomnia, obesity, decreased insulin sensitivity, depression, and *reduced immune function*.

If the stress is not resolved, the exhaustion stage develops and the body becomes very prone to developing chronic and life endangering diseases.

Dr. Don Colbert, a *New York Times* best-selling author, described the stress reaction this way:

> God designed the hormonal emergency alarm system to save our lives. But what happens if a person activates this system too many times for too many reasons? The alarm is turned upside down into something that destroys life . . . The first line of defense is to come to grips with our mental and emotional habits.[2]

Dr. Ryke Geerd Hamer of Germany, former head internist in the oncology clinic at the University of Munich, Germany spent years studying the mind body connection to cancer and disease. He theorizes that disease is caused by a "conflict shock" like a death or loss of job and identity that catches an individual completely off guard. Every disease, he theorizes, is controlled from its own specific area in the brain and linked to a very particular, identifiable "conflict shock."

When unresolved and chronic emotions such as anger, grief, lack of forgiveness, self-pity, and frustration are experienced, the brain sends out wrong signals to the body and cancer cells develop. Dr. Hamer studied visible concentric brain lesions seen in specific locations of the brain in cancer patients that relate to an emotional wound. He also noted image changes after the conflict was resolved.

Dr. Bernie Siegel's 1986 best-selling book, *Love, Medicine & Miracles*, changed many people's lives. Siegel, a surgeon, showed us that the power of healing stems from the human mind.

> When we don't deal with our emotional needs, we set ourselves up for physical illness. We are comfortable saying we're being driven crazy, but not that we're being driven to illness.

> Depression's effects on the immune system often appear very quickly if some remnant of a previous disease remains . . . Depression as defined by psychologists generally involves

quitting or giving up. Feeling that present conditions and future possibilities are intolerable, the depressed person "goes on strike" from life, doing less and less, and losing interest in people, work, hobbies, and so on. Such depression is strongly linked with cancer.

Dr. Siegel also taught us that exceptional cancer patients make time in their lives to seek the help they need to maximize their healing choices.

Dr. Dalal Akoury of South Carolina counsels her patients that cancer is an energy disease. "Do not surround yourself with people who drain your energy," she said. "Always forgive, make peace, be grateful, and believe in your healing. Claim your energy back."

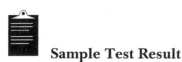

How to Obtain the Test

This test is not one found in a lab. You guessed it – it is found in your own heart.

The first step is to realize that there is an emotional connection to disease and then seek out a path to healing. This may begin by breaking the isolation and speaking honestly with someone – friend or professional.

Sample Test Result

Ask yourself:

* Are my words pleasant?
* Do I allow negative and destructive thoughts to take hold in my mind?
* Do I jump to conclusions and allow my mind to predict the worst possible outcome without all of the facts?
* Do I always expect people to treat me in a way that I approve of? This belief will lead to constant frustration and anger. Learn that not everyone has the same moral

compass. You may be expecting more from someone than they have to give.

- Do I need for everyone to like me? Believe me, you can never please all of the people all of the time. This need to be universally liked creates wounds in your heart and leads to low self-esteem.
- Do I speak positive affirmations to myself? Such as:
  - o I am a kind, loving and worthy?
  - o Freely I have been forgiven and freely I forgive.
  - o My body has miraculous healing power within it.
- Am I angry? Anger can come from feelings that are hard to show such as fear, helplessness, panic, frustration, or anxiety. If you feel angry, don't pretend that everything is okay. Talk with your family and friends about it.
- Do I have a habit of worrying? Research has shown that 90 percent of the things that most people worry about never happen.
- Is there anyone I need to forgive? Author and Pastor Michael Barry published a book in 2010 describing his discovery that the immune system and forgiveness are very much connected. In *The Forgiveness Project: The Startling Discovery of How to Overcome Cancer, Find Health, and Achieve Peace* he tells the stories of five cancer patients whom he coached to identify and overcome barriers that were preventing their healing. A somewhat different take on the act of forgiveness is championed by www.theforgivenessproject.com.
- Am I carrying guilt?
- Do I have fear?
- Do I feel worthy and loved?
- Am I easily offended? Change your thought patterns and refuse to be offended.
- Do I look at all things through loving eyes? I especially find comforting this passage from 1 Corinthians 13:4-8:

Love is patient, love is kind. It does not envy, it does not boast, it is not proud. It does not dishonor others, it is not self-seeking, it is not easily angered, it keeps no record of wrongs. Love does not delight in evil but rejoices with the truth. It always protects, always trusts, always hopes, always perseveres. Love never fails . . .

- Do the people in my life lift me up and encourage me? Get new friends if you need to.
- Do I know my limits? Learn to say NO in a respectful way. By doing this you can reduce and protect yourself from stress. Simply say something like, "I can't take on that responsibility right now," or "I'm not available to do that right now."
- Do I believe that my heart can be healed?
- Do I believe that poor health or a terminal diagnosis can be turned around?
- Do I believe that I should not die from a premature or unnatural death?
- Am I thankful?
- Do I believe that I have to take action to gain my healing? I remember being told a story about a man who was tossed into the sea after a shipwreck. He prayed to God to save him. A large buoyant plank floated by. He continued to pray even louder, his hands reaching toward the Heavens. Another large piece of flotsam from the wreck floated by. He continued to pray, but now he was getting very tired from treading water. A life preserver floated by. Still he continued to pray, imploring God to save him. Finally, he succumbed to the tiredness and drowned. When St. Peter greeted him at the gates to Heaven, the man asked why God had allowed him to drown. St. Peter said, "We sent you help several times, even a very recognizable life preserver, but you chose not to use them." God gives us "life preservers" in the people around us. It is our job to open our eyes and use the gifts that come our way.
- Do I have strong faith? If not strengthen it.

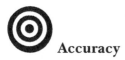 **Accuracy**

Accuracy of emotional conflict can be demonstrated by the manifestation of healing and the restoration of personal peace.

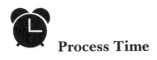

Cost

The monetary cost can be as little as "zero," but the benefits of conflict resolution and healing of the heart can be priceless! Many churches and social clinics offer no or low cost counseling.

Process Time

Healing can be gradual and can take some time to be completed. The key is to discover and face the issues.

Benefits

- Increased immune function resulting in healing and proper body functioning.
- Increased overall internal peace.

Limitations

There does not seem to be any limitations to reducing stress and healing emotional wounds of the heart. Do yourself a favor and give it a try.

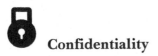

Confidentiality

Dealing with emotional issues is a very personal experience. Confide only in trusted friends and counselors. There are times when it may be necessary to speak to a person with whom a conflict or stress has originated to resolve the issue.

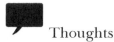 Thoughts

Americans consume billions of dollars of anti-depressants, tranquilizers, anxiety reducing drugs, and pain relievers each year. The majority of these medications are taken to deal with stress, depression, and the resulting physical pain. The problem is not just the emotional issue but more importantly, how we react to it. We must change and manage our perceptions, reactions, and create new thought habits. Perception is key and working to change your thought patterns is absolutely necessary. It is very important that we transform negative thoughts and experiences into neutral or positive feelings. We need to examine issues from a different perspective.

Know that we cannot change the past, but we can ask God to heal our heart. He can do it, but we must be an active participant. Talking with someone may be the first step to relieve the pressure you may be feeling.

I heard Lori Bakker on the Jim Bakker show say: "Do not allow your heart to be hardened, but allow people to love you. Feel that love, and then love yourself."

And in loving yourself, take steps to heal not only your body, but your mind and spirit.

Keep your heart with all Diligence, for out of it spring the issues of life.

– Proverbs 4:23

Footnotes

1   Burton Goldberg website. The Link Between Heart Disease, Cancer and Your Emotions. Retrieved January 4, 2015 at: www.burtongoldberg.com/page85.html.

2   Colbert D. *Stress Less: Break the Power of Worry, Fear, and Other Unhealthy Habits*. Siloam, 2008. p, 27.

Chapter 33

SpectraCell Analysis

Micronutrient Test

SpectraCell Laboratories, Inc.
Micronutrient Testing
10401 Town Park Drive
Houston, Texas 77072
800-227-5227
Fax: 713-621-3234
E-mail: spec1@spectracell.com
www.spectracell.com

*The following information was obtained from
SpectraCell Laboratories. Check their website for updates.*

TEST

Summary and Explanation

SpectraCell's micronutrient test (MNT) measures the function of 35 nutritional components including vitamins, antioxidants, minerals and amino acids within white blood cells

The test utilizes a functional intracellular analysis to identify specific micronutrient deficiencies. Unlike other methodologies, SpectraCell's MNT uses the patient's own cells (metabolically active peripheral lymphocytes) and measures cell growth (DNA synthesis) in a patented, chemically-defined culture medium to identify functional intracellular deficiencies that limit mitogenic responses or cell-mediated immune functions.

Instead of measuring how much of a vitamin or mineral is present in the blood (static), MNT measures how well a nutrient works in its natural cellular environment. Quantities of nutrients measured outside the cell, as in extracellular fluid & blood plasma, do not necessarily reflect their interactive function inside the cell.

Thus it is possible to uncover deficiencies that standard serum tests may miss. If not corrected, such deficiencies could impair health by contributing to the development and/or progression of chronic disease. The technology used was developed at the University of Texas, by the Clayton Foundation for Research, as a diagnostic blood test for helping clinicians assess the intracellular function of essential micronutrients.

MNT uses the patient's own cells as a control, which is consistent with the philosophy of biochemical individuality, thus taking into consideration individual differences in absorption, nutrient transfer across cell membranes, and personal metabolic requirements. Since each person is biochemically unique, it is important to take into consideration differences in diet, lifestyle, past or present illness or injury, prescription drug usage, exercise level, genetics, age, and other factors that contribute to a person's biochemical individuality. Because the MNT uses a person's own cells, and it is a functional test, these personal differences are fundamentally taken into account. This technique takes evaluation of vitamin status to a higher, more functional level. It is also a good way to verify how much of what you should take, and whether or not you are actually absorbing, assimilating, and metabolizing your supplements and natural health products.

A SpectraCell analysis can provide a roadmap to repairing the body and ensuring that the cells have the needed nutrients at the basic cellular level. Symptoms such as low energy, allergies, migraines, arthritis, fibromyalgia, and depression are often signs of a nutrient deficiency.

Cancer has long been known as a disease of deficiency, therefore it is important to identify and correct identified problems.

SpectraCell Laboratories, established in 1993, is a CLIA-accredited clinical testing laboratory. It is the leader in intracellular micronutrient analyses and holds the exclusive world-wide license to perform the patented functional intracellular analysis.

The following items are included in the test:

- **Vitamins:** vitamin A, vitamin B1, vitamin B2, vitamin B3, vitamin B6, vitamin B12, biotin, folate, pantothenate, vitamin C, vitamin D, vitamin K.
- **Minerals:** calcium, magnesium, manganese, zinc, copper.
- **Amino acids:** asparagine, glutamine, serine.
- **Antioxidants:** alpha lipoic acid, coenzyme Q10, cysteine, glutathione, selenium, vitamin E.
- **Carbohydrate metabolism:** chromium, fructose sensitivity, glucose-insulin metabolism.
- **Fatty acids:** oleic acid.
- **Metabolites:** choline, inositol, carnitine.
- **SPECTROX™:** antioxidant function.
- **IMMUNIDEX™:** immune response score.

 How to Obtain the Test

- Find a SpectraCell provider by searching their "Clinician" database at www.spectracell.com/clinicians
- Order directly and utilize an independent lab to facilitate the blood draw. If ordering directly, SpectraCell can recommend a clinician for report interpretation and treatment plans. It is not recommended that you interpret your own lab results. With any medical report, best clinical outcomes are achieved when results are reviewed with a professional. If you prefer to place your order over the phone, call the "Client Services" department at 800-227-5227.

Note: If you are ordering lab tests without going through a physician, you cannot submit the test fee to your insurance for payment or reimbursement. Specimens cannot be collected and lab results cannot be mailed to MD, MA, NJ, NY, and RI residents.

Sample Test Result

SpectraCell Laboratories, Inc.   Accession Number: H55964
Laboratory Test Report   Thomas Doe

Micronutrients	Patient Results (% Control)	Functional Abnormals	Reference Range (greater than)
B Complex Vitamins			
Vitamin B1 (Thiamin)	100		>78%
Vitamin B2 (Riboflavin)	64		>53%
Vitamin B3 (Niacinamide)	98		>80%
Vitamin B6 (Pyridoxine)	74		>54%
Vitamin B12 (Cobalamin)	9	Deficient	>14%
Folate	47		>32%
Pantothenate	7	Deficient	>7%
Biotin	36		>34%
Amino Acids			
Serine	54		>30%
Glutamine	57		>37%
Asparagine	56		>39%
Metabolites			
Choline	22		>20%
Inositol	75		>58%
Carnitine	61		>46%
Fatty Acids			
Oleic Acid	71		>65%
Other Vitamins			
Vitamin D (Ergocalciferol)	90		>83%
Vitamin A (Retinol)	74		>70%
Minerals			
Calcium	41		>36%
Zinc	35	Deficient	>37%
Copper	57		>42%
Magnesium	43		>37%
Carbohydrate Metabolism			
Glucose-Insulin Interaction	49		>38%
Fructose Sensitivity	41		>34%
Chromium	58		>40%
Antioxidants			
Glutathione	57		>47%
Cysteine	53		>41%
Coenzyme Q-10	95		>86%
Selenium	83		>74%
Vitamin E (A-tocopherol)	91		>84%
Alpha Lipoic Acid	92		>81%
Vitamin C	77		>40%
SPECTROX™			
Total Antioxidant Function	65.8	Deficient	>65%

SAMPLE REPORT

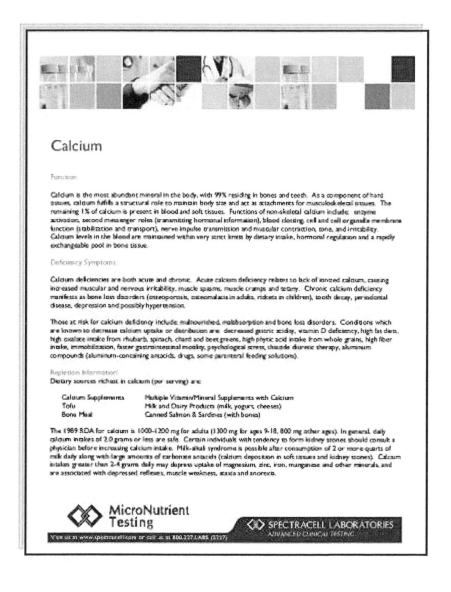

Calcium

Function

Calcium is the most abundant mineral in the body, with 99% residing in bones and teeth. As a component of hard tissues, calcium fulfills a structural role to maintain body size and act as attachments for musculoskeletal tissues. The remaining 1% of calcium is present in blood and soft tissues. Functions of non-skeletal calcium include: enzyme activation, second messenger roles (transmitting hormonal information), blood clotting, cell and cell organelle membrane function (stabilization and transport), nerve impulse transmission and muscular contraction, tone, and irritability. Calcium levels in the blood are maintained within very strict limits by dietary intake, hormonal regulation and a rapidly exchangeable pool in bone tissue.

Deficiency Symptoms

Calcium deficiencies are both acute and chronic. Acute calcium deficiency relates to lack of ionized calcium, causing increased muscular and nervous irritability, muscle spasms, muscle cramps and tetany. Chronic calcium deficiency manifests as bone loss disorders (osteoporosis, osteomalacia in adults, rickets in children), tooth decay, periodontal disease, depression and possibly hypertension.

Those at risk for calcium deficiency include: malnourished, malabsorption and bone loss disorders. Conditions which are known to decrease calcium uptake or distribution are: decreased gastric acidity, vitamin D deficiency, high fat diets, high oxalate intake from rhubarb, spinach, chard and beet greens, high phytic acid intake from whole grains, high fiber intake, immobilization, faster gastrointestinal motility, psychological stress, thiazide diuretic therapy, aluminum compounds (aluminum-containing antacids, drugs, some parenteral feeding solutions).

Repletion Information

Dietary sources richest in calcium (per serving) are:

Calcium Supplements	Multiple Vitamin/Mineral Supplements with Calcium
Tofu	Milk and Dairy Products (milk, yogurt, cheeses)
Bone Meal	Canned Salmon & Sardines (with bones)

The 1989 RDA for calcium is 1000-1200 mg for adults (1300 mg for ages 9-18, 800 mg other ages). In general, daily calcium intakes of 2.0 grams or less are safe. Certain individuals with tendency to form kidney stones should consult a physician before increasing calcium intake. Milk-alkali syndrome is possible after consumption of 2 or more quarts of milk daily along with large amounts of carbonate antacids (calcium deposition in soft tissues and kidney stones). Calcium intakes greater than 2-4 grams daily may depress uptake of magnesium, zinc, iron, manganese and other minerals, and are associated with depressed reflexes, muscle weakness, ataxia and anorexia.

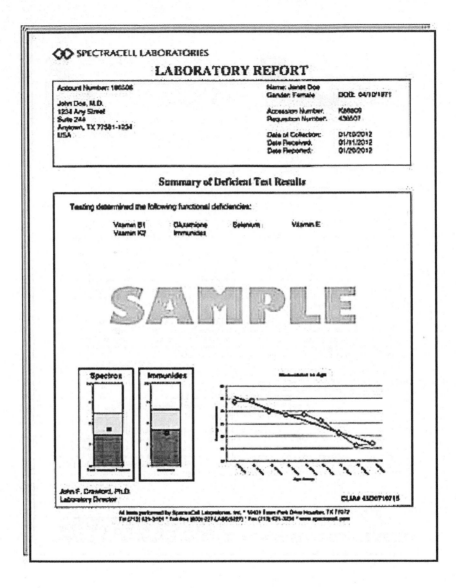

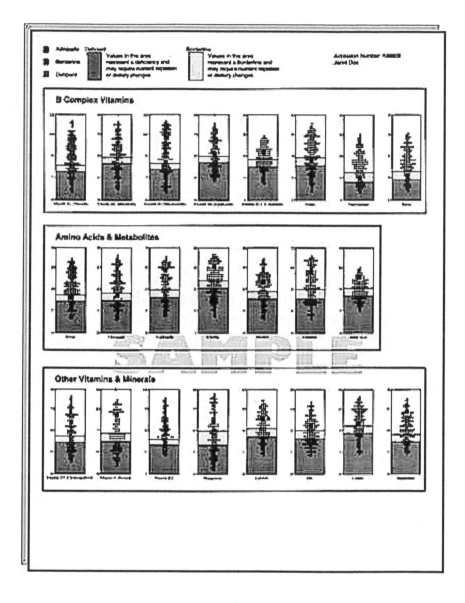

Interpretation

From the blood sample, white blood cells (lymphocytes) are extracted and then stimulated to grow. These immune cells are bathed in 35 different nutrient media, and it is the response to these media (metabolic changes) that are measured as values against reference ranges established for the general population.

For example, if lymphocyte growth in a medium lacking thiamine (vitamin B1) is less than the growth in a complete medium, then a deficient thiamine status is ascertained. Or, if B12 is removed from the medium and cell growth is not sufficient, this suggests that the lymphocyte cells being tested have a functional intracellular deficiency of B12.

Results include an overview page with all deficiencies listed, numeric and graphic reports easily identifying deficiencies and supplementation recommendations.

Results are reported as: Adequate, Borderline, or Deficient.

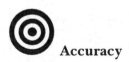

Accuracy

Each nutrient is tested in triplicate to ensure accuracy.

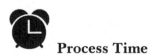

Cost

Micronutrient testing is $390. Price includes the kit for comprehensive testing of 35 components, return shipping, and results with nutrient information.

Process Time

An easy-to-read test report is will be received within 3 weeks.

BENEFITS

Benefits

* Ability to identify and address a problem before symptoms develop.
* Results are individual and specific for the person tested.
* Repeat testing can be utilized to monitor efforts to correct deficiencies.
* It is a long term nutritional marker that assesses the previous 4-6 months nutritional status.

LIMITATIONS

Limitations

Can only identify deficiencies in the tested nutrients.

Confidentiality

Results are reported directly to the ordering consumer or practitioner.

Thoughts

We are all looking for methods to not only manage illness, but to prevent it. Unfortunately a multivitamin does not always meet every nutritional requirement. Each person's body is unique and a SpectraCell nutrient analysis can provide a personalized treatment outline. With the complexity of the human body, and the challenges of today's lifestyle, an individualized healthcare approach seems to be the best way to achieve optimal results. You can be deficient in micronutrients and not even know it. Since the technology is available, take a peek inside your cells and take steps to make sure that they are functioning optionally.

Detect cellular deficiencies, a known problem with cancer, and prevent a potential systemic breakdown before you have a major problem.

Reference

Case studies, research data, and articles are available at www. spectracell.com/clinicians/clinical-education-center.

Chapter 34

Spinal Alignment Analysis

Maximized Living
1170 Celebration Blvd., Suite 100B
Celebration, FL 34747
321-939-3060
www.maximizedliving.com

Information on this test was provided by
Maximized Living and research done by the author.

TEST

Summary and Explanation

Cancer, and other conditions, can be defined by changes in cellular energy and energy flows through the spinal column.

When optimal organ and immune function is your goal, it is vital to work with a corrective care chiropractor who actively fosters the health and regeneration of the spine and nervous system, rather than just addressing pains and symptoms. Occasional visits to the chiropractor will not usually get the job done.

A spinal analysis requires a few simple X-rays and a physical exam. Additional tests may be used to measure the electrical activity of muscles and nerves.

There are several primary areas assessed during the exam. First, is the spine straight? Curvatures to the side are called scoliosis. Next, are there subluxations, misaligned vertebra? Subluxations put pressure on the spinal column and compress nerves. Lastly, a side view of the spine should reveal three well placed arcs that are vital to proper immune, organ, and nerve function. A careful examination will often reveal a health issue that is impacted by a decrease in the electrical energy supplied through the nerves.

Interpretation

X-rays document the amount of deviation from a normal spinal position.

From the front, the spine should be straight, with the head, shoulders, hips, and feet lined up. From the side, the ears should be back over the shoulders, and the shoulders should be back over the pelvis.

Deviations from normal are reported in percentages. With proper corrective therapy, most patients achieve a high percentage of correction.

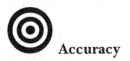

How to Obtain the Test

Log on to www.maximizedliving.com and click on the "Find a Doctor" tab to find a qualified Maximized Living Health Center in your area.

Maximized Living chiropractors have clinics throughout the United States and the world. They have a program specific to cancer patients; in fact, they have produced a book entitled *Cancer Killers*.

Accuracy

Chiropractic is a particular talent and outcomes vary with the skill of each doctor. For sustained immune response, a program of correction – not just treatment – must be initiated.

Cost

The initial consultation, exam, X-rays, and other testing can run anywhere from $150 - $350. Most offices accept insurance.

Additionally, many corrective care offices have reduced rates available through classes offered in the community.

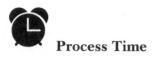

Process Time

The exam and interpretation takes about 30 minutes. The active spinal correction program is usually completed in about 2-3 months. At that point, progress is re-evaluated. A maintenance program will be required.

Benefits

Remembering that cancer starts when cells can no longer hold a healthy energetic charge, the restoration of the nervous system and its pathways is a way to reduce energetic blocks and reverse a downward spiral. The correct operation of the nervous system is an often overlooked, but basic foundation of health.

* Increased immune function.
* Increased function with daily activities.

Limitations

* A program of maintenance must be followed.
* 100 percent correction is not always possible. The goal of this work is to see improvement and keep as much energy flowing to the cells as possible.

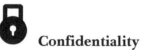

Confidentiality

Results are reported directly to each patient and become part of the clinics medical record.

A note from Dr. Brian Anderson, B.Sc., D.C., C.C.W.P. Life Essentials Chiropractic, Missouri City, TX

The brain and nervous system house the very power or intelligence that animates and controls all human life and function. Remove your heart, kidneys, liver, circulatory system, immune glands or any organ from the nervous system and they're dead. It's like unplugging a lamp. They've got to stay plugged in so that the power can get to them and allow them to express life. While the body can go days without water, weeks without food, and minutes without oxygen, it cannot live even a second without the power provided through nerve supply.

To experience maximum nerve supply to your body, you've got to look at your spine. The spine is created as a shield of bony armor to protect the nervous system. Unfortunately, in today's unnatural world there is a whole lot of physical, chemical, and emotional trauma that God did not intend for you to endure. These traumas can move the spine out of place so that rather than shielding the nervous system, the spine is actually damaging it. A spine out of its proper alignment is going to put pressure on nerve roots and disrupt life from getting to organs and tissues of the body. The end result is malfunction. When malfunctioning, rather than the cells being in a state of balance or ease, you end up in a state of disease. As this continues, abnormal cell growth, symptoms and eventually disease will result. In fact, sometimes the first symptom is the disease itself or even death, not pain.

In order to maximize nerve supply, it requires spinal correction, not just symptom management. Maximized Living doctors are trained to correct the spinal to the point of its maximum function. You just don't know whether or not you are well until your spine and nervous system have been examined by a trained Corrective Care Chiropractor.

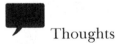 Thoughts

We all start as embryos with a tiny spinal cord and our organs grow off of that spinal cord. Could it be that cancer patients are unknowingly walking around with impaired nerve function to the very organs that have cancer? Wouldn't it be worth checking this out? I think so.

I am confident that a spinal assessment and correction is one of the final and necessary pieces of the puzzle when working to heal from cancer or prevent it.

If this concept is new to you, you could read *The Cancer Killers, the Cause Is the Cure* or *Cruise Ship or Nursing Home*. Both books are loaded with patient testimonies.

Reference

Patient testimonials are available at www.maximizedliving.com.

Chapter 35

Thermography Exam

TEST

Summary and Explanation

Breast thermography is a diagnostic procedure that images the breasts to aid in the early warning of breast cancer. It was approved by the FDA in 1982 for breast cancer risk assessment. This test is non-invasive, requires no compression, and uses no radiation.

The test is based on the principle that as a tumor develops, it builds a network of blood vessels. That extra activity generates heat which can be seen on a thermogram. Thermography uses ultra-sensitive infrared cameras and sophisticated computers to detect, analyze, and produce high-resolution diagnostic images of these temperature and vascular changes. The images visually map the body temperature and reveal a pattern of where infrared radiation is being emitted from the body surface. Higher temperature readings indicate higher levels of inflammation, which can indicate cancer or lead to cancer.[1] In this way, thermography can detect cancer's formation up to 10 years before a lump is big enough to be pictured on a mammogram. It is a better early detection screening.

Breast thermography is a screening and detection procedure, which when added to a woman's breast health examination, can substantially increase the ability to detect areas of concern associated with the breast. It is especially useful to younger women under 50 whose denser breast tissue significantly reduces the effectiveness of mammograms.[2]

Len Saputo, M.D., explains:

Breast thermograms have highly specific thermal patterns in each individual woman. They provide a unique "thermal signature" that remains constant over years unless there is a change in an underlying condition. Thus, over time, it is possible to differentiate between cancers and benign conditions.[3]

 Interpretation

The images produced reveal red-colored areas caused by heat in tissue that has increased inflammation, blood flow, or a probable cancer. Cooler areas are indicated by a blue or darker colors. If images show areas of high inflammation, the area may need further evaluation.

By carefully examining changes in the temperature and blood vessels of the breasts, signs of cell growth may be detected up to 10 years earlier than they would typically be discovery through mammogram or palpation.

Some clinicians will also look for any connection between the mouth and the breast as breast cancer is believed to be related to infections in the mouth. If that is the case, the images will show a red spot/infection in the mouth and a red spot/cancer or developing cancer in the breast(s). There may be a thin red line between the two spots.

Comparisons of past thermography images will be used to look for stability and symmetry over time, which is why it is recommended that patients get a thermography exam at regular intervals. The first set of images is used as a baseline.

How to Obtain the Test

Thermography exams are available in most cities. Check your local listings or refer to one of the following organizations:

- The International Academy of Clinical Thermology: www.iact-org.org/links.html.
- Breast Thermography: www.breastthermography.com/find-a-center.htm.
- The American College of Clinical Thermology: www.thermologyonline.org/Breast/breast_thermography_clinics.htm.

Pre-examination instructions are very specific and must be followed (i.e., no lotions, powders, or deodorant can be worn, no hot showers less than 2 hours prior to exam, no caffeine or alcohol or sunbathing 24 hours prior to exam). It's very important that you check with your testing center for additional test preparation instructions.

- Upper body clothing and jewelry must be removed and a gown is worn.
- Testing is performed after waiting in a cool room for approximately 15 minutes. This is to allow the skin surface temperatures to stabilize prior to the test.
- Images are taken, similar to the taking of a photograph, with the camera positioned several feet in front of the area being examined.
- Images will be taken from several different positions and only take a few minutes.
- Approximately 8 images will be taken.

Cost

$150-$250 is the average cost for the first breast thermography test. A second exam may be less and is recommended to be done 3 months after the initial exam. The two sets of images are compared for vascular and other changes.

Only a few insurance companies provide coverage for thermography. Please check with your provider.

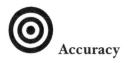

Accuracy

Breast thermography is very accurate, but only in the hands of a Certified Clinical Thermographer using sophisticated infrared cameras.

A 1998 study reported that thermography has an accuracy and sensitivity record in the 90% and above range.[4]

In 2003, the *American Journal of Radiology* reported that thermography had 99 percent sensitivity in identifying breast cancer with single examinations and limited views. "Thus, a negative thermogram (Th1 or Th2) in this setting is powerful evidence that cancer is not present." The report goes further to suggest that a negative thermogram can give women greater reassurance they don't have breast cancer.[5]

A Word About Mammograms

A number of prominent studies have come out in recent years that find mammography is an overhyped, poor screening technique for breast cancer (see the Statistics – Misconceptions of Reality chapter).

This brings up the sticky issue that mammography is particularly weak when it comes to "seeing through" dense breasts. The radiologist and the woman's physician are aware when a patient has dense breasts, but the patients routinely are not told. And almost half of all women have dense breast tissue. This prompted a push for new laws in many states. But heavy resistance has come from the American College of Radiology, which defends lack of disclosure because the information may create "undue anxiety." Women's groups call it an egregious violation of ethical guidelines that continues because the ACS desires to maintain the status quo of mammogram screenings from which it makes money.[6] The FDA approved in 2012 the much better Automated Breast Ultrasound System (ABUS) for women with dense breasts, but the government kept the radiologists happy by advising doctors to use it in combination with mammography.[7]

Newer 3-D mammography can spot smaller tumors in dense breasts. But 3-D comes with two significant downsides:

1. It requires that the breast be compressed for about twice as long which increases the potential for spreading an existing mass. When a cancerous mass is squeezed, the membranes which contain cancerous cells can be damaged, releasing cancer cells into the body.
2. The dose of radiation is higher than with conventional mammography. And again, radiation is carcinogenic.

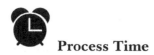

Process Time

The entire appointment should last no more than 30 minutes with the actual test taking just a few minutes.

Benefits

- Unlike conventional mammography, thermography is completely safe for pregnant women, women with breast implants, and women with large, dense, or sensitive breasts.
- There is no compression of breast tissue.
- There is no radiation exposure. Pre-screening with thermography prevents radiation exposure caused by mammograms.
- In patients without cancer, the examination results are used to indicate the level of possible future cancer risk.
- Detects physiologic changes.
- Can be used to monitor benign breast tumors, effectiveness of cancer treatment, breast mastitis, fibrocystic breast disease breast, and for cancer risk assessment.
- Thermography is able to detect angiogenesis (a group of blood vessels formed by the tumor for food and oxygen).
- Shown to find changes in the breast tissue up to 10 years before a cancer diagnosis.

Limitations

- Thermography does not have the ability to pinpoint the exact size and location of a tumor. It only indicates the area of concern. A mammogram is typically used then to locate the tumor more precisely.
- Requires additional testing, such as a biopsy, to officially diagnose cancer.

- Can cause concern as hot areas may indicate unhealthy tissue, inflammation, infection, stagnant lymphatic flow, cystic activity, scar tissue, an injury, or a hormonal imbalance.
- Not effective on slow-developing cancers or encapsulated tumors that produce little heat.

Confidentiality

Results are given directly to the patient and images become part of your medical record.

Thoughts

Since it has been determined that about 1 in 8 women will get breast cancer, and every woman is at risk, every means possible should be used to detect a tumor when there is the greatest chance for survival. Adding a thermography exam greatly increases the capacity for early detection without the risk of radiation exposure.

Breast self-exams and physician exams are important too. Typically, mammograms are not recommended for women under 40 and are not effective in detecting cancer in women with dense breast tissue. Also, the age at which women are being diagnosed is getting younger and younger. The opportunity for early diagnosis is often missed in these younger women. Thermography can fill this gap. Therefore, it is important to begin breast cancer screening long before age 40. Because thermography is safe, an initial test can be started on young women in their early twenties.

These tests provide a baseline or bench mark early on in life that can be used to identify changes sooner rather than later. Thermography has been underutilized because of politics – the makers of mammography machines have forged relationships with radiology groups and breast cancer groups to promote mammogram screenings. For example, General Electric, one of the biggest manufacturers of mammography machines, partners with the Susan G. Komen organization that adamantly recommends mammograms. These factors have stifled consumer education and the ability to have insurance cover thermography.

The cost of thermography is a small price to pay compared to the expense of a cancer diagnosis. The exam is as simple as getting your picture taken, so smile for the camera and save your breasts.

This chapter is dedicated to two of my very special and dear friends, Janet Ely and Faye Weatherbe. Both died at a much too young age after being diagnosed with breast cancer tumors that were large enough, even though small, to be visible on a scan. This early detection test could have saved their lives.

Footnotes

1 Lin QY, Yang HQ, et al. Detecting early breast tumour by finite element thermal analysis. *J Med Eng Technol*. 2009; 33(4):274-280.
2 Rhodes DJ, Hruska CB, et al. Dedicated dual-head gamma imaging for breast cancer screening in women with mammographically dense breasts. *Radiology*. 2011 Jan; 2011 Jan; 258(1):106-118.
3 Saputo L. Overview-Beyond Mammography. *Townsend Letter*. 2004 June.
4 Keyserlingk MD, et al. Infrared imaging of the breast: initial reappraisal using high-resolution digital technology in 100 successive cases of stage I and II breast cancer. *Breast J*. 1998 Jul; 4(4):245-251. doi: 10.1046/j.1524-4741.1998.440245.x.
5 Parisky YR, Sardi A, Hamm R, et al. Efficacy of computerized infrared imaging analysis to evaluate mammographically suspicious lesions. *AJR Am J Roentgenol*. 2003 Jan; 180(1):263-269.
6 Alternet website. A Basic Fact About Breasts that Could Save Your Life: And The Forces Trying to Keep It Under Wraps. October 20, 2013. Retrieved January 3, 2015 at: www.alternet.org/personal-health/basic-fact-about-breasts-could-save-your-life-and-forces-trying-keep-it-under-wraps.
7 FDA website. Press release September 18, 2012. FDA approves first breast ultrasound imaging system for dense breast tissue. Retrieved January 18, 2015 at: www.fda.gov/NewsEvents/Newsroom/PressAnnouncements/ucm319867.htm.

Chapter 36

Viral Screening

TEST

Summary and Explanation

Viral screenings are lab tests that check for the presence of a past or current infection. Samples of blood, urine, stool, organ tissue, spinal fluid, and saliva can be used for the tests; however, blood is most commonly utilized and is the type of test that we will discuss here.

Some of the most common viruses implicated with cancer are the human papilloma virus (HPV), Epstein-Barr virus (EBV), cytomegalovirus, hepatitis B (HBV), hepatitis C (HCV), human immunodeficiency virus (HIV), human herpes virus 8 (HHV-8), and the human t-lymphotrophic virus-1 (HTLV-1).

The American Cancer Society recognizes the link between viral, bacterial, and parasitic infections. They report infections account for around 10 percent of cancers in the United States and approximately 25 percent in developing countries.

Viruses are simple organisms that consist of genetic information in the form of DNA or RNA that is wrapped in a protective protein coating. Viruses enter a living cell and takeover the cell's activities by inserting their viral DNA and RNA. The cell has now become a factory for producing more viral cells. Some viruses are able to remain dormant in the infected cells and produce no new viral particles. In some cases, this type of latency in infected cells predisposes the cells to cancer.

It is important to know that viruses associated with cancer are found in many people in the healthy population, not just in the people who develop cancer. Viral infections create long term inflammation and suppress the immune system and that makes it easier for cancer to grow. They can also cause mutations at the cellular level and produce chronic infections in certain areas of the body that can lead to cancer.

The body's immune system makes antibodies to fight a specific viral infection. These antibodies attach to an infected cell allowing immune system cells to attack the virus. Viral testing looks for antibodies to a specific viral infection. If an antibody is found, this test can show whether a person was infected recently or in the past.

The evidence that a cancer is viral-related can be confirmed by the cancer tissue. When positive, often every cancer cell within a tumor will carry the same viral genetic information.[1] The viral antibody test is the most commonly utilized testing method and a test must be ordered for each specific virus. Viral antigen, culture, DNA or RNA detection tests are also available and are used less frequently.

A study by the International Agency for Research on Cancer in France reported on the global burden of cancers attributable to infections in 2008:

Of the 12.7 million new cancer cases that occurred in 2008, the population attributable fraction for infectious agents was 16.1%, meaning that around 2 million new cancer cases were attributable to infections. This fraction was higher in less developed countries (22.9%) than in more developed countries (7.4%), and varied from 3.3% in Australia and New Zealand to 32.7% in sub-Saharan Africa. Helicobacter pylori, hepatitis B and C viruses, and human papillomaviruses were responsible for 1.9 million cases, mainly gastric, liver, and cervix uteri cancers. In women, cervix uteri cancer accounted for about half of the infection-related burden of cancer; in men, liver and gastric cancers accounted for more than 80%. Around 30% of infection-attributable cases occur in people younger than 50 years.[2]

Identification of a virus can be an indicator that you may want to address the infection in the form of anti-viral drugs, vaccines, homeopathic remedies, or natural and herbal therapies.

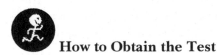 **How to Obtain the Test**

The viral antibody test is a simple blood test and it is available at most laboratories. The test requires no special preparation and you can eat and drink normally before the test. For insurance reimbursement, a doctor's order is usually needed.

Direct to consumer lab testing is available at www.requestatest.com for the cytomegalovirus, Epstein-Barr virus, hepatitis virus, herpes virus, and human immunodeficiency virus antigens. To order the test, log onto the site and create a user name and password. Testing locations are located around the country. You will be given a secure profile in which to view your results when available.

The test for the human t-lymphotrophic virus-1 (HTLV-1), associated with human T-cell leukemia/lymphoma and tropical spastic paraparesis, is not readily available so consult your physician. The test for human papilloma virus (HPV) is done as part of a cell swab taken during a gynecological exam.

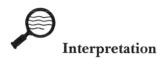 **Interpretation**

The antibody test is interpreted by looking at two different measurements.

* IgM antibodies usually develop within a couple of weeks after initial infection and are no longer detectable after several months. A positive result indicates a recent infection.
* IgG antibodies typically begin to develop several weeks or months after infection and remain present for the life of the person. After an initial infection, the virus will normally become inactive but may reactivate later in a person's life. Additional IgM antibodies are produced when a latent infection becomes active.

Normal value ranges may vary slightly among different laboratories.

Cost

Medicare and insurance usually cover the test when ordered by a physician. Check with your provider.

Direct to consumer pricing is available at www.requestatest. com for the cytomegalovirus, Epstein-Barr virus, hepatitis virus, herpes virus, and human immunodeficiency virus antigens. Prices range from $59 - $79 per test.

Process Time

Viral antibody tests results are usually available with 24 – 48 hours.

Benefits

- Individuals with a chronic viral infection are at an increased risk to develop cancer. A viral related cancer often takes years, even decades, to develop after a person gets an infection. Early detection of a viral condition with subsequent treatment may keep you from getting a cancer diagnosis later.
- Treatment of a viral infection can free up the immune system to fight other conditions such as cancer.

Limitations

Incubation periods, the development of an infection inside the body to the point at which the first signs of disease become apparent, may affect results and vary for each virus.

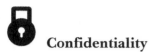 **Confidentiality**

Tests ordered by a physician will become part of your medical record. Tests ordered from a direct to consumer lab will be reported to you.

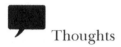 Thoughts

The viruses that are associated with cancer can often times be debilitating or at other times be quite insidious. By insidious, I mean that they can slowly and subtly cause harm and be destructive to your health. Often individuals are not even aware that they have an infection.

Since viral detection and treatments are available, I encourage you not to overlook this testing.

Footnotes

1   Cancer Research UK. Infections and cancer-an overview. Updated 1/01/12. Retrieved January 1, 2012 at: www.cancerresearchuk. org/cancer-info/cancerstats/causes/infectiousagents/virusesandcancer/viruses-in-general. This information is no longer available.

2   de Martel C, Ferlay J, Franceschi S, et al. Global burden of cancers attributable to infections in 2008: a review and synthetic analysis. *Lancet Oncol.* 2012 Jun; 13(6):607-615.

Chapter 37

Direct to Consumer Lab and Imaging Testing

Costs can vary significantly on laboratory and imaging services. Many of us are not aware of this because with insurance, we don't pay the bills; we may not be aware of what the lab charged or the amount that insurance actually paid to the lab. And those prices typically vary a lot.

You may have noticed that if you walk into a lab and pay for a standard lab test such as a vitamin D level, without a doctor's order or without having insurance, the cost is substantially higher than what insurance companies pay.

Insurance companies have leveraged their clout to get a better deal with labs such as LabCorp and Quest. You have seen the same concept at work when you book a hotel room. Hotels offer discounted rates if you are in their "rewards program" or if you have a membership in AAA (American Automobile Association) or some such affiliation. Insurance companies and direct-to-consumer lab testing companies don't pay "full price" either because they negotiated lower rates.

If you don't have insurance, or if you want a test your doctor has not ordered, you can use a direct-to-consumer company that makes their negotiated pricing available to you as a consumer. You can order the test yourself, usually online, pay for it, and get the results sent to you. Also, many imaging centers are offering discounted cash pricing on MRIs, PET, and CT scans.

Many people tell me they can't afford to get basic testing because they have no insurance or a huge deductible. Today, you have options with low cost testing. And if a problem is noted, the lab report alerts you to see a doctor. The earlier a problem is detected, the easier and more likely it is to be treatable.

We now have direct access to clinical laboratory testing across the U.S. for those important blood chemistry and wellness tests such as a complete blood count, urinalysis, liver function panel, cholesterol, allergy, C-reactive protein, hormones, HIV, and more.

Laboratory testing is available to the public at reduced pricing. The benefits are:

- No insurance is needed.
- Scheduling and payment are available online.
- Results are confidential.
- Many results are available in 24 hours.
- No medical exam is needed.
- No medical records required.
- No prescription is needed.
- No co-pay.
- No referral needed.

Getting standard lab tests is as easy as 1-2-3.

1. Order your tests and pay online, then print your requisition form.
2. Visit a laboratory location to have the sample collected. Be sure to bring a photo ID.
3. View your confidential results. Usually you can arrange to have the results emailed or faxed or mailed directly to you.

Tests are ordered online and pre-paid. Most of these companies accept Visa, MasterCard, American Express, Discover, and PayPal. Check their website for specials and coupons. Most labs require that you be 18 years old to purchase their services.

Tests may not be available in Maryland, New York, New Jersey, Rhode Island, and Massachusetts because state laws inhibit third party billing.

As always, if you find a problem, seek professional advice.

Direct-to-Consumer Laboratory Services In the United States:

www.LEF.org
800-208-3444

www.requestatest.com
888-732-2348

www.healthtestingcenters.com
877-511-5227

www.anylabtestnow.com
800-384-4567

www.personallabs.com
888-438-5227

www.directlabs.com
800-908-0000

www.walkinlab.com
800-539-6119

Imaging Services - Nationwide

NextImage Direct is a radiology management service company that offers you high-quality, low-cost imaging solutions. Savings can be as high as 70 percent for those who are uninsured, have a high deductible health plans, or wish to self-pay. CTs, MRIs, and ultrasounds are available. A prescription is required.

www.nextimagedirect.com
888-608-6099

MD Aligne offers telephone doctor consultations if you need a prescription for an imaging test. They offer 24 hour access to nurses and doctors. No prescription is necessary. Current cost is $65.00 for a phone consultation. Their doctors and nurses are U.S. licensed.

www.mdaligne.com
888-738-5574

Another option is to conduct an Internet search in your area for "cash pricing for medical imaging." Many cities have facilities that offer reduced cash pricing.

Consider taking advantage of the significant discounts offered by these companies. The days of the uninsured getting stuck paying exorbitant fees are soon fading. You have options.

Part 4

Additional Information to Consider

Chapter 38

Cancer – Beat It, Don't Feed It

We will know that America is serious about reducing the incidence of cancer when we see the American Cancer Society and the Susan G. Komen Foundation wage a "war on sugar."

I recently saw an invitation from a major hospital in the Houston area to attend "A Survivor's Celebration of Life." The program included culinary creations from local bakeries and a cake decorating contest. Since we know that many of these survivors will have a recurrence and that cancer cells use sugar for their metabolism, it is simply wrong for the people entrusted to cure these survivors to turn around and feed them something that will fuel their disease. I was speechless.

Along the same lines, I attended a luncheon for breast cancer survivors. As each woman left the luncheon, she was handed a beautifully wrapped iced cake pop. Pink of course. You can safely assume that I declined the parting gift.

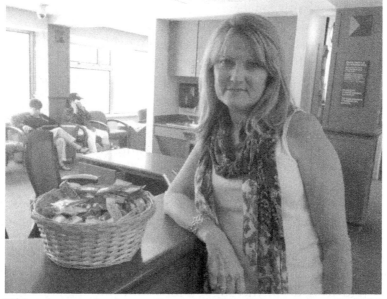

This photo – that's me, Jenny Hrbacek – was taken in 2013 in the surgical waiting area of one of Houston's well known cancer treatment centers. A large basket of candy awaits everyone at the desk.

I have other photos of the sugary items offered in the hospital cafeteria, such as at the pastry and beverage counters; however, I felt that the photo above made my point. To be fair, I did find a small basket of red and green apples near the register.

How can the medical establishment say it is waging a war on cancer while passing out candy? Simply, it cannot. The establishment has not taken what is arguably the first step in fighting cancer which is to wage war on sugar.

On February 4, 2014 front page newspaper headlines said, "Too much sugar tied to heart problems." The accompanying articles explained that a major CDC study – the biggest of its kind – concluded that consuming added sugar clearly increases risk of death from heart disease. People who consumed the highest amounts of added sugars were more than twice as likely to die from cardiovascular disease.[1]

Wow. That is straight to the point. Perhaps finally we are turning the corner and coming to a more enlightened approach to heart disease than blaming it on cholesterol, something the body makes and needs to survive and thrive.

But not so with cancer.

The same day, news headlines proclaimed: "Cancer to sky-rocket worldwide; imminent disaster; World Health Organization report faults smoking, obesity, rise in population."[2]

The American Cancer Society posted an essay for World Cancer Day 2014 and said:

> Avoiding tobacco, maintaining a healthy body weight, eating right and getting enough exercise, and getting appropriate cancer screening tests can all make a significant difference.[3]

No wow there. As usual, smoking leads the list. I agree that quitting smoking is a great preventive thing in terms of avoiding cancer, but since only 18 percent of Americans smoke anymore, that advice does not apply to 4 out of 5 people. Eating added sugar applies to many, many more people. Are the powers that be afraid to take on the sugar lobby and put sugar front and center in the war on cancer?

Are We Serious About Beating Cancer?

It is well known that lifestyle choices have proven to be an overwhelming factor in cancer development. If we removed artificial sweeteners, high fructose corn syrup, inflammatory vegetable oils, excess refined salt, genetically modified foods, antibiotics, hormones, pesticides, etc., from the standard American diet, I predict cancer rates would drop substantially.

Unfortunately, eating in today's world has become more about convenience and pleasure than it is about eating for nutrition. I have to admit, with the bounty of easily accessible processed foods with their attractive packaging, it is challenging to give your body what it needs in terms of quality fats, proteins, and carbohydrates on a daily basis. It can seem like a treasure hunt to find nourishing foods while avoiding toxic, empty calorie foods.

Encarta Dictionary defines food as, "material that provides living things with the nutrients they need for energy and growth." Check out your local vending machine and see if you think the items in it meet the definition of food. (Hint: they don't.)

In the 2010 American Cancer Society Annual Report, the organization touted the rollout of their new "Choose You" prevention program, aimed at getting women to think about their own health. And who sponsored this prevention effort? A major soft drink company whose product contains carbonated water, citric acid, natural flavors, potassium citrate, potassium benzoate, aspartame, and acesulfame potassium. Let's see . . . potassium benzoate is a preservative that forms benzene when it is combined with vitamin C (ascorbic acid) and sodium. The ACS calls benzene a carcinogen; European governments have banned its use in products such as pediatric medications. And aspartame, an artificial sweetener whose approval was very controversial and political, has been linked to cancer.[4]

Headlines were generated by the Susan G. Komen organization when they took money from chocolate candy makers (sugar), a fried chicken restaurant chain (fried foods are linked to cancer), and a number of companies that make processed foods. No organization serious about winning a war on cancer would pick these kinds of sponsors.

Sugar Acts As Fertilizer for Cancer

It has been known for decades that sugar is a major enemy of your body's immune system. And cancer is the ultimate immune system disorder. A 1973 study showed that simple sugars (including fructose, glucose, sucrose, honey, and even orange juice) can decrease the white blood cells' ability to fight infection for up to five hours after ingestion.[5] This study used high dosages of sugar, but the evidence strongly suggests that chronic consumption of sugar may suppress immunity. We all need a robust immune system to recognize and be able to kill cancer cells.

In 1800, the average person consumed about 18 pounds of sugar per year. Today, it's about 76 to 100 pounds a year, depending on who produces the statistic.[6] Sugar needs to be removed from the vocabulary, pantries, and diets of anyone who wants to be cancer free.

On a personal note, I want to encourage anyone who is not worried about the risk that sugary foods create, to be sensitive to anyone with cancer. The fight is tough enough without watching the people around you drinking sodas and eating candy bars, cookies, and chips.

I cannot emphasize enough how important diet is, whether you are in treatment, recovering, or trying to prevent cancer. Starchy carbohydrates and processed sugar have become a toxic addictive staple of most of our diets.

I understand that these foods are comforting to the patients and that the doctors don't take time to address diet because they are busy with tests results, chemo, surgery, etc. But this practice of turning a blind eye must end if we are going to reduce the incidence of cancer. So right now, it is up to you. You must take charge of all aspects of your health, even those that are not addressed by your doctor or covered by insurance.

A little eye-opening tidbit is that a seemingly harmless slice of whole wheat toast will raise your blood sugar at least as much as eating a small candy bar. Many people incorrectly believe toast is good for us, but the body rapidly breaks this grain down into sugar.

Processed Foods, a Poor Nutritional Choice

Processed foods are easy to recognize – they are nearly always in a package to make them more convenient. They have usually been heated, milled, irradiated, and contain artificial additives. Foods are usually processed to extend their shelf life. This is important for food that travels long distances or sits in supermarkets for long periods. For example, the natural fats in many oils go rancid within a few days, so removing them and replacing them with inexpensive, stable trans fats can extend shelf life by months. But their changed molecular structure links them to diseases like heart disease and cancer. For decades, the American Heart Association advised people to eat trans fats to prevent heart disease. The FDA is belatedly now, at the time of this writing, poised to revoke their "Generally Recognized As Safe" (GRAS) status.

Artificial sugars, flavorings, corn syrup, and salt are often added to improve the flavor and disguise the taste of low fat and low quality, inexpensive ingredients. Each step of the processing removes nutrients. Refined bread is "enriched" for example because so many vitamins are removed in processing. Much has been written warning of the synthetic, fractionated vitamins used to "fortify" flour and milk. There is little or no nutritional content in most of what you find in bag or box.

You can check the label on most processed food and find high levels of the infamously addictive trio: fat, salt, and sugar. Dr. David Kessler, former head of the FDA, said food companies have literally captured our brains to keep us coming back for more processed food products. Remember that marketing jingle for potato chips – you can't eat just one? Well, Dr. Kessler told us that is because food companies scientifically experiment with taste, texture, color, smell, look – and above all sugar, fat, and salt – to come as close as possible to eating's "bliss point," where the brain's reward system is captured by this immensely complex, artificially designed food that is as powerful as a drug.[7]

At some point, you have to just say NO.

Recently, several Latin American countries essentially said "NO" in an attempt to lessen the obesity epidemic. In 2014, Brazil released dietary guidelines that warned against processed foods. "Limit consumption of ready-to-consume food and drink products," the guidelines say. "When you eat out, choose restaurants that serve freshly made dishes and meals. Avoid fast food chains."[8] The city of Buenos Aires installed vending machines with fruit. And Mexico, which leads the most populous countries in obesity statistics, passed a groundbreaking soda tax that is expected to prevent up to 630,000 cases of diabetes by 2030. Billboards across Mexico City ran photographs of a man with amputated feet as a consequence of diabetes. They warned that a roughly 20-ounce bottle of soda contained 12 teaspoons of sugar, and asked, "Would you eat 12 spoonfuls of sugar? Why do you drink soda?"[9]

Reducing Sugar - Ketogenic Diet As an Option

The ketogenic diet is becoming a popular approach to removing sugar from the diet. It involves eliminating carbohydrates and replacing them with healthy beneficial fats and limited amounts of organic/grass fed protein. The principle behind this replacement is that since cancer cells need glucose (sugar) to thrive, and carbohydrates turn into glucose in your body, then cutting out processed carbs literally starves the cancer cells by taking their fuel source away. All cells including cancer cells use glucose for metabolism.

An important difference is that cancer cells cannot adapt to a fat or ketone burning mode while healthy cells can. The basic goal of the diet is to get the body to use fat for fuel rather than carbs. Some of the diet's good fats include olive oil, coconut oil, butter, avocados, egg yolks, and raw nuts. Protein recommendations are usually set at around 50 grams per day. Always consult an enlightened nutritionist or doctor when considering a diet change.

In my research into a nutrition plan that would deprive cancer cells of the sugar that they need to survive, I met Ellen Davis and read her book on the ketogenic diet. It is well researched and referenced. I highly recommend it; it will help you make a dietary change. It is available as an ebook at www.ketogenic-diet-resource.com.

Ms. Davis told me:

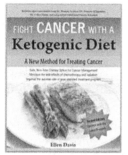

Making the statement that "cancer feeds on sugar" sounds like a fringe chant from some alternative health guru on television, but I can assure you, that statement is backed up with real scientific evidence from as far back as the early 1920s.

In 1924, Dr. Otto Warburg, a Nobel Prize winning biochemist, proposed the hypothesis that cancer is a metabolic disease. Dr. Warburg showed in his studies that cancer cells exhibit a preference for the fermentation of sugar as a fuel, even when the oxygen that normal cells use for energy creation is available. He wrote:

Cancer, above all other diseases, has countless secondary causes. But, even for cancer, there is only one prime cause. Summarized in a few words, the prime cause of cancer is the replacement of the respiration of oxygen in normal body cells by a fermentation of sugar.

Until recently, Dr. Warburg's hypothesis has been marginalized by the persistent belief in the oncology profession that cancer is a genetic disease. However, in the new book *Cancer As a Metabolic Disease: On the Origin, Management, and Prevention of Cancer*, Dr. Thomas Seyfried has begun to shed light on the hypothesis that cancer is instead a metabolically based disease, and that the genetic markers which the cancer research community has focused on for so long are really just downstream effects of the cancer cell's broken metabolism.

What does it mean to say that cancer is a metabolic disease? Metabolic diseases are conditions in which the metabolism, or the making of energy from the food we eat, is broken or abnormal in some way.

Normal body cells are able to create energy by using the food we eat and the oxygen we inhale to complete normal cellular "respiration" and make ATP (adenosine triphosphate), our main cellular energy source. Most of this energy production happens in the mitochondria, tiny organelles which are the "powerhouses" of the cell. There are two primary types of food-based fuels that our cells can use to produce energy:

- The first cellular fuel is glucose, which is also called by the common name of blood sugar or blood glucose. Glucose is a product of the starches and sugars, (carbohydrates) in our diet, and it is converted into energy in our cells via a process called glycolysis. In normal cells, glycolysis is a source of other molecules which flow into the mitochondria to complete normal oxygen dependent cellular respiration.
- The second type of cellular fuel comes from fatty acids. There are various kinds and they come from fats we eat or from the release of stored fat in our fat cells. When blood glucose is low, these fats are used to make up the fuel deficit. They are broken down by the liver into products called ketone bodies. This process is called ketogenesis, and the shift in metabolism that favors using fats as the primary source of energy is called ketosis.

When glucose levels are low, most normal cells will switch to using ketone bodies for fuel. Even the brain and nerve cells, which are normally dependent on glucose, can utilize ketone bodies for fuel. This ability of most normal cells to use ketones when glucose is unavailable indicates that the cell's mitochondria are healthy and functioning properly.

In contrast, cancer cells are less able to utilize ketones for energy. They have dysfunctional mitochondria which don't allow for this metabolic flexibility. That leaves cancer cells dependent on glucose and other less efficient forms of cellular energy.

Ketones allow normal cells to be metabolically flexible, so to speak. This metabolic flexibility is exactly why a ketogenic diet can exploit metabolically compromised cancer cells: by forcing them to literally "run out of fuel."

The ketogenic diet is a powerful tool for fighting cancer. But for all its metabolic power, it has very few side effects, and instead of being toxic to normal cells, it actually strengthens the body. People who adhere to the ketogenic diet have reported less physiological stress when undergoing mainstream chemotherapy and radiation treatments.

In fact, a ketogenic diet is an effective tool for just about any disease system involving metabolic derangement. This is why I have dedicated my www.ketogenic-diet-resource.com website to educating the public about the power of this diet. I want you to have all of the options.

Footnotes

1   Yang Q, Zhang Z, et al. Added Sugar Intake and Cardiovascular Diseases Mortality Among US Adults. *JAMA Internal Medicine.* 2014 Apr; 174(4):516-524.

2   CNN.com website February 4, 2014. Hume T, Christensen J. WHO: Imminent global cancer 'disaster' reflects aging, lifestyle factors. Retrieved January 19, 2015 at: http://www.cnn.com/2014/02/04/health/who-world-cancer-report/index.html.

3   American Cancer Society. World Cancer Day 2014. Retrieved January 27, 2014 at: www.cancer.org/cancer/news/world-cancer-day-2014.

4   Schernhammer ES, Bertrand KA, et al. Consumption of artificial sweetener – and sugar-containing soda and risk of lymphoma and leukemia in men and women. *Am J Clin Nutr.* 2012 Dec; 96(6):1419-1428. Erratum in *Am J Clin Nutr.* 2013 Aug; 98(2):512.

5   Sanchez A, Reeser JL, Lau HS, et al. Role of sugars in human neutrophilic phagocytosis. *Am J Clin Nutr.* 1973; 26(11):1180-1184.

6   Strom S. U.S. Cuts Estimate of Sugar Intake. *New York Times.* October 26, 2012.

7   Kessler D. *The End of Overeating: Taking Control of the Insatiable American Appetite.* Rodale. 2009.

8   Food Politics website. Brazil's new dietary guidelines: food-based! English translation retrieved January 14, 2015 at: www.foodpolitics.com/2014/02/brazils-new-dietary-guidelines-food-based.

9   Guthrie A. Health Battle Over Soda Flares in Mexico. *The Wall Street Journal.* August 29, 2013.

Chapter 39

Nutrients – Critical Components

G. Edward Griffin in his 2010 eye-opening book, *World Without Cancer*, asks the question: Why hasn't orthodox medicine embraced non-drug approaches to healing and health? He says the answer is to be found, not in science, but in politics, and is based upon the hidden economic and power agenda of those who dominate the medical establishment:

> There is a great deal of evidence supporting the nutritional-deficiency concept of cancer – more than enough to convince most people that the thesis is proven. But the word *proven*, when used by the FDA, has an entirely different meaning. It is a technical definition. When the FDA says a therapy is *proven*, it means only that its promoters have complied with the testing protocols set by the agency to demonstrate safety and effectiveness. It is important to know, however, that the successful completion of those tests does not mean, as the terminology implies, that the therapy is *safe* and effective. It merely means that tests have been conducted, the results have been evaluated, and the FDA has given its approval for marketing, often *in spite of t*he dismal results . . .

> No substance from nature will ever be legally available for cancer or *any other* disease unless its source can be monopolized or its processing can be patented. No matter how safe and effective it may be, and no matter how many people are benefited, it will forever be relegated to the category of "unproven" therapies. As such, freely available cures from nature will always be illegal to prescribe, to promote, and in many cases even to use.[1]

The FDA's system of establishing the efficacy of things is not designed to take into account the impact of nutrition and lifestyle changes. And we wonder why we have lost the war on cancer? We never addressed it very fully. We went down a singular road of surgical and chemical attack and left many other roads relatively untraveled.

Anti-cancer Natural Substances

Many substances that enter the body are potentially carcinogenic, depending upon what happens when they interact with enzymes in the liver. Some phytonutrients – beneficial substances in plants – enhance the production of enzymes that render potentially carcinogenic substances harmless. Garlic, onions, broccoli, and cauliflower are examples of foods with beneficial phytonutrients.[2]

Integrative oncologists have been using food and natural substances to treat cancer for many decades. Many of the most common items are available at your local grocery store or farmers markets.

Dr. William Li, president and medical director of the Angiogenesis Foundation, has done a tremendous amount of research on the health benefits of natural foods. He has found that some foods have the ability to inhibit the process through which cancer cells create new blood vessels by boosting our bodies' natural ability to produce angiogenesis inhibitors. Without blood vessels to supply them with the nutrients necessary for growth, microscopic cancers find it difficult to grow and spread. Li explains in his lectures that healthy cells have a natural system of checks and balances to regulate the growth of blood vessels. He refers to this as angiogenesis stimulators and inhibitors. However, we know that cancer cells make errors in DNA replication and this somehow allows these cells to hijack the body's system of checks and balances, using angiogenesis stimulators to create the blood supply they need for survival and growth. It has been reported that a tiny microscopic tumor, given a steady supply of blood, can grow to up to 16,000 times its original size in as little as a few weeks. This brings us back to the potential for circulating tumor cells (CTCs) to escape the tumor and travel through the blood and start a new metastasis.

If a substance is anti-angiogenic – tumeric, cinnamon, parsley, garlic, berries, apples, green tea, olive oil, bok choy, and kale to name it few – it has the ability to interfer with cancer cells' ability to create a blood supply. And if it is an apoptosis agent – such as marine oils, omega 3s, onions, radishes, resveratrol, berberine – it promotes cancer cell death.

If you wish to avoid cancer, or if testing indicates that you are about to be diagnosed with it, accept the benefits that nature has to offer. Incorporate some of these naturally occurring inhibitors into your diet.

What follows here is a list and the functional description for some of the top anti-cancer substances in nature. Many of these items are included in the nutient sensitivity testing offered by R.G.C.C. and Biofocus labs. It is important to note that no treatment should be undertaken without the supervision of a physician.

Cancer does not have an instruction book and everyone is different. That is why nutrient sensitivity testing can be helpful. Also, my experience is that it is best to use a multifaceted approach, meaning not just shooting one bullet at the target but firing a whole round of different kinds of bullets. You too can learn more about how these natural assets hit the cancer cell from every possible angle:

Vitamin C (Ascorbic Acid)

Intravenous vitamin C may be one of the best documented natural cancer treatments. Vitamin C is selectively toxic to cancer cells and tumor-toxic levels of vitamin C can be attained using intravenous administration.[3] Vitamin C kills cancer because cancer cells do not have the enzyme catalase to break down hydrogen peroxide (H_2O_2) into water and oxygen. Oral vitamin C is an antioxidant and is not effective; however, IV vitamin C is a pro-oxidant, because it generates hydrogen peroxide (H_2O_2) in the extracellular space. The result is that the tumor is killed from the inside out by the resulting H_2O_2.

Curcumin

Curcumin is a perennial herb in the ginger family and the major component in curry powder. It is the active ingredient in turmeric and in high concentrations can be very useful adjunct in cancer treatment. Studies of this herb have shown immense therapeutic potential in preventing breast cancer metastasis. It has been shown to inhibit proliferation of cancer cells by arresting them at various phases of the cell cycle. Curcumin-induced apoptosis mainly involves a mitochondria-mediated pathway.[4]

Vitamin D

The hormonally active form of vitamin D, calcitriol 1,25-dihydroxyvitamin, also called D(3), is being widely used for cancer prevention and treatment. It has been proven to inhibit the growth of many kinds of cancers.[5] It is a promoter of apoptosis, inhibits the invasion of other tissues, inhibits metastasis, and is anti-angiogenic. Vitamin D also has anti-inflammatory properties and interferes with estrogen synthesis.[6] New genes are frequently discovered that vitamin D either up-regulates or down-regulates in the body's attempt to keep us healthy.

Beta Glucan

Beta glucan is a natural extract from baker's yeast. It has shown anti-tumor activity in many cancers. Studies show that it enhances the production of immune cells in the bone marrow. Also, phagocytes, "eating cells," have been shown to engulf more invaders and digest them faster with beta glucan bound to their receptor cites. Beta glucan is often described as the substance that puts microscopic glasses on your immune cells.

Mistletoe

This is a semi-parasitic plant that grows on some types of trees. Mistletoe extract is called Iscador. In some European countries, extracts made from European mistletoe are among the most prescribed therapies for cancer patients. Extracts of mistletoe have been shown to kill cancer cells in the laboratory and to boost the immune system.[7] The FDA has not approved the use of mistletoe as a treatment for cancer and does not allow injectable mistletoe extracts to be imported or used except for clinical research.

Salvestrol

Salvestrols are a new class of natural chemicals found in plants and can be safely eaten in the diet. They are reported to have the ability to recognize and enter cancer cells. Once inside the cancer cell, they undergo a process of molecular activation by a special enzyme, CYP1B1, and thereby cause the cells to cease growing or die. CYP1B1 is pronounced "sip one bee one" and is an intrinsic component of cancer cells. Salvestrols are available in fruits, vegetables, and herbs such as strawberries, blueberries, broccoli, bell peppers, basil, parsley, and mint.[8,9] The attention that salvestrol receives confirms why a plant-rich diet has traditionally been considered to offer protection against cancer.[10]

Artemisinin

Artemisinin or wormwood extract comes from a Chinese herb. It has been used for thousands of years for treating malaria and more recently, cancer. Artemisinin becomes cytotoxic (cell killing) in the presence of ferrous iron. Once inside the cell, artemisinin reacts with the iron inside the cell, spawning highly reactive chemicals called "free radicals." The free radicals attack other molecules and the cell membrane, breaking it apart and killing the cells. The process selectively targets cancer cells, leaving healthy cells alone.[11] Dr. Robert Rowan says artemisinin is a close cousin to oxygen therapy in that it delivers a knockout oxidative stress to cancer cells.[12]

Iodine

Iodine is an essential trace element, a vitally important nutrient that is detected in every organ and tissue of the human body. Many, if not most of us, are deficient. We may not get enough in our food, and our body's ability to use iodine is compromised by environmental toxins like fluoride and perchlorate. Iodine-deficient breast tissue shows alterations in DNA and increases in estrogen receptor proteins.[13] Breast cancer cells avidly absorb iodine, which in turn suppresses tumor growth and causes cancer cell death.

Lycopene

Lycopene is a carotenoid, a pigment made by plants. Lycopene is found in fruits and vegetables like tomatoes, carrots, apricots, and watermelons. Studies have shown that supplementing with lycopene can reduce PSA levels in men; prostate cancer cells treated with lycopene had changes in their cell division cycle, leading to less cancer cell growth.[14]

Berberine

Berberine is a natural alkaloid found in a wide variety of traditional herbs including goldenseal, barberry and Oregon grape. It demonstrates important benefits for cancer modulation, glucose metabolism, maintenance of healthy lipid levels, insulin sensitivity, cardiac support, weight management, gastrointestinal health, immune modulation, and cognitive support.[15]

Haelan 951

Haelan 951 is a unique liquid dietary supplement used by many naturopaths and integrative oncologists. It is made from non-genetically modified *fermented* soy. It is used to boost the immune system and suppress cancer cell progression. It is usually used to supplement to an existing cancer treatment protocol. To read more about and the studies done on it, go to www.haelanproducts.com.

Quercetin

Quercetin is a type of plant-based chemical, or phytochemical, known as a flavonoid. Findings suggest that quercetin displays antitumor activity by triggering apoptosis. It has been shown to down-regulate the expression of an anti-apoptosis protein and up-regulate the expression of pro-apoptosis protein. It also shows activation of a mitochondrial pathway to induce apoptosis (cell self-destruction). Good sources include grapefruit, apples, onions, red wine, and black tea.

Paw Paw

This is an edible bean-shaped fruit native to North America also called Asimina triloba. In vitro studies demonstrated that Paw Paw extract has cytotoxic properties against cancer cell lines including those resistant to Adriamycin® (a chemo drug) and has anti-angiogenic properties. Another reported mechanism of action is that it causes a drop in the ATP or energy of the cell, thus promoting apoptosis/cell death.[16]

Amygdalin B17 (Laetrile)

Laetrile is a partly man made (synthetic) form of the natural substance amygdalin. Amygdalin is a plant substance found naturally in raw fruit seeds, particularly apricot kernels. Laetrile works by targeting and killing cancer cells and building the immune system. BioFocus reports that amygdalin B17 is capable of down regulation of the expression of Cox2, a human protein that is evaluated in their lab test. The use of laetrile for cancer is not legal in the United States, although studies in the 1970s verified its safety and effectiveness, according to Ralph Moss.[17]

Inositol Hexaphosphate (IP6)

IP6 is a chemical found in beans, brown rice, corn, sesame seeds, wheat bran, and other high-fiber foods. It is a powerful antioxidant, immune system enhancer, and booster of natural killer cells. It has been called a "natural cancer fighter" and scientific studies suggest that it slows or reverses the growth of various forms of cancer, including breast, colon, and prostate cancers.[18] The pioneer in the study of IP6 is Dr. Abulkalam Shamsuddin, a scientist at the University of Maryland School of Medicine. He discovered IP6 can control the rate of abnormal cell division and normalize the sugar production of cancerous cells, thereby altering their gene expression toward a more healthful state.

C-statin

C-statin is a group of proteoglycan molecules isolated from a common garden weed called bindweed. It acts as an anti-angiogenesis factor meaning it stops new blood vessels from growing. Cancer is surrounded by many small blood vessels (angiogenesis). If the angiogenesis is inhibited, cancer cells will be starved.

Di-Indoly Methane (DIM)

DIM is a phytonutrient (plant nutrient) found in cruciferous vegetables (such as broccoli, cabbage, cauliflower, kale, turnips and mustard greens). It specifically promotes beneficial estrogen metabolism and helps restore a healthy hormonal balance. This is important because estrogen is known to promote cancer cell growth. According to Memorial Sloan-Kettering Cancer Center, DIM has been found to help prevent and treat breast and prostate cancers. Studies done on animals also found DIM to prevent the replication and spreading of cancer cells.

Genistein

Genistein is the predominate isoflavone found in soy products. The primary known activity of genistein is as a tyrosine kinase inhibitor, mostly of the epidermal growth factor receptors (EGFR) of cancer cells. There is a growing body of evidence that it modulates cell activity increasing apoptosis.

Resveratrol

Resveratrol is found in the skin on red grapes and other fruits. Resveratin has both resveratrol and quercetin. Resveratrol acts to induce apoptosis. It is also a powerful antioxidant and neutralizes free radicals. Free radicals can lead to cancer by causing mutations in a cell's DNA or by promoting inflammation.

Medical Cannabis

There has been at great deal of research done on the chemical compounds secreted by the oils of cannabis flowers. THC is most well-known of its compounds, or cannabinoidsas they are called, because it produces the "marijuana high." But that is just one of at least 85 compounds in this plant. Another compound, CBD, is the primary focus of medical cannabis. Studies have shown that some cannabinoids have anti-tumor effects, including induction of cell death, inhibition of cell growth, and inhibition of tumor angiogenesis, invasion and metastasis. Cannabinoids work by binding to receptors throughout the body. Therefore, it is critical to aim the right cannabinoids at the right receptors. I strongly encourage anyone considering medical cannabis to not buy blindly. With cancer and other conditions, it is critical that the correct ratio of cannabinoids be utilized; there are different ratios for different cancers and conditions. United Patients Group (UPG), based out of California (415-524-8099 www.UnitedPatientsGroup.com), is a leader in information and education for cannabinoid therapeutics, including CME courses for physicians. UPG provides the essential guidance needed to make critical decisions that may affect your life. A consultation with their oncology nurse or nurse-practitioner is approximately $150. They will review your records, labs, and scans and discuss your options.

Modified Citrus Pectin

Citrus pectin is the naturally occurring soluble fiber that joins the cells of fruit together. Modified citrus pectin (MCP) is made from pectin purified from the inner pith of citrus peel. This kind of pectin is indigestible and passes through the intestinal tract. A great deal of research has been done on the benefits of MCP. It has been shown to prevent abnormal cellular growth including cancer, modulate immune function, remove heavy metals and toxins from the body, and block the creation of fibrotic scar tissue. MCP has also been shown to inhibit galectin-3 activity in the extracellular matrix and blood stream. Cancer patients typically have elevated levels of a protein called galectin-3 and this can increase the probability of metastasis. Refer to Galectin-3 Test chapter for information on the galectin-3 test. There are many forms of MCP and I want to caution you not to buy blindly. The molecular weight and structure of the pectin molecules must be extremely small so they can enter the blood stream and be effective at the cellular level. I had the opportunity to visit with Isaac Eliaz, M.D., of Santa Rosa, California; virtually all the clinical trials in the last two decades have used his formulation, PectaSol-C by ecoNugenics. I have personally added his formulation to my anti-cancer regime.

Poly-MVA

Poly-MVA® is a one-of-a-kind powerful liquid nutritional supplement. I was introduced to it because it showed a positive response on my R.G.C.C. nutrient sensitivity test. I am impressed by the case studies and positive reports shared by patients and doctors with whom we have spoken and interviewed.

Poly-MVA is a bit expensive but worth it, especially if you are dealing with or have had cancer or a degenerative disease. Note: as the rates of cancer are increasing in pets, Poly-MVA is available for them also.

I want to share a bit of information on Poly-MVA because of its usefulness in cancer and many other chronic medical conditions.

The following information is provided with permission from AMARC Enterprises, Inc. Statements have not been evaluated by the Food and Drug Administration, and the product is not intended to diagnose, treat, cure or prevent any disease.

- What Poly-MVA Is and How It Works

  Poly-MVA is a patented and uniquely-formulated liquid dietary supplement. It contains a proprietary complex of the mineral palladium bonded to alpha-lipoic acid and vitamin B1 along with a proprietary blend of B2 and B12; formyl-methionine; N-acetyl cysteine; plus trace amounts of molybdenum, rhodium, and ruthenium. "MVA" stands for minerals, vitamins, and amino acids.

  This formulation is designed to provide energy for compromised body systems by changing the electrical potential of cells and facilitating aerobic metabolism within the cell. In other words, it shuttles energy for proper metabolism. As a nutritional supplement, Poly-MVA works at the cellular level in the electron transport chain, supporting the mitochondria while protecting the cell and it's DNA/RNA.

  Poly-MVA travels easily throughout the body, and can cross the blood-brain barrier. Poly-MVA is showing great promise in cases where other means of supporting cell nutrition are ineffective and in combination with many other protocols.

  In more scientific terms, the proper transfer and movement of energy/electrons is how cells process all their various functions, communicate, and survive. Normal cells use oxygen and energy/electron transfer one way, and abnormal cells a different way. PolyMVA targets this cellular pathway and therefore can support ALL normal cell functions. This electron dysfunction in abnormal/anaerobic cells is how many chemotherapeutics and radiation therapies try to target abnormal cells, and the effort requires the presence of electrons. Lipoic acid palladium complexes can generate and shuttle energy/electrons; it therefore can be used in some cases as adjunctive support to potentiate – make stronger – various therapies. This polymer/complex not only protects the cell, but will also donate energy to the normal cells electron transport chain via the mitochondria which in turn provides energy to the cell by supporting the ATP cycle where by whereby it can stabilize and support the metabolic needs of the cell.

The benefits of the lipoic acid palladium complex in Poly-MVA may include:

o Discourage abnormal cell growth.
o Support oxygenation of cells and tissue.
o Support the liver in removing harmful substances from the body.
o Improve metabolic function – enhance proper cellular function for normal cells, and provide underperforming cells (compromised mitochondrial function) with more energy.
o Slow the aging process from cellular breakdown.
o Support cellular function and raise energy levels.
o Support appetite.
o Protect cellular DNA.
o Convert free radicals into an energy source.
o Support nerve and neurotransmitter function.
• Ongoing Research
Poly-MVA has undergone numerous cell line studies, safety, animal, and human tests since 1992 when it was formulated. Among those:

o Board certified oncologist Dr. James W. Forsythe M.D., H.M.D., of Nevada conducted an outcome study on various stage IV adult cancers with 500+ patients over a 7 year period, observing a 70 percent overall positive response rate. He concluded that Poly-MVA is an essential component of his patients' protocols for improved results, health, and overall outcomes:

In stage IV adult cancers of any origin, improvement in quality of life issues is directly proportional to improvement to overall response rate. Even stable disease can be effectively managed and improved into a chronic livable condition. Poly-MVA has been a key part of this protocol since 2004 and we look forward to its ongoing integration into various types of other protocols for mitochondrial dysfunction.

o   Ongoing research by independent laboratories has confirmed the effectiveness of Poly-MVA in multiple cancer types, including: brain, lung, breast, skin, prostate, and liver.
o   Ischemia studies demonstrated that acute, post, and prophylactic administration of Poly-MVA limits damage and protects cellular function.
o   Phase I human safety trials have been conducted in the PUNCH Study (Poly-MVA Utilized as Neuroprotection against Chronic Hypertension), paving the way for a glioblastoma study, multiple myeloma and M/S studies.
o   A 1000-patient animal study with a veterinary oncologist resulted in an 86 percent improved quality of life response in the animals' health.

Poly-MVA has been approved by the FDA's review process for further investigation in human clinical use for efficacy in cancer and degenerative disease care.

⌘⌘⌘

I encourage you to see the "Doctors Reviews" and "Customers Experiences" tabs at www.polyMVA.com and www.polymva-survivors.org. Numerous articles, studies, and in-depth data are available on their website.

. . . do you not know that your body is the temple of the Holy Spirit within you, whom you have from God? You are not your own, for you were bought with a price. So glorify God in your body.

– 1 Corinthians 6:19-20

NUTRIENTS – CRITICAL COMPONENTS 369

Footnotes

1 Griffin GE. *World Without Cancer: the Story of Vitamin B17*. American Media, Second edition, 2010.

2 Tortora GJ, Derrickson B. *Essentials of Anatomy and Physiology*. 9th edition. 2013; p. 70.

3 Orthomolecular Medicine News Service press release September 22, 2005: Intravenous Vitamin C is Selectively Toxic to Cancer Cells. Retrieved January 14, 2015 at: http://orthomolecular.org/resources/omns/v01n09.shtml.

4 Karunagaran D, Rashmi R, Kumar TR. Induction of apoptosis by curcumin and its implications for cancer therapy. *Curr Cancer Drug Targets*. 2005 Mar; 5(2):117-129.

5 Garland C, Garland F, et al. The role of vitamin D in cancer prevention. *Am J Public Health*. 2006 Feb; 96(2):252-261.

6 Vuolo L, Somma CD, et al. Vitamin D and Cancer. *Front Endocrinol* (Lausanne). 2012; 3:58.

7 Choi SH, Lyu SY, Park WB. Mistletoe lectin induces apoptosis and telomerase inhibition in human A253 cancer cells through dephosphorylation of Akt. *Arch Pharm Res*. 2004 Jan; 27(1):68-76.

8 Murray G, Taylor M, et al., Tumor-specific expression of cytochrome P450 CYP1B1. *Cancer Res*. 1997; 57:3026-3031.

9 Potter GA, Patterson LH, et al. The cancer preventative agent resveratrol is converted to the anticancer agent piceatannol by the cytochrome P450 enzyme CYP1B1. *Br J Cancer*. 2002 March 4; 86(5):774-778. doi: 10.1038/sj.bjc.6600197.

10 Schaefer B. *Salvestrols: Nature's Defence Against Cancer: Linking Diet and Cancer*. CreateSpace Independent Publishing Platform. 2012.

11 Lai HC, Singh NP, Sadaki T. Development of artemisinin compounds for cancer treatment. *Invest New Drugs*. 2013 Feb; 31(1):230-246.

12 Rowan RJ. Artemisinin: From Malaria to Cancer Treatment. *Townsend Letter*. December 2002.

13 Eskin BA. Iodine and mammary cancer. *Adv Exp Med Biol*. 1977; 91:293-304.

14 National Cancer Institute. Prostate Cancer, Nutrition, and Dietary Supplements. Q&A About Lycopene. Updated 11/25/13. Retrieved January 29, 2015 at: www.cancer.gov/cancertopics/pdq/cam/prostatesupplements/Patient/page4.

15 Tan W, Li Y, et al. Berberine hydrochloride: anticancer activity and nanoparticulate delivery system. *Int J Nanomed*. 2011; 6:1773-1777.

16 Coothankandaswamy V, Liu Y, et al. The alternative medicine pawpaw and its acetogenin constituents suppress tumor angiogenesis via the HIF-1/VEGF pathway. *J Nat Prod*. 2010 May 28; 73(5):956-961.

17 Consumer Health Organization of Canada website. Moss R. Why We Are Losing the War on Cancer. June 1990. Retrieved January 15, 2015 at: www.consumerhealth.org/articles/display. cfm?ID=19990831140122.

18 Shafie NH, Esa NM, et al. Pro-Apoptotic Effect of Rice Bran Inositol Hexaphosphate (IP6) on HT-29 Colorectal Cancer Cells. *Int J Mol Sci*. 2013 December; 14(12):23545-23558.

Chapter 40

What to Do Now

I hope that by this point in the book you have learned that cancer is more than just a tumor; it is an outward manifestation of a sick body. The causes – cellular toxicity and deficiency – must be addressed.

I am a big believer in the ability of the body to heal if it has the necessary building blocks. Every day is a new day and you can birth healthy cells tomorrow. Those healthy cells will come forth from a body that has the necessary fats, minerals, vitamins, and amino acids from proteins to function properly.

This may require a change in thought process. Instead of living to eat, you eat to live. I am personally doing this and I invite you to join me.

If your testing is positive for cancer
or tells you that it may be developing,
what should you do?

The relatively new science of epigenetics tells us that only 3 percent to 5 percent of cancers are genetically driven, meaning caused by the genes over which we have no control. The vast majority of cancers are epigenetically driven, meaning caused by environmental factors that turn some of our genes on or off.

When the Human Genome Project was finished in 2003, we finally had a map of the human genes. Many experts were surprised to find that humans have just 25,000 genes, not the 100,000 as was expected. This pretty much put an end to the idea that one gene gone wrong was the cause of any one disease. Something else and more complex was at work. Scientists began to focus on the epigenome, a network of chemical switches that tweak how our genes express.

We inherit one copy of a gene from Mom, and one from Dad. We may inherit one bad gene, but we likely inherit at least one good gene. That is enough for most people to live their lifetime with that one good gene expressing.

For example, the BRCA1 mutation makes a person more susceptible to breast cancer, but not everyone with this mutation will have breast cancer? Why? Epigenetics. Our network of chemical messengers is affected by an extra dose of vitamins, exposure to toxins like pesticides and radiation, a critical stress like divorce or job loss . . . Vitamin D speaks to our genes, so does the spice curcumin. Food and environment tweak the chemical messengers and affect whether some genes turn on or off.

There is a lot we can do to encourage good expression and discourage cancer.

Assemble a Team and Test

Cancer is a formidable opponent and will require that you assemble a team of experts. Use the resource section in this book as a starting place. Get on the phone and Internet and research to connect with nutrition minded integrative professionals. Interview their patients and ask about real survival outcomes. Interview doctors and ask lots of questions. Find a physician who believes in the "support and heal" philosophy, not just the "attack and kill" approach.

Commit to beating the disease and measure the progress of your treatment with one or more of the tests in this book. Make adjustments when needed. If you are not getting positive results, reevaluate and try something else.

Good Nutrition Is Critical

Know that many of your food preferences were established when you were a young child and they continue to be influenced by your present environment – an environment where almost one out of two people get cancer.

Look at your thoughts; employ your brain, not just your taste buds. Instead of thinking how delicious a piece of thick chocolate cake looks, take a minute and consider the fats, sugar, empty calories, and artificial chemicals that will permeate your body if you eat it. Tell yourself that your body deserves better. Love yourself enough to feed your body according to its needs.

Our diet, heavy on processed foods, is making us fat and sick. We need to go back to basics. If the label has a lot of ingredients, and ones you cannot pronounce, move on to something more natural and healthy.

This is probably a good time to mention that I look at labels that say "natural" with a raised eyebrow, because the term does not have any legal meaning and food producers love to use it on everything. You can buy hamburger that comes from cattle given hormones and steroids and antibiotics and fed an unnatural diet of genetically modified corn and soy. The meat counter may have a sign saying "all natural," but God would say otherwise.

I encourage you to invest in your health and healing by seeking out a holistic nutrition specialist, one who will incorporate many of Mother Nature's benefits through the use of purposeful supplementation. Consider more than a multivitamin – consider whole foods, properly prepared.

It is my opinion that cancer treatments will produce marginal benefits if nutrition is not addressed. Please don't leave out this important aspect.

Here is a thought from Paul Zane Pilzer, an economist who earned his first $10 million before the age of thirty. Pilzer says the American sickness-based health insurance system will be replaced by a new wellness-based system that will pay for weight reduction, exercise plans, nutritional advice, vitamins, minerals, and hundreds of other wellness-related or preventative treatments. He predicts that a wellness revolution is coming, a shift to proactive wellness that will reshape our lives as much as the automobile and the personal computer did. It would be none too soon for those who are about to become a cancer statistic.

So You Want to Prevent Cancer or Support Your Body to Defeat It

You eat at least three times a day. It matters what you eat. Feed yourself like you want to live to see your grandchildren grow up – or whatever in life is fulfilling for you.

Before I begin this section, I need to define what I mean by the term "food." Basically, it is things that will rot, spoil, and decay because they have life in them and can give life to us when we eat them. Digestion of "empty" carbs depletes the body's reserves of vitamins, minerals, and enzymes. That concept takes most of our readily available processed food products out of the discussion. So with that defined, please read on.

How do you start? I'll share a few things that I learned along the way and wish I had known at the start:

Don't Eat 4 Hours Before Bedtime

This may seem hard, but let me first say that you can have a 100-calorie snack before bed. If you understand why this is important, it may be a bit easier. When we go to bed with a full stomach, digestion gets priority and the nutrients and energy that would be used for nighttime detox and healing will be spent on digestion. Also, the bi-product of digestion is acid waste, waste that would be removed by the kidneys during the day, but during the night, the kidneys are trying to rest, leaving the body to rest in all that acid waste. Remember, most cancer thrives in an acidic body.

Hydrate

Drink lots of clean water. Proper hydration will open up the body's detoxification pathways and assist with alkalinity. If you have a reverse osmosis system that gets rid of chlorine and fluoride, that's great. But add minerals because reverse osmosis strips the water of minerals and electrolytes. Start the day with a cup of warm lemon tea. I squeeze the juice of a fresh lemon in warm water for an alkalizing drink. I try to drink one ounce of water for every two pounds of body weight.

Green Juice

Many advocate for green juices, but I want to express a caution. Many people "chug" the juice and that is an unnatural way to digest it. Vegetables are a carbohydrate and they want to be primarily digested by the amylase enzyme in the saliva in the mouth. In other words, they want to be chewed; they want to be in contact with the amylase enzyme. Organic green vegetable juice can fill the gap many people have because they don't eat enough vegetables. If you can't make it from scratch, substitute with a green food supplement. I use "Green Power" from Welltrients. It is a capsule, easier to take. But again a word of caution, you need fiber and that comes from real vegetables.

Enzyme Supplementation

As we age, our natural enzyme levels are reduced and most people will benefit from supplementation. Take digestive enzymes with meals to help with digestion. This will aid in the complete digestion of food and reduce acid producing fermentation in the colon. This may seem like a needless and laborious step, but it can make a huge difference.

According to Dr. Jonathan Wright, most of us don't make enough stomach acid, hydrochloric acid (HCL) to break down our foods well. It may seem counterintuitive because so many people take antacids to relieve what they think is too much stomach acid. But actually, when you have too little acid, food ferments and those gasses come up into the esophagus (i.e., heartburn). The stomach was meant to be an acid chamber to break down proteins especially. My Welltrients supplement includes both HCL and a wide variety of digestive enzymes.

Proteolytic enzymes (protein-eating) work differently. For cancer patients, these enzymes are typically used to weaken the protein coating around cancer cells that protects them. Proteolytic enzymes can also reduce inflammation; kill off bacteria, viruses, molds, and fungi; clean the blood of debris and fibrin; and work on large undigested proteins that made their way into the bloodstream where they trigger allergies and autoimmune disease. These enzymes can be taken on an empty stomach (two hours after a meal or in the middle of the night).

High Quality Protein

Cancer patients in particular need adequate amounts of protein to prevent muscle wasting. But it is a balancing act. You need enough protein to build, repair, and maintain the body, but not so much that you inadvertently feed the growth of cancer cells. I keep my protein consumption to about 6 – 7 ounces per day. This is important because excess protein is believed to stimulate the mammalian target of rapamycin (mTOR) pathways, which facilitate the building of muscles. However, this can be detrimental when treating cancer, as the mTOR pathway increases cellular proliferation because it increases growth hormone and IGF-1. Interestingly, the pharmaceutical drug Metformin, which has anti-cancer activity, also inhibits the mTOR pathway.

I calculate my needed daily protein consumption by dividing my weight in pounds by 2.2 to convert it to kilograms, and then I multiply by 0.8. This gives me my total daily amount of protein in grams. As a general rule of thumb, I keep the serving to about the size of a deck of cards.

Protein sources should be nutrient dense and high quality – eggs and chicken from pastured farms, beef that is grass fed, and fish that is never farm-raised. Do not consume meat from animals slaughtered in large feedlots where they were fed drugs and an unnatural diet. The hormones and antibiotics these animals were given to make them grow fast also fuel cancer.

Avoid charring your meats. Acrylamide, a carcinogen, is created when starchy foods are baked, roasted, grilled or fried and has been found to increase cancer risk.

Essential Fatty Acids

Many nutrition experts are saying that the biggest dietary mistake we have made in the last 50 years came when we turned our back on butter, coconut oil and other natural, unprocessed fats that fed mankind for centuries. Instead, we were erroneously told to embrace vegetable oils, and it did sound healthy, didn't it? But mankind never ate these oils before. Processed oils (corn, soy, canola) are high in omega-6 fatty acids and that throws off our balance. They are often pumped with hydrogen so they have a longer shelf life. These are a source of lethal trans fats. Most of us need to increase omega-3 fats with avocados, walnuts, wild caught salmon (not farmed), or sardines. Good oils to use are coconut oil, avocado, and extra virgin olive oil. You might supplement with organic flax and evening primrose oils, two tablespoons of each a day. Omega-3 deficiencies are a common underlying factor for cancer. Some 50 percent of our cell membranes are made up of fat – make it the best quality possible so nutrients and oxygen can get into the cells and waste products can leave.

Increase Consumption of Living Food

Eat about half of your food in its natural or fermented state, which means before any cooking or freezing. The living enzymes are great for the immune system. Learn how to ferment foods. Check out the book *Wild Fermentation* by Sandor Ellix Katz.

Gluten

Wheat – the staff of life, it was called. But no more. In the last 50 years, much cross-breeding and gene splicing has taken place to produce greater yields. The result is "dwarf wheat," a mutant plant with a genetic code that never existed in nature before, and an inflammatory gluten content that is upwards of 50 times greater than wheat of Biblical times. Dr. William Davis, in his book *Wheat Belly*, writes modern wheat is a high glycemic index carb that produces documented effects of exaggerated blood sugar swings, exposure to brain-active exorphins, triggered glycation processes that underlie aging, and sets in motion disordered immune responses. Two slices of wheat toast will raise your blood sugar more than two tablespoons of sugar. A lot of candy bars would raise the blood sugar less than two slices of toast. Few foods have as high a glycemic index as wheat. Whole wheat is worse. Go gluten-free; it is much more than a fad.

GMOs

Genetically modified organisms (GMOs) have altered DNA and are risky; avoid them. GMO corn and cottonseed oil have been genetically altered to produce their own systemic insecticide which breaks open the stomach of insects to kill them. The same insecticide enters your gut when you eat those foods. Almost all corn, soy, cotton, canola, and sugar is GMO – another reason to avoid sugar. Not to mention that most seeds are hybridized to increase profits. These hybrid seeds are not the same ones that our creator intended for us to eat. Studies keep warning us of the hazards of glyphosate and other pesticides heavily used in GMO crops. In 2015, the International Agency for Research on Cancer, an arm of the World Health Organization, declared glyphosate "a probable human carcinogen."[1] It does not make sense to eat food produced with toxic chemicals imbedded within its structure.

Pesticides

Get friendly with non-toxic fertilizers for your back yard, and select fruits and vegetables that are pesticide-free. If you have a gardener, talk to him about the products he uses. Buy organic in the produce isle to reduce the intake of pesticides that have been absorbed by fruits and vegetables. Environmental Working Group puts out a list of what they refer to as the "Clean 15" and the "Dirty Dozen"; see www.ewg.org. Pesticides can damage DNA and disrupt hormonal activity.

Soy

The topic of soy is very controversial. My advice: Avoid *unfermented* soy products because they are high in plant estrogens or phytoestrogens (also known as isoflavones). In studies, unfermented soy appears to work along with human estrogen to increase breast cell proliferation.

Restrict Dairy Products

The lactose in daily products is a milk sugar that can suppress the immune system and most people have a difficult time breaking down the casein protein. I attempt to limit my dairy consumption to organic butter and heavy whipping cream. The Weston A. Price Foundation, Dr. Ron Schmid, and others have pointed out the many problems with modern pasteurized and homogenized milk "products." Many people find that raw milk, butter, and cheeses are good for them; however, they are difficult to find in the grocery store.

Avoid Fructose and Sugar

This is especially important for anyone currently undergoing cancer treatment: You absolutely MUST avoid all forms of sugar. There is a strong relationship between, sugar, insulin and insulin-like growth factor. All provide fuel for and signal growth of cancer cells. When consuming fruit, stick to those that are lower in sugar, such as green apples, berries, and cherries. Dr. Ray Hammon says that for every serving of fruit you consume, you should have two servings of a vegetable. It's a rare day that I consume the sugary foods of yesteryear – alcohol, desserts, beverages, corn, wheat, bread, pasta, potatoes, and rice. Also, remember that carbohydrates like bread, potatoes, and rice break down into sugar so consume them sparingly.

Avoid Artificial Sweeteners and MSG

Don't be fooled by the "zero calorie" marketing. These products are not beneficial to your health. Also, studies have shown repeatedly that diet beverages make you gain weight faster than non-diet. Avoid all glutamate additives like monosodium gluta-mate (MSG), monopotassium glutamate, hydrolyzed vegetable protein, and hydrolyzed plant protein because these additives can stimulate tumor growth and invasion.

Avoid Alcohol

The sugar and yeast in alcohol are fertilizers for cancer. Also the alcohol breaks down to acetelhyde (a carcinogen). If it sounds hard to give up that evening cocktail, try having a little bit of kombucha tea. It is a fermented beverage that can help you digest meals while giving you that "something special" at the end of the day. It is sold in most health food stores, and after a while, you might want to make it from scratch.

Spices

Learn to use quality spices, not the ones at the grocery store that may not be fresh and may have been irradiated. Turmeric, for example, is the subject of some 5,000 peer reviewed studies which are finding this time-honored Indian spice does an amazing job of fighting cancer and a growing number of chronic illness.

Maintain a Healthy Body Weight

Excess body fat produces estrogen that fuels cancer. Obesity has been linked to cancer. The excess sugar in the modern diet can be fuel for the growth of cancer.

Exercise

Exercise can lower your risk of cancer. It increases oxygen, detoxification, and reduces elevated insulin and blood sugar levels. All of these discourage the growth and spread of cancer cells. Exercise often because it increases the release of endorphins in the brain creating a sense of well-being and elevating your mood.

Not into exercise you say? Anybody can walk for 15 minutes after lunch or dinner and it doesn't cost a dime. Advance to the point you give it 30 minutes a day. Include aerobic and muscle building. Start out slow and build up strength and endurance. Exercise is potent medicine for chronic disease because it optimizes your insulin and leptin receptor sensitivity.

Sweat Every Day for Detox

This can be accomplished during exercise. I also use a far infrared sauna. This type of sauna raises the core body temperature and triggers deep-sweating.

Take Probiotics

Supplement your diet with a good multi-strain probiotic. The immune system is based in your gut so good bowel function is key.

Optimize Vitamin D and K2 Levels

Try to maintain your vitamin D levels over 50. I try to keep mine around 75. There is a free one hour presentation on the subject at www.Mercola.com. Find the search box and type in "vitamin D lecture." Vitamin D and K2 go together like a horse and saddle. So increase vitamin K2 for proper vitamin D function.

Enjoy the Sunlight

Spend at least 20 minutes in the mid-day sun daily with at least 40 percent of your skin exposed. This increases your vitamin D and elevates your mood. Vitamin D was meant to be made by your skin, not swallowed as a pill and processed by the stomach. But if you cannot get out in the sun, then use the pill. Vitamin D is cancer preventive. One of the big mistakes in American health happened in the 1980s when we got sold on the idea it was not safe to go outside without slathering on sunscreen. Turns out, the sunscreen had toxic chemicals in it and vitamin D levels plummeted as a result of blocking the body from creating it naturally.

Take Professional-grade Nutritional Supplements

In today's world it is hard to get all the nutrients you need, even from organic food; the soil is depleted, which means there are less minerals in the plants. Avoid the seduction of cheap vitamins at the big-box stores. Quality matters. For me, I use www.welltrients.com because I think they are head and shoulders above most other options, they work synergistically together, and I have seen so many success stories in people who changed their diet and used these nutrients. I know many people who have chosen to put themselves in "Nutritional Intensive Care" using Welltrients' products with amazing results.

I want to caution you not to run out and purchase individual herbs and vitamins. I have learned that it is important to have these items free of preservatives, broken down to a form that the body can easily use, and combined with the necessary co-factors. For example, don't take just magnesium; the body loves balance and it wants a balance of all minerals.

Make Sure You "GO" Everyday

Enzyme supplementation with meals and probiotics should do the trick, but if you are not having at least one good bowel movement every day, add a fiber supplement at bedtime.

Parasites and Yeast

Do a parasite and yeast cleanse several times a year. Both are implicated in cancer. However, I must caution that you make sure that you are in good health before doing a cleanse. Parasites feed on dying and dead parasites, and you don't want to feed the problem.

Iodine Supplementation

Have your iodine levels checked because this trace mineral has been removed from much of the standard American diet. Add it to your supplements if necessary. Iodine is critical for thyroid function and metabolism. It is best to use a sea based iodine from the kelp plant.

Avoid Electromagnetic Fields

I enjoy walking barefoot on the grass, a great way of transferring electrons and grounding yourself! Pick up a copy of Clint Ober's book, *Earthing*. He explains that when a person's bare skin touches the ground, the contact provides a neutralizing charge to the body and naturally protects the nervous system from extraneous electrical interference. Electrons enter the body and work like antioxidants, disarming the free radicals that age us and set the state for illness. Consider Earthing products like a grounded bed sheet or computer pad to ground yourself while sleeping and working.

For more information on the hazards of electromagnetic fields (EMF), check out www.blakelevitt.com or the writings of Camilla Rees, founder of www.ElectromagneticHealth.org, for a well-rounded take on everything from cell phones and smart meters, to dirty electricity and DNA damage. Learn how to protect yourself from man-made, unnatural frequencies at night when your body does the bulk of its detoxing activities.

Bio Feedback

Dr. Royal Rife was an inventor who discovered in the 1930s that every living organism vibrates at its own, unique frequency. He identified the frequency of many microorganisms, including cancer, and was able to destroy them with targeted frequencies. Think of the opera singer who is able to hit just the right note long enough to shatter glass. Likewise, if you transmit the exact frequencies that cancer cells use, you can kill them.

Every organ in our body vibrates with a unique frequency that can be measured. Unhealthy organs put out too much or too little vibration. Stress, toxins, nutritional deficiencies, and age can alter the frequencies, causing organs to either underperform or overperform.

There are a variety of machines on the market that can scan the body and measure the many frequencies being emitted. Some can also direct energy back into the organs to balance them. The right machine can eliminate electromagnetic chaos and restore energy at the cellular level.

A few words of caution here: there can be a world of difference between an original machine and a knock off, and an experienced practitioner makes a huge difference.

I was lucky to be trained by Janine Kennedy, R.N., in the use of the BioScan Pro (www.BioScanPro.com). I like that it gives a choice of areas I want to scan, and it gives me a good graphical representation on a computer screen. It gives a fast assessment of my stresses so I can better manage my body's needs. I use this machine several times a week for frequency therapy. Instead of sending a destructive frequency to the body, the BioScan Pro sends the precise frequency that each cell and organ need to function correctly.

Avoid Synthetic Hormone Replacement

Birth control pills are comprised of synthetic hormones and have been linked to cervical and breast cancers. Bioidentical hormone replacement appears to be safer.

Avoid BPA, Phthalates, and Other Xenoestrogens

These are estrogen-like compounds that have been linked to increased breast cancer risk and are found in plastics, cosmetics, children's toys, non-stick cookware – pretty much everywhere around us today. Try to store food in glass containers and drink out of glass bottles.

A great source of information about environmental toxins can be found in a free PDF download entitled *State of the Evidence* at: www.breastcancerfund.org/media/publications/state-of-the-evidence. It is produced by the Breast Cancer Fund, one of the few organizations who make it their mission to prevent cancer. The title suggests it is about breast cancer, but the information applies to pretty much to any manner of cancer.

Get a Good Night's Rest

Sleep boosts the immune system, lowers cortisol levels, and aids the production of important hormones. Night time is when our body does a lot of detoxification and repair work. Get to bed at a reasonable hour and considering wearing an eye mask to black out all light.

Relax, Smile, and Laugh

Find time each day to de-stress. If someone or some situation is causing chronic stress, take steps to remove the source. Stress is strongly implicated in cancer.

Check out a book by Brenda Stockdale, *You Can Beat the Odds: Surprising Factors Behind Chronic Illness & Cancer.* She is a pioneer in psychoneuroimmunology and its practical applications. Her stress-reducing techniques have been implemented in hospitals, cancer centers, and primary care settings around the United States.

Consider a Cancer Consultant

There are a lot of qualified people working and treating cancer with great success, so put on your investigative "hat" and gather information. In my opinion, when dealing with a life threatening disease, two heads are better than one. Some of the people I am familiar with include Ralph W. Moss, Ph.D.; Bill Henderson; and Dr. Janey Little (South Africa). These consultants offer telephone consults and their approach is integrative. Or you can contact me at www.CancerFreeAreYouSure.com.

Having an advocate in your corner can be very valuable. I wish that I had found such a person at the time of my diagnosis. Remember, you don't get answers if you don't ask questions. These people have already asked many of the questions that you have, and they have enlightened answers.

⌘⌘⌘

Steve Steeves, CCN, CNT, author of *The Trinity Diet* had this to say:

We must stop long enough to consider if our behavior is constructive for the kingdom of God, and if what we are doing as active agents for the Lord is beneficial to our bodies, our families and our communities that depend on us. Eating mindfully and worshipfully is a discipline worth striving for.

Oh, how my heart rejoiced to read his words, so eloquently and perfectly written. I have struggled for years to put the pieces together. I have watched so many precious people die while I struggled to relate to them the importance of healing the heart and the physical body, not just cutting out or poisoning the cancer.

We live in a world that is heavy in stress, loaded with toxins, and our food supply is highly processed and lacking the much needed nutrients that the body needs for optimal health. I believe that if you implement a healthy lifestyle, you will have a much better chance of avoiding or beating cancer.

And just as important, if you have already gone the route of surgery, chemotherapy, and radiation, and have been pronounced "Cancer Free," I encourage you to use one of more of the tests in this book to validate that proclamation.

Take great care of yourself. Live purposefully and consider your choices wisely. See cancer coming early. Don't let it hang around for up to 5 or 10 years before it is discovered. Find it early, when it is treatable and beatable. You will find that making a positive impact on your health is hard work. I don't disagree, but you are worth the effort and life is worth living, and boy is it a lot more fun when you are in good health!

I have learned a great deal through my personal cancer journey. Gregg Matte of Houston's First Baptist Church summed up my purpose for writing this book when he said:

"Make your misery your ministry and your test your testimony."

I have experienced misery and have been tested. I pray that my resulting ministry and testimony will lighten your load and bring about abundant blessings to you and everyone that you love.

– Jenny Hrbacek, R.N.

Find CANCER before it manifests!

Get TESTED!

Footnotes

1 Guyton KZ, Loomis D, et al. Carcinogenicity of tetrachlorvinphos, parathion, malathion, diazinon, and glyphosate. *The Lancet Oncology*. 2015. Retrieved March 30, 2015 at www.thelancet.com/journals/lanonc/article/PIIS1470-2045%2815%2970134-8/abstract

Resources

Organizations

International Organization of Integrative Cancer Physicians (IOICP)
Directory of IPT and integrative cancer physicians in the United States and around the world.
www.ioicp.com

Best Answer for Cancer Foundation
Providing prevention, education, awareness, options, and support to patients and physicians dealing with cancer.
www.bestanswerforcancer.org

Oncology Association of Naturopath Physicians (OncANP)
Naturopathic physicians specializing in naturopathic oncology. OncANP initiated a credentialing process for naturopathic doctors in 2006.
www.oncanp.org

National Center for Homeopathy
Directory of physicians who take an integrative approach, tailored to the individual situation: (1) post treatment recovery, (2) preventing recurrence, and (3) symptom relief in terminal situations and an improved quality of life for as long as possible. Homeopaths determine remedies that fit the particular patient at a particular point in time.
www.nationalcenterforhomeopathy.org

Cancer Control Society
Holds a large annual conference with more than 50 speakers on alternative cancer treatment. This conference is for professionals and the public. Presentation videos are available online. They offer a "green sheet" with alternative physicians and a "white sheet" with patient testimonials.
www.cancercontrolsociety.com
323-663-7801

The Annie Appleseed Project

Features information on natural therapies and substances, lifestyle issues, complementary and alternative medicine (CAM) from a patient's perspective. Features a yearly conference for the public.
www.annieappleseedproject.org

The Cure Research Foundation

An additional source for information on alternative treatments, integrative practitioners, and open-minded oncologists. Provides a partial list of clinics inside and outside the U.S.
www.cancure.org
800-282-2873

Alternative Cancer Doctors and Clinics

Source of many health articles. Partial directory of practitioners U.S. and worldwide.
www.whale.to/cancer/doctors.html

CANHELP, Inc.

Information and support service for lifesaving alternative cancer therapies and complementary cancer treatments.
www.canhelp.com
800-364-2341

Center for Advancement In Cancer Education

Providing research-based education on how to prevent, cope with, and beat cancer through diet, lifestyle, and other immune-boosting approaches.
www.beatcancer.org
888-551-2223

American College for Advancement in Medicine (ACAM)

"The voice of integrative medicine." This long-established organization is focused on advancing the cause of integrative medicine and disseminating cutting edge information on the prevention and remission of disease. Also has a substantial directory of natural practitioners.
www.acam.org
888-439-6891

The American Academy of Environmental Medicine (AAEM)
Non-profit medical society committed to educating physicians
on the cause and effect relationship between environment and
ill-health.
www.aaemonline.org
316-864-5500

Foundation for Alternative and Integrative Medicine
FAIM disseminates information on new frontiers in science and
medicine and encourages adoption of cost effective therapies
through global networking, conferences, publishing books, and
Internet website postings. Under the "Investigations and Activities" tab, click CANCER.
www.nfam.org
info@FAIM.org

Cancer Tutor
A grassroots website with information on alternative and natural
approaches to cancer.
www.cancertutor.com

People Against Cancer
A grassroots website describing treatment options for people with
cancer.
www.PeopleAgainstCancer.org
800-662-2623

Integrative Health International
Integrative education to help prevent, heal, and reverse degenerative diseases. Features a yearly "Integrative Health Conference"
for the public.
info@integratedhealthinternational.com
888-848-0142

Breast Cancer Fund
Its mission is to "expose and eliminate the environmental
causes of cancer. We can stop this disease before it starts." Has
a free, downloadable report, "State of the Evidence," that is
updated periodically and is an excellent source of environmental

considerations for cancer.
www.breastcancerfund.org
866-760-8223

Breast Cancer Choices, Inc.
A nonprofit organization scrutinizing and reporting the evidence for breast cancer procedures and treatments.
www.breastcancerchoices.org

Tahoma Clinic Foundation
A nonprofit organization in Tukwila, Washington "dedicated to promoting the enormous potential of nutritional therapy and natural medicine." Dr. Wright has clinics in the Puget Sound area. Founded by Jonathan V. Wright, M.D.
www.tahomaclinic.com/tahoma-clinic-foundation

The Gerson Institute
A non-profit organization in San Diego, California "dedicated to providing education and training in the Gerson Therapy, an alternative, non-toxic treatment for cancer and other chronic degenerative diseases." They have clinics in Tijuana, Mexico, and Hungary.
www.gerson.org

Life Extension Foundation
"Global authority on nutrition, health, and wellness." A good source of tests you can order without a doctor's referral. Partial directory of doctors with an interest in innovative and alternative therapies.
www.lef.org/health-wellness/innovativedoctors
800-678-8989

The Weston A. Price Foundation (WAPF)
A non-profit organization dedicated to "restoring nutrient-dense foods to the human diet through education, research, and activism" and teaching the optimum characteristics of human diets.
www.westonaprice.org

The Price-Pottenger Nutrition Foundation (PPNF)
A non-profit education foundation "committed to reversing the trend of declining health in our modern world. We teach both the public and health professionals the proven principles from nutrition pioneers Dr. Weston A. Price, Dr. Francis M. Pottenger, Jr., and other leading health experts." Provides a directory of healthcare practitioners who are PPNF members.
www.ppnf.org
800-366-3748

Food Matters
Online nutritional information: DVDs, videos, detox, recipes, clinics, juicing, etc.
www.foodmatters.tv

Environmental Working Group (EWG)
A health research and advocacy organization with top-notch reports. Check out the "Skin Deep Database." It provides safety information about more than 72,000 products and their ingredients. If a product is not listed, simply enter the ingredient in question. Also, see their guides to pesticides and cleaning products, and their "Body Burden" studies on the chemicals inside us.
www.ewg.org

The Organic Center
Numerous downloadable reports on nutritional quality of organic versus conventional food, the impact of GMOs and pesticides, identifying smart food choices, and more.
http://organic-center.org/scientific-resources/publication-archive

The Cornucopia Institute
This organization works to "empower farmers and consumers in support of ecologically produced local, organic, and authentic food." Produces reports – scorecards – on how much integrity exists in the "organic" label, which corporations own organic brands, and more.
www.cornucopia.org/category/reports

Organic Consumers Association
"We are the only organization in the U.S. focused exclusively on promoting the views and interests of the nation's estimated 50 million organic and socially responsible consumers." Has a substantial directory of green and organic businesses throughout the United States, everything from food and home furnishings, to holistic dentists and travel sites.
http://organicconsumers.org/btc/BuyingGuide.cfm

Eat to Beat Cancer
Founded in 1994, the Angiogenesis Foundation is "the world's first nonprofit organization dedicated to conquering disease using a new approach based on angiogenesis, the growth of new capillary blood vessels in the body. Find information on cancer fighting foods based on the latest medical science."
www.eattobeat.org

Insulin Potentiated Therapy

- www.bestanswerforcancer.org
- www.IPTforcancer.com
- www.iptq.com

Cancer Clinic Tours

Cancer Control Society – Tijuana Clinic Tours
frankcousineau@yahoo.com

Cancer Health Tours – Available by Appointment
getwell@healthtours.com
619-475-3834

Biological Dentistry

International Academy of Oral Medicine and Toxicology (IAOMT)
Members promote the use of mercury-free dentistry and therapeutic approaches. Check out the short video entitled

"Smoking Teeth" which demonstrates the release of mercury vapor from amalgam fillings. See the video at: http://iaomt.org/mercury. www.iaomt.org

International Academy of Biological Dentistry and Medicine
Directory of network physicians and allied health professionals who acknowledge the whole body effects of dental materials, techniques, and procedures. Members are committed to fluoride-free, mercury-free, and biocompatible dental materials.
www.iabdm.org
281-651-1745

Huggins Applied Healing
Dr. Hal A. Huggins discovered that standard dental practices, such as root canals and the use of mercury fillings, are the cause of many unexplained diseases and symptoms. Find a dentist utilizing the famed protocol of Dr. Huggins.
www.hugginsappliedhealing.com
866-948-4638

Talk International
"The source for the mercury toxicity issue since 1997." Discusses health concerns about mercury and fluoride. Provides an international directory for holistic dentists, mercury free dentists, and biological dentists as well as a partial directory of holistic physicians and alternative health care practitioners in the U.S., Canada, and the Bahamas.
www.talkinternational.com
310-208-1158 or 888-708-2525

Books / Reports / Websites

Cancer As a Metabolic Disease - On the Origin, Management, and Prevention of Cancer
By Dr. Thomas N. Seyfried, 2012

The Emperor of All Maladies: A Biography of Cancer
By Siddhartha Mukherjee, 2011

Cancer Killers: The Cause Is the Cure
By Dr. Charles Majors, Dr. Ben Lerner, and Sayer Ji; 2012

Cancer - Step Outside the Box
By Ty Bollinger, 2006

Cancer Free - Your Guide to Gentle, Non-toxic Healing
By Bill Henderson and Carlos M. Garcia, M.D.; 2006

Cancer and Vitamin C: A Discussion of the Nature, Causes, Prevention, and Treatment of Cancer with Special Reference to the Value of Vitamin C, Updated and Expanded
By Ewan Cameron and Linus Pauling, 1993

Cruise Ship or Nursing Home
By Ben Lerner, Greg Loman, Charles Majors, Chris Pellow, and Eric Shuemake; 2009

Beating Cancer with Nutrition
By Patrick Quillin, 2005

World Without Cancer
By G. Edward Griffin, 2010

Cancer Is a Fungus
By Dr. T. Simoncini, 2007
www.cancerisafungus.com

German Cancer Breakthrough
The first English language guide to German cancer clinics.
By Andrew Scholberg, 2008

Cancer Breakthrough USA!
A guide to outstanding alternative clinics.
By Frank Cousineau with Andrew Scholberg, 2007
www.cancerdefeated.com/ABCD/vsl-way.php

Adios! Cancer
How the rich and poor alike beat cancer at clinics south of the boarder; available as a book and digital download.

By Frank Cousineau and Andy Scholberg, 2010
www.cancerdefeated.com/amish-secret

Stage Four Cancer Gone!
By Shirley Williams, 2014
http://shirleymwilliams.com/book

Defeat Cancer Now: A Nutritional Approach to Wellness for Cancer and Other Diseases
By Tamara St. John, 2013
www.tamarastjohn.com/#!books/cnec

The Germ that Causes Cancer
By Doug A. Kaufmann, et al; 2005

The Cancer Journal – Heal Yourself!
By Lisa Gail Robbins, 2013

Cancer Cure and Survivor Stories
By Lisa Gail Robbins, Elaine Cantin, et al; 2013

Knockout
By Suzanne Somers, 2010

Healing the Gerson Way: Defeating Cancer and Other Chronic Diseases
By Charlotte Gerson, Beata Bishop, et al; 2009

Customized Cancer Treatment: How a Powerful Lab Test Predicts Which Drugs Will Work for You – and Which to Avoid
By Ralph Moss, 2010

The Complete Guide to Alternative Cancer Treatments
A publication of the Alternative Cancer Research Institute, 2011
www.cancerdefeated.com

The Moss Report (Available for specific types of cancer)
www.cancerdecisions.com

Mercola.com

Dr. Joseph Mercola sends out a daily email that re-examines many aspects of standard medical practice. The site has a huge archive of articles; search it for almost any subject and you will access a great wealth of enlightened information. This is the most accessed alternative-health website on the Internet.
www.Mercola.com

GreenMedInfo.com

Run by Sayer Ji, this is "the world's most widely referenced, open access, natural medicine database,"were you can access studies and summaries. They also send out a daily email about timely health issues.
www.greenmedinfo.com

Cancer Tutor.com

This site has hundreds of articles including complete protocols for advanced cancer patients.
www.cancertutor.com

Reducing Environmental Cancer Risk – What We Can Do Now

2010 candid report by The President's Cancer Panel "meetings to assess the state of environmental cancer research, policy, and programs addressing known and potential effects of environmental exposures on cancer."
http://deainfo.nci.nih.gov/advisory/pcp/annualReports/pcp08-09rpt/PCP_Report_08-09_508.pdf

Living Downstream – An Ecologist Looks At Cancer and the Environment

By Sandra Steingraber, 1997

The Secret History of the War on Cancer

By Devra Davis, 2007

Fight Cancer with a Ketogenic Diet – A New Method for Treating Cancer

By Ellen Davis
eBook available at www.ketogenic-diet-resource.com

Beta Glucan
By Vaclav Vetvicka, Ph.D.; 2011

Nourishing Traditions: The Cookbook that Challenges Politically Correct Nutrition and the Diet Dictocrats
By Sally Fallon and Mary Enig, Ph.D.; 2003

Nutrition and Physical Degeneration
By Weston A. Price, D.D.S.; 2009

Pottenger's Cats
By Dr. Francis M. Pottenger, Jr.; 1995

The Disease Delusion
By Dr. Jeffrey Bland, 2014

The Rosedale Diet
By Ron Rosedale, M.D.; 2004

Why Stomach Acid Is Good for You
By Jonathan Wright, M.D., and Lane Lenard, Ph.D.; 2001

Salt Sugar Fat: How the Food Giants Hooked Us
By Michael Moss, 2013

The End of Overeating: Taking Control of the Insatiable American Appetite
Dr. David Kessler, 2010

The Fat Switch
By Dr. Richard J. Johnson, 2012

The Untold Story of Milk
By Dr. Ron Schmid, 2003

Farmer John's Cookbook: The Real Dirt on Vegetables
By Farmer John Peterson and Angelic Organics, 2006

Holy Cows and Hog Heaven: The Food Buyer's Guide to Farm-Fresh Food
By Joel Salatin, 2005

7-Day Detox Miracle
By Peter Bennett, N.D., and Stephen Barrie, N.D.; 2001

You Can Beat the Odds: Surprising Factors Behind Chronic Illness & Cancer
By Brenda Stockdale, 2009

The Trinity Diet – Lifestyle Balancing Body, Mind and Spirit
By Steve Steeves, 2013

The Believer's Authority
By Kenneth E. Hagin, 1985

Healing Is Voltage: The Handbook (3rd Edition)
By Dr. Jerry Tennant, 2010

Earthing: The Most Important Health Discovery Ever?
By Clint Ober, Dr. Stephen Sinatra, Martin Zucker; 2014

Videos

Cancer Conquest: The Best of Conventional and Alternative Medicine
www.burtongoldberg.com

The Beautiful Truth – The All-Natural Treatment for Cancer and Chronic Disease
www.gersonmedia.com

Heal Yourself, Heal the World – The Legacy of Dr. Max Gerson
www.gersonmedia.com

Cut, Poison, Burn – In the War on Cancer, the Disease Is Only Half the Battle
http://cutpoisonburn.com

Why Are We Losing the War on Cancer?
http://products.mercola.com/cut-poison-burn-dvd

Truly Heal from Cancer
www.trulyheal.com

Doug Kaufmann's Know the Cause
Doug Kaufman is the host of the TV show, "Know The Cause." Find information about fungus and ill health. Also, the Phase One-Phase Two-Life Phase diets were developed to starve the body of parasitic fungi, while simultaneously providing proper nutrition.
www.knowthecause.com

Skin Cancer/Sunscreen - the Dilemma
From University of California, San Diego
www.youtube.com/watch?v=eeXtGHSt-5o

Cancer Doesn't Scare Me Anymore!
www.drday.com

Healing Cancer from Inside Out
www.ravediet.com/caDVD.html

Fat, Sick & Nearly Dead
www.fatsickandnearlydead.com

Detoxing for Health
www.JuiceladyCherie.com

Hungry for Change – Your Health Is in Your Hands
Food Matters – You Are What You Eat
www.foodmatters.tv

Genetic Roulette – The Gamble of Our Lives
www.GeneticRouletteMovie.com

The Ten Americans
By Ken Cook of Environmental Working Group
www.ewg.org/news/videos/ken-cook-environmental-working-group-presents-ten-americans-part-1
www.ewg.org/news/videos/ken-cook-environmental-working-group-presents-ten-americans-part-2

Fluoridegate – An American Tragedy
www.fluoridegate.org

Farmers Markets

Local Harvest
Use this website to find farmers' markets, family farms, and other sources of sustainably grown food in your area, where you can buy produce, grass-fed meats, and many other goodies.
www.localharvest.org

Eat Wild
Author Jo Robinson's website "has been providing information about the benefits of choosing meat, eggs, and dairy products from pastured animals since 2001." Has a state-by-state listing of where to find food from "animals and the land that are well-treated, that their products are exceptionally high in nutrition, and free of antibiotics and added hormones." Many farmers ship to other states.
www.eatwild.com/products/index.html

I invite you to join me!

Log on to www.NoLumpOrBump.com

to show your support for a public awareness campaign

to spread the word that "TRUE" early detection tests are available.

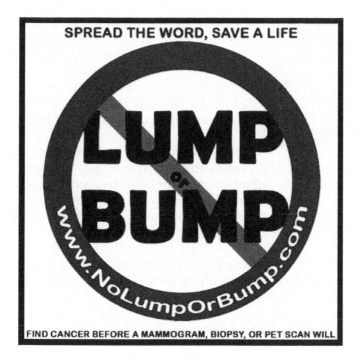

It has often been said the United States does not

have a health care system;

we have a disease-management system

focused on expensive drugs and invasive surgeries.

**Through public awareness let's ask that the system
do more to promote health.**

Let's make the insurance industry aware of these state-of-the-art tests

and that we want medical plans to cover our use of them.

Jenny Hrbacek, R.N.

Jenny set out on a life changing journey when she was diagnosed with breast cancer in April 2009. Today, Jenny spends time communicating with other newly diagnosed patients, offering 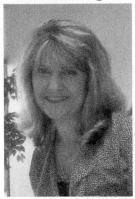 them guidance, encouragement, and hope. She has developed a presentation entitled "KNOWLEDGE IS POWER" as a result of several years of research into alternative health therapies, nutrition, and diagnostic testing. Jenny discusses tools and tests that can be implemented to improve health and reduce the risk of a cancer reoccurrence. The information she presents was not given to her by her U.S. oncology team, but was discovered through her quest for health.

She is married with three adult children, lives in Sugar Land, Texas and is active in her community and many charitable organizations. She spent several years serving as a board member for "Reconstruction of a Survivor," a faith based organization that provides cancer support group sessions throughout the greater Houston metropolitan area.

She has been a registered nurse since 1990 and is available for speaking engagements and health coaching. Contact her at www.CancerFreeAreYouSure.com

Mary Budinger, NTC, Editor

Mary Budinger is an Emmy award-winning broadcast journalist and certified nutritional therapy consultant. After overcoming 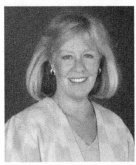 an autoimmune disease, she made her professional life about integrative medicine and nutrition. She completed nutrition training through the Nutritional Therapy Association of Olympia, Washington. Her first book venture, *An Alphabet of Good Health*, was awarded the 2011 Readers Views 1st place award for both Health & Fitness, and Self-help. She lives in Phoenix, Arizona.

CPSIA information can be obtained
at www.ICGtesting.com
Printed in the USA
LVOW04s0705101115

461698LV00001B/1/P